D1613899

# HEALTH FITNESS MANAGEMENT

## Third Edition

# HEALTH FITNESS MANAGEMENT

## Third Edition

**Mike Bates, MBA**
University of Windsor
Refine Fitness Studio

**Michael J. Spezzano**
Mike Spezzano Consulting

**Guy Danhoff, Assistant Professor**
Missouri Baptist University

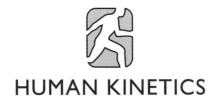

HUMAN KINETICS

**Library of Congress Cataloging-in-Publication Data**

Names: Bates, Mike, 1972- author. | Spezzano, Michael J., author. | Danhoff,
   Guy, author.
Title: Health fitness management / Mike Bates, MBA, University
   of Windsor, Refine Fitness Studio, Michael J. Spezzano, Mike Spezzano
   Consulting, Guy Danhoff, Assistant Professor, Missouri Baptist University.
Description: Third edition. | Champaign, Illinois : Human Kinetics, [2020] |
   "This book is a revised edition of Health Fitness Management, published in
   2008 by Mike Bates"--T.p. verso. | Includes bibliographical references and
   index.
Identifiers: LCCN 2018021718 (print) | LCCN 2018023642 (ebook) | ISBN
   9781492574989 (ebook) | ISBN 9781450412230 (print)
Subjects: LCSH: Physical fitness centers--United States--Management. |
   Physical fitness--Study and teaching--United States.
Classification: LCC GV428.5 (ebook) | LCC GV428.5 .H43 2020 (print) | DDC
   613.7/068--dc23
LC record available at https://lccn.loc.gov/2018021718

ISBN: 978-1-4504-1223-0 (print)

This book is a revised edition of *Health Fitness Management*, published in 2008 by Mike Bates.

The web addresses cited in this text were current as of October 2018, unless otherwise noted.

**Senior Acquisitions Editor:** Amy N. Tocco; **Managing Editor:** Anna Lan Seaman; **Copyeditor:** Karla
Walsh; **Indexer:** Nan Badgett; **Permissions Manager:** Dalene Reeder; **Senior Graphic Designer:** Joe
Buck; **Cover Designer:** Keri Evans; **Cover Design Associate:** Susan Rothermel Allen; **Photograph
(cover):** RusianDashinsky/Getty Images; **Photographs (interior):** © Human Kinetics, unless otherwise
noted; **Photo Asset Manager:** Laura Fitch; **Photo Production Manager:** Jason Allen; **Senior Art Manager:** Kelly Hendren; **Illustrations:** © Human Kinetics, unless otherwise noted; **Printer:** Sheridan Books

Printed in the United States of America

10 9 8 7 6 5 4 3 2 1

The paper in this book is certified under a sustainable forestry program.

**Human Kinetics**
P.O. Box 5076
Champaign, IL 61825-5076
Website: www.HumanKinetics.com

In the United States, email info@hkusa.com or call 800-747-4457.
In Canada, email info@hkcanada.com.
In the United Kingdom/Europe, email hk@hkeurope.com.

For information about Human Kinetics' coverage in other areas of the world,
please visit our website: **www.HumanKinetics.com**

E5485

# Contents

Preface   ix

## Part I   Human Resources                                             1

### 1   Recognizing the Importance of Leaders and Managers . . . . . . . . 3
Exploring Management and Leadership Theory. . . . . . . . . . . . . . . . . . . . . . . . 4
Acknowledging the Difference Between Managing and Leading. . . . . . . . . . . . 6
Struggling as a Manager: Pitfalls to Avoid . . . . . . . . . . . . . . . . . . . . . . . . . 14
Succeeding as a Manager: A Strategy to Manage Talent . . . . . . . . . . . . . . . 16

### 2   Understanding Organizational Design . . . . . . . . . . . . . . . . . . . 19
Growth and Management Positions . . . . . . . . . . . . . . . . . . . . . . . . . . . . . . 21
Roles and Responsibilities . . . . . . . . . . . . . . . . . . . . . . . . . . . . . . . . . . . . . 22
Writing Job Descriptions. . . . . . . . . . . . . . . . . . . . . . . . . . . . . . . . . . . . . . 22
For-Profit Organizations . . . . . . . . . . . . . . . . . . . . . . . . . . . . . . . . . . . . . . 23
Not-For-Profit Community Facilities. . . . . . . . . . . . . . . . . . . . . . . . . . . . . . 30
Hospital-Based Fitness Centers . . . . . . . . . . . . . . . . . . . . . . . . . . . . . . . . . 33
Corporate-Based Fitness Organizations . . . . . . . . . . . . . . . . . . . . . . . . . . . 36

### 3   Recruiting the Best Staff for Your Facility . . . . . . . . . . . . . . . 43
Analyzing Staffing Needs . . . . . . . . . . . . . . . . . . . . . . . . . . . . . . . . . . . . . 44
Utilizing Job Descriptions . . . . . . . . . . . . . . . . . . . . . . . . . . . . . . . . . . . . . 45
Designing the Appropriate Recruiting Vehicle . . . . . . . . . . . . . . . . . . . . . . . 48
Developing Interview Strategies . . . . . . . . . . . . . . . . . . . . . . . . . . . . . . . . 51
Selecting the Best Candidate for the Position . . . . . . . . . . . . . . . . . . . . . . . 55

### 4   Training and Developing Staff . . . . . . . . . . . . . . . . . . . . . . . . 61
Five Steps to Creating Internal Training Programs . . . . . . . . . . . . . . . . . . . 62
Outside Resources for Training and Development . . . . . . . . . . . . . . . . . . . . 72
Assessment of Training Costs . . . . . . . . . . . . . . . . . . . . . . . . . . . . . . . . . . 73

### 5   Managing Staff Performance. . . . . . . . . . . . . . . . . . . . . . . . . . 77
Role of the Manager in Staff Performance . . . . . . . . . . . . . . . . . . . . . . . . . 78
Steps in Managing Performance . . . . . . . . . . . . . . . . . . . . . . . . . . . . . . . . 81
Employee Termination . . . . . . . . . . . . . . . . . . . . . . . . . . . . . . . . . . . . . . . 94

### 6   Developing a Compensation Program . . . . . . . . . . . . . . . . . . . 97
Forms of Compensation . . . . . . . . . . . . . . . . . . . . . . . . . . . . . . . . . . . . . . 98
Compensation and Management . . . . . . . . . . . . . . . . . . . . . . . . . . . . . . . 102
Compensation Program Basics . . . . . . . . . . . . . . . . . . . . . . . . . . . . . . . . 105
Performance-Based Pay . . . . . . . . . . . . . . . . . . . . . . . . . . . . . . . . . . . . . 110

## Part II   Member Recruitment, Retention, and Profitability   115

**7   Marketing Your Program** . . . . . . . . . . . . . . . . . . . 117

Developing Strategic Marketing Plans . . . . . . . . . . . . . . . . . . 118
Marketing Research . . . . . . . . . . . . . . . . . . . . . . . . . . . 119
Identifying Target Markets . . . . . . . . . . . . . . . . . . . . . . . 122
Defining Marketing Goals and Objectives . . . . . . . . . . . . . . . . 123
Planning the Company Brand and Program Brand . . . . . . . . . . . . 125
Social Media Marketing . . . . . . . . . . . . . . . . . . . . . . . . . 127
Best Practices in Modern Marketing . . . . . . . . . . . . . . . . . . 131
Writing an Effective Marketing Plan . . . . . . . . . . . . . . . . . . 132
Evaluating Marketing Programs . . . . . . . . . . . . . . . . . . . . . 133

**8   Increasing Membership Sales** . . . . . . . . . . . . . . . . . 137

Fostering a Partnership Between the Reception Desk and the Membership Staff . . 138
Telephone Best Practices . . . . . . . . . . . . . . . . . . . . . . . . 142
Maximizing the Face-to-Face Selling Process . . . . . . . . . . . . . . 144
Corporate and Group Membership Sales . . . . . . . . . . . . . . . . 160

**9   Focusing on Customer Service** . . . . . . . . . . . . . . . . 163

Recognizing the Importance of Customer Service and Loyalty . . . . . . 164
Identifying Your Customer . . . . . . . . . . . . . . . . . . . . . . . 165
Understanding What the Customer Wants . . . . . . . . . . . . . . . . 166
Training Staff for Exceptional Customer Service . . . . . . . . . . . . . 169
Dealing With Difficult Customers . . . . . . . . . . . . . . . . . . . . 174
Customer Service Best Practices . . . . . . . . . . . . . . . . . . . . 174
Monitoring the Effects of Customer Service . . . . . . . . . . . . . . . 176

**10   Retaining Members Through Program Management** . . . . . . . 179

Membership Retention . . . . . . . . . . . . . . . . . . . . . . . . . 181
Establishing the Purpose of Programming . . . . . . . . . . . . . . . . 182
Diversification of Activities . . . . . . . . . . . . . . . . . . . . . . . 184
Progression of Programs . . . . . . . . . . . . . . . . . . . . . . . . 184
Promotion of Programs . . . . . . . . . . . . . . . . . . . . . . . . . 184
Reliability of the Schedule . . . . . . . . . . . . . . . . . . . . . . . 184
Accountability for Growth and Retention . . . . . . . . . . . . . . . . 185
Programming by Logical Progression . . . . . . . . . . . . . . . . . . 185
Developing a Successful Program . . . . . . . . . . . . . . . . . . . . 190
Recognizing the Importance of Program Directors . . . . . . . . . . . . 192

**11   Generating Revenue Through Profit Centers** . . . . . . . . . . 195

Development and Organization of Profit Centers . . . . . . . . . . . . 197
Five Common Profit Centers . . . . . . . . . . . . . . . . . . . . . . 198

## Part III   Operations and Facility Management     221

### 12  Understanding Financial Management . . . . . . . . . . . . . . . 223

Cash Versus Accrual Accounting . . . . . . . . . . . . . . . . . . . . . . . . . . . 224
Financial Statements . . . . . . . . . . . . . . . . . . . . . . . . . . . . . . . . . . . 225
Budgeting . . . . . . . . . . . . . . . . . . . . . . . . . . . . . . . . . . . . . . . . . . 230
Income Management . . . . . . . . . . . . . . . . . . . . . . . . . . . . . . . . . . 234
Accounts Receivable . . . . . . . . . . . . . . . . . . . . . . . . . . . . . . . . . . . 234
Sales Analysis . . . . . . . . . . . . . . . . . . . . . . . . . . . . . . . . . . . . . . . . 236
Expense Management . . . . . . . . . . . . . . . . . . . . . . . . . . . . . . . . . . 237
Tax Considerations . . . . . . . . . . . . . . . . . . . . . . . . . . . . . . . . . . . . 241

### 13  Risk Management: Addressing Health and Safety Concerns . . . 245
**Anthony Abbott and Mike Greenwood**

Creating a Safe Environment . . . . . . . . . . . . . . . . . . . . . . . . . . . . . 246
Screening Before Activity . . . . . . . . . . . . . . . . . . . . . . . . . . . . . . . 252
Administering Physical Fitness Assessments . . . . . . . . . . . . . . . . . . 259
Designing Safe Exercise Programs . . . . . . . . . . . . . . . . . . . . . . . . . 264
Providing Safety Orientation . . . . . . . . . . . . . . . . . . . . . . . . . . . . . 266
Supervising Members . . . . . . . . . . . . . . . . . . . . . . . . . . . . . . . . . . 267
Managing Emergencies . . . . . . . . . . . . . . . . . . . . . . . . . . . . . . . . . 268
Risk Management Documentation . . . . . . . . . . . . . . . . . . . . . . . . . 281

### 14  Maintaining Your Facility . . . . . . . . . . . . . . . . . . . . . . . . . 285
**Mike Greenwood and Anthony Abbott**

Maintenance Activities . . . . . . . . . . . . . . . . . . . . . . . . . . . . . . . . . 286
Four Areas of Maintenance Management . . . . . . . . . . . . . . . . . . . . 289
Determining Maintenance Needs . . . . . . . . . . . . . . . . . . . . . . . . . . 289
Performing a Needs Assessment . . . . . . . . . . . . . . . . . . . . . . . . . . 290
Planning the Facility Maintenance Program . . . . . . . . . . . . . . . . . . 293
Personnel . . . . . . . . . . . . . . . . . . . . . . . . . . . . . . . . . . . . . . . . . . . 294
Implementing a Maintenance Program . . . . . . . . . . . . . . . . . . . . . . 300
Evaluating Facility Maintenance . . . . . . . . . . . . . . . . . . . . . . . . . . 304
Developing a Preventive Maintenance Program . . . . . . . . . . . . . . . 307

### 15  Understanding Legal and Insurance Issues . . . . . . . . . . . . . 311
**John Wolohan**

Civil Versus Criminal Liability . . . . . . . . . . . . . . . . . . . . . . . . . . . . . 312
Tort Law . . . . . . . . . . . . . . . . . . . . . . . . . . . . . . . . . . . . . . . . . . . 312
Contracts . . . . . . . . . . . . . . . . . . . . . . . . . . . . . . . . . . . . . . . . . . . 320
Employment Law . . . . . . . . . . . . . . . . . . . . . . . . . . . . . . . . . . . . . 324
Insurance Considerations . . . . . . . . . . . . . . . . . . . . . . . . . . . . . . . 327

**16** **Strategic Planning and Evaluation** . . . . . . . . . . . . . . . . . . . . . . **333**

Strategic Planning. . . . . . . . . . . . . . . . . . . . . . . . . . . . . . . . . . . . . . . 334

Evaluation . . . . . . . . . . . . . . . . . . . . . . . . . . . . . . . . . . . . . . . . . . . . 336

Health and Fitness Evaluation Model. . . . . . . . . . . . . . . . . . . . . . . . . . . 337

Location Analysis . . . . . . . . . . . . . . . . . . . . . . . . . . . . . . . . . . . . . . . 339

Industry Evolution and Differentiation. . . . . . . . . . . . . . . . . . . . . . . . . . 342

**Appendix   349  •  References   353  •  Index   359**

**About the Authors   371  •  Contributors   373**

# Preface

If you are looking for a fast-paced, constantly changing profession that will give you the opportunity to make a difference in the lives of thousands of people, then this book is for you. If you love interacting with people and motivating them to be the best they can be, then this book is for you. If you want to be a part of one of the fastest-growing and most challenging industries in the world, then this book is for you. If you are interested in a 9-to-5 desk job, you should probably stop reading right now, because this book is definitely not for you.

This third edition of the popular reference and textbook *Health Fitness Management* is written for everyone who has an interest in managing a health and fitness facility. The contributors to this text are some of the most experienced and knowledgeable people in the fitness industry. Whether you are a student learning about this topic for the first time or you are a seasoned veteran, we are confident you will find this text helpful. This new edition offers updated information, more practical examples, case studies on legal issues, and new best practices to take your social media game to the next level, making this the best text on the topic.

The manager of the health and fitness club is the single most important person in determining the long-term success of the club. This is the person who gets the call at 5 a.m. when a staff member has overslept and the club has not opened on time. This is the person who is often left dealing with the most difficult and challenging customers. The club manager is the one who assembles the team of sales, service, programming, and maintenance staff. He or she is also the one who pays the price when things go wrong with the staff.

On the other hand, the manager is the one who gives people an opportunity to succeed in an extremely satisfying industry. This is the person who coaches staff until they are able to overcome some of their greatest fears and challenges. The manager's job is an extremely rewarding one that comes with a significant amount of responsibility and enjoyment.

This book is divided into three parts. Part I, on human resources, will give you all the information you need to get started with organizational development, hiring, evaluation, and compensation. This part, consisting of chapters 1 through 6, is potentially the most important part of the book. As a manager, your job is to hire, train, and retain the best people you can find. These six chapters will help you understand all of these areas.

Part II covers member recruitment, retention, and profitability. In order for your club to be successful, you need to be able to attract new members and keep current members. And, in order to make a profit, you'll need to effectively market to sell products, programs, and services to those members.

Part III covers operations and facility management—information that you'll need to know in order to run a successful club. As a manager, you need to know how to read financial statements and how to implement systems that ensure your club is well maintained. You also need to have a solid understanding of the risks that are associated with running a fitness club, both for your staff and the general public. (Not learning this side of the business is something you may regret forever once an accident occurs at your facility.) Also important is a manager's understanding of legal issues and insurance. Part III ends with a chapter on how to properly evaluate a fitness business.

Within each chapter you'll find various tools that enhance the overall learning experience. Each chapter begins with a list of learning objectives to help you focus on what you should be learning while you're reading. After the objectives, you'll read a scenario that illustrates the main topic of the chapter. These stories, which are largely based on the authors' actual experiences, are a great way to get students involved in a class discussion. Additional real-world scenarios are integrated throughout the chapters so that you'll know how to apply the material. Throughout each chapter, The Bottom Line features summarize and emphasize the most important topics in the text. Key terms—words and phrases that readers should be familiar with—are also boldfaced in the text.

For instructors who are using this as a course textbook, this third edition comes with a test package and an instructor guide. The test package features multiple-choice questions that are based on material from each chapter. The instructor guide includes summaries of each chapter and various teaching tools that will help the instructor prepare for lectures and class discussions. The instructor guide also has assignments for instructors to assign their students. These assignments are practical in nature and will allow students to apply the information presented in the text.

If you think you are ready for a career in the fitness industry, we applaud you for your interest. The true test will be how you use the information in this book to make your club or fitness center the best it can be for you, your staff, your members, and the public.

# HUMAN RESOURCES

Human resources are often the most overlooked aspect of running a fitness club. Throughout this book, we talk about the importance of member retention—keeping the members you have from year to year. Equally as important is staff retention. Keeping staff members motivated and challenged will have a positive impact on member retention levels: Members like to see the same people when they come in to your facility, and the relationships that members form with staff members will make them want to keep coming back. If the facility is constantly losing staff, the result will be the eventual loss of members. Successful clubs realize that spending time on developing their human resources will pay off in the long run.

In chapter 1 you will discuss the importance of the leader within the fitness club. As with any business, a strong leader is necessary to build a great team. This chapter will examine common mistakes among managers and what it takes to become a great manager.

In chapter 2, you will learn how various fitness businesses are organized. You will see that there are many potential ways to design your organizational structure. It is critical that each person on the team knows the role that he or she plays and how the role contributes to the company's goals.

Chapter 3 will help you get the most out of your staff by addressing important topics such as recruiting and hiring. Sections on building job descriptions and designing appropriate interview questions are included. Each of these areas is a critical component of all successful businesses.

In chapter 4, you will see that the most successful clubs differentiate themselves by offering staff training programs that build great employees. One common denominator among successful fitness businesses is their investment in people and their consistent training and development programs.

In chapter 5, you will learn how to properly evaluate your staff and give them feedback so that they are working at the highest level possible. Giving employee feedback and conducting formal evaluations can be very complicated. This chapter will guide you in designing a performance appraisal system. This chapter includes the sensitive topic of terminating employees; although this is never fun, it is important to the business and the employee that managers understand how to do this properly.

Part I concludes with chapter 6, in which you will learn how to design a compensation program that motivates employees and rewards the best performers. Various industry approaches to compensation are discussed. Once you have an understanding of each approach, you will be able to discuss the advantages and disadvantages of each.

# Recognizing the Importance of Leaders and Managers

## Learning Objectives

After studying this chapter, you will be able to

- understand basic management and leadership theory,
- identify the roles of the manager and the leader,
- recognize the critical skills required to be a successful manager,
- identify behaviors that limit the ability to be a successful manager, and
- develop a strategy for managing talent.

Sean Greely is the president of Net Profit Explosion (NPE), a company that focuses on empowering fitness business owners to take control of their organizations by providing them with tools, coaching, and education. Sean started out as a personal trainer and grew his small personal training business into a multiple-location business in a very short time. After this successful venture had run its course, Sean recognized a need in the marketplace and a personal desire to help other fitness business owners achieve their dreams. NPE has been on the Inc. 500 list numerous times; this list includes some of the fastest-growing companies in the world. Sean has seen massive growth in NPE, and he and his team have helped hundreds of fitness business owners turn their businesses around.

Sean is a tremendous leader who has created an extremely devoted client following. The NPE culture is primarily focused on getting clients results and exceeding expectations. NPE's clients regularly give testimonials, speak at events, and help one another through the various online forums NPE has created. Sean often needs more coaches due to business growth, and he has consistently been able to hire them from a pool of clients who have flourished using his **systems**.

Recently, a group of Sean's VIP clients started a scholarship program for struggling fitness business owners. NPE matches the funds contributed by the clients. At the company's annual event, Mega Training, eight scholarships were awarded. The scholarships allow people to attend an NPE educational event free of charge.

As the business grew, Sean recognized that he needed to remove himself from the day-to-day operations. This allowed him to work on the business rather than in it. To do this,

The author acknowledges the significant contributions of Dr. Jane Riddell to this chapter.

he hired great people and developed great systems. Doing this allowed Sean to continue to expand the vision and scope of business that NPE can take on. This never would have happened if Sean had focused on day-to-day operations. This is not to say that he does not know what is going on within the business; rather, he focuses on bigger picture things, such as developing key employees, building a great culture, and setting the longer-term vision for the company. This is a difficult but critical lesson for all fitness business owners to learn.

---

As you read in the opening, great leaders need to be sure they are focused on the long-term aspects of the business. It is easy to get caught up in the day-to-day business operations. When this happens, too often the organization does not hit its long-term goals. Dr. Stephen Covey (2008) says these long-term activities are important but not urgent. Things such as planning, relationship building, and seeking new opportunities are not pressing matters that require immediate attention, but if you don't address them, the business is not likely to be successful long term.

## EXPLORING MANAGEMENT AND LEADERSHIP THEORY

Over the years, there has been intense interest in the what makes managers and leaders effective and whether there are differences between the roles of managers and leaders. The following overviews of management theory and leadership theory will allow you to draw your own conclusions about the answers to these important questions and to understand current thinking regarding these subjects.

### Management Theory

There are three approaches to management theory:

1. *Scientific management approach.* This theory defines the relationship between incentive and performance and advocates rewarding people based on their output rather than hours worked. An example would be rewarding salespeople via commission and bonuses (commonly termed *incentive pay*) rather than paying them an annual salary or hourly rate. Although this approach was developed almost a century ago by Frederick Taylor

(1911), it is still effectively used today by many club operators.

2. *Human relations management approach.* This theory evolved in the late 1920s and early 1930s from studies on more than 20,000 workers that demonstrated that if employees felt valued, they became more productive. Mayo (1933) hypothesized that when employees felt important, they had higher levels of job satisfaction, which in turn led to higher levels of productivity. The theory has been supported and augmented by several other researchers since Mayo, most notably Maslow (1954), Herzberg (1966), and McGregor (1960).

3. *Process (or administrative) approach to management.* Originally developed in the 1930s by Gulick and Urwick (1937) and since refined by Hersey, Blanchard, and Johnson (2001) as well as Koontz, O'Donnell, and Weihrich (1984), this approach has a broader perspective on the way managers take actions and make decisions. Five processes revolve around the central constructs of taking actions and making decisions: planning, organizing, directing, staffing, and controlling or evaluating (see figure 1.1). Decisions made in one of the five processes always affect the other four; in other words, the five processes are interrelated. At the risk of stating the obvious, planning is most often done first. An effective manager, however, will most likely perform more than one process simultaneously.

According to Mintzberg (1973, 1990), the typical manager assumes 10 distinct roles (i.e., sets of expected behaviors associated with a managerial position) that are divided into the following three categories:

1. Interpersonal roles
   - Figurehead who acts in symbolic and ceremonial ways
   - Leader who influences and coordinates the work of followers to achieve the goals of the organization

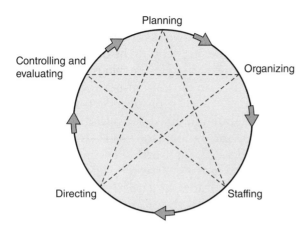

**Figure 1.1** The process approach to management.

Reprinted by permission from P.M. Pedersen, and L. Thibault, *Contemporary Sport Management*, 6th ed. (Champaign, IL: Human Kinetics, 2019), 97.

- Liaison who develops and cultivates relationships with people and groups outside the organization

2. Informational roles
   - Monitor who scans the environment for information about trends and events that can affect the organization
   - Disseminator who transmits information to stakeholders in the organization
   - Spokesperson who transmits information to people or groups outside the organization

3. Decisional roles
   - Entrepreneur who searches for opportunities to improve the organization
   - Disturbance handler who responds to unexpected situations that may disrupt normal operations
   - Resource allocator who determines how to best allocate resources to achieve the goals of the organization
   - Negotiator who confers with people or groups outside the organization to obtain concessions or gain agreement on important issues

## Leadership Theory

Understanding leadership theory will provide greater insight into how leadership has been viewed from a historical perspective. More impor-

tant, this understanding will allow you to make decisions about your personal leadership style, which will help you maximize your effectiveness. Leadership theory is divided into the following three approaches.

## Trait Leadership Theory

Trait leadership theory is based on the premise that leaders can be identified by physical, intellectual, or personality attributes and is perhaps best summed up by the statement "leaders are born, not made." Although it was discredited for some time, this school of thought generated renewed interest when Kirkpatrick and Locke (1991) demonstrated that core traits such as drive, desire to lead, honesty and integrity, self-confidence, cognitive ability, and knowledge of the business are assumed to be good predictors of the potential to lead, although they do not guarantee successful leadership.

## Behavioral Leadership Theory

Behavioral leadership theory hypothesizes that if critical behaviors of leaders can be identified, then a blueprint for successful leadership can be created and duplicated (Likert 1961). This analysis focuses on what leaders do, whereas trait theory focuses on their attributes and characteristics. Behavioral theory categorizes leaders as job centered (concerned with attaining personal or organizational goals) or employee centered (concerned with building good relationships with peers and followers). These two categories are not mutually exclusive; indeed, leaders and managers are most effective when they are focused on getting the job done and building relationships.

## Situational Leadership Theory

Situational leadership theorists observed that a variety of leadership styles could be used simultaneously in response to changing situations. There are several models of situational leadership theory, but the following are four of the most well-known:

1. *Fiedler's contingency model.* Fiedler (1967) theorized that the effectiveness of a leader depends on the leader's personal style and the amount of control the leader has over the situation. In this model, the leader is primarily task oriented or

relationship oriented. Fiedler believed that the environment can be manipulated to match leaders' personal styles (which he believed could not be easily changed) by either assigning followers who are compatible with the leaders' personal styles or seeking out situations that match the leaders' styles, thereby allowing for a higher probability of success.

2. *Path–goal model.* This model suggests that followers are motivated by their estimates of the probability that their behaviors will result in a valued outcome and by the level of personal satisfaction they will experience based on their work. Evans (1970) proposed that the primary role of the leader is path clarification, whereby the leader describes the behaviors that will lead to the reward. According to House and Mitchell (1997), leaders who are aware of the personal characteristics of their followers and of the environment can modify their behavior to maximize motivation under the given circumstances.

3. *Situational leadership model.* This model was developed by Hersey and Blanchard (1969) and suggests that leaders' behaviors depend on the mix of task (directive) and relationship (supportive) styles that are required to adapt to the situation as quickly as possible to benefit everyone involved. There are four behaviors: telling, selling, participating, and delegating. Telling is considered the most direct form of leadership because the leader simply informs the group on how and what to do. Selling requires the leader needing to convince some of the group to follow their way. Participating is about the leader building relationships with group members and sometimes not making all of the decisions but rather deferring to someone who possesses more knowledge or experience in a specific situation. Finally, delegating refers to the leader assigning responsibilities for a project or task to team members. Another aspect of this model is how ready the follower is to perform the task, which is aptly termed *readiness.* Once the leader can identify the follower's readiness level, the model can be used to select the most appropriate style and communication pattern for that follower.

4. *Full range of leadership model.* This model encompasses three leadership styles: transactional, laissez-faire, and transformational. Transactional leadership is a negotiated and agreed-on deal between leaders and followers that outlines rewards and punishments for levels of perfor-

mance by the followers (Bass 1985). Laissez-faire leadership is, as one would expect, the do-nothing approach to leading people. This is the least effective of all leadership styles. Transformational leadership focuses on the four Is: idealized influence, inspirational motivation, intellectual stimulation, and individualized consideration (Avolio, Waldman, and Yammarino 1991). These leaders are considerate, trustworthy, encouraging, and willing to take risks. Research suggests that the most effective leaders engage in all three styles to different degrees—transformational leadership most often, transactional leadership occasionally, and laissez-faire leadership seldom if at all (Bass and Avolio 1994).

## ACKNOWLEDGING THE DIFFERENCE BETWEEN MANAGING AND LEADING

It will not come as a surprise that every successful organization needs a leader. A leader's role is to formulate the vision for the organization, provide clarity for what the future will look like, and inspire group members to align themselves with the vision. Essentially, the leader sets the course for the group. Recently, more than 200 Canada geese were found dead in a frozen Manitoba wheat field. Initially, it was thought they had been poisoned; however, autopsies on the birds revealed that their breastbones were shattered and their necks were broken. It was concluded that the leader had become disoriented during a dark, moonless night and had flown at full speed into the frozen ground, and the rest of the flock had obediently followed. There are two morals to this story. The first is that you need to choose your leader wisely. The second is that if you are going to lead people, you had better do a good job; if you don't, the consequences can be dire.

Leaders, by definition, must have followers. To get people to believe in your leadership capability and therefore follow you, you need to develop good relationships with your key people. They need to trust you and believe that you genuinely care about them. The best leaders are those who take the time to learn about their associates so they understand what motivates them, what they are proud of, what their goals are, and who or what is important to them. The most effective leaders are fully engaged in the performance of their people and continually coach and provide timely, constructive feedback. Leaders provide vision, create clarity, foster hope by telling their people that they believe in them, and, of course, deliver results.

With the exception of providing vision, all of this sounds like what managers are expected to do. So, is there a difference between managing and leading? The literature in this area is controversial. On the one hand, Peter Drucker (1998), one of the most respected management gurus of the modern era, supports the notion that leadership and management are identical. On the other hand, Marcus Buckingham (2005), who is equally respected, tells us that the core activities of the leader and the manager are totally different.

Buckingham (2005) believes that the manager looks inward—into the processes, the systems, and, most important, the people. The leader, on the other hand, looks outward—to industry trends, external factors such as competitive influences, and best practices from other companies and industries. Thus, managers and leaders perform distinct but complementary roles within the organization.

It is possible to be a great leader and a great manager; in fact, the best managers must also be good leaders. In the book *Jack Welch and the GE Way*, Welch says leaders speed things up and managers slow things down (Slater 1999). This, as Martha Stewart would say, is a very good thing. Leaders are all about vision and forward thinking, and the sooner they can get the organization to the goal, the better. From the leader's perspective, if it could happen tomorrow that would be okay, but today would be better and yesterday would have been ideal. Leaders are not interested in the *how*; most great leaders regard details as necessary evils. Managers, on the other hand, are intensely interested in the *how* because they are charged with the responsibility of making the goal happen. They have to marshal the people and the resources to accomplish the task and formulate the action plan.

Using the analogy of the ready, aim, fire sequence, the leader is essentially concerned with fire, whereas the manager is all about ready and aim. Great managers must have the ability to organize people around achieving the common vision or goal. They must be able to inspire their group to work hard, smart, and together, and this is where leadership comes into the manager's world. It is impossible for a manager to achieve

significant success without good leadership skills. The reality is that in a small organization, you (and probably others on your team) will need to don the leadership hat from time to time. Great organizations grow leaders at all levels. Organizations such as Southwest Airlines and Starbucks empower their associates to make decisions to preserve their well-deserved reputation for outstanding customer service. The good news is that most research shows us that anyone can become a great leader; it is not a genetic gift.

## The Bottom Line

Some of the best leaders of our time were brought up through the military ranks. Military experts will be the first to tell you about the critical role training plays in developing strong leaders. This reinforces the notion that great leaders were not born this way.

# Characteristics of Great Leaders

This section outlines a few of the most important characteristics that great leaders share. It focuses on culture as a critical component for the success of the leader and the organization.

## Great Leaders Create the Group Culture

In an intensely competitive industry such as ours, arguably the only **sustainable competitive advantage** you have is culture. In other words, when everyone in the industry has access to the same knowledge and technology, the only way to achieve a long-term edge on the competition is through the culture developed within the company. Great leaders carefully craft the culture of the organization and then promote and protect it at every turn. If you don't consciously create the culture, it will be created for you—and it may not be one you find desirable.

What is that elusive quality called *culture*? It is the combination of values and beliefs that guide behavior. It is reflected in how associates treat members, each other, and themselves. If your culture is strong, you will attract like-minded people to your company. They will feel comfortable operating within the values and beliefs espoused by the group. When their behavior is consistent with the culture of the company, it will be rewarded, recognized, and reinforced by leaders, managers, and peers. Similarly, those who cannot internalize the culture of the company will leave, either voluntarily or with a gentle push. When your culture is strong, members will experience consistent treatment from your associates even if a manager is not present.

## The Bottom Line

Culture is one of those fluffy terms than many people don't quite understand. The reality is that to develop and sustain a strong organizational culture, you must have clear plan. One of the most important parts of building culture is making sure the members of your team buy into the culture you are setting. People who truly match an organization's culture are totally on board with what the organization is all about. The result is a high-performing business with low employee turnover and happy customers. If your culture is about having fun, getting results, and sharing information, then you need to hire people who fit these characteristics and have ongoing systems in place to make sure this culture continues.

How can you create culture?

- Clearly define your values and communicate them tirelessly.
- Champion and reward positive behaviors and discourage and eliminate negative behaviors.
- Have all key people in the organization walk the walk and talk the talk all the time.
- Create **cultural heroes,** which are associates who, through actions consistent with the values of the company, create an amazing experience for a member. These heroes are then held up to the rest of the organization as shining examples of what appropriate behavior looks like, and they are rewarded accordingly.

## Great Leaders Inspire Trust

Great leaders don't necessarily have to be charismatic, larger-than-life figures. Some of the best leaders are those who quietly toil behind the scenes building great teams that are capable of extraordinary performance. Regardless of their personal characteristics, all great leaders can rally people to them because people feel they are trustworthy. They believe that such leaders will deliver on their promises because they have a proven history of doing so. If you truly want to become a great leader, be sure you can fulfill your commitments. Before verbalizing a promise, understand what you must do to keep it. Great leaders under promise and over deliver. You will quickly build a reputation for being trustworthy if you always deliver on your promises.

Finally, when great leaders don't have the answers, they don't fabricate them. When Mayor Rudy Giuliani was asked questions he didn't know the answers to in the terrible days after September 11, 2001, he replied honestly and with great compassion. In so doing, he won the trust of the nation.

## Great Leaders Communicate the Goals of the Organization

Great leaders understand that people are drawn toward the vision of success. If the vision is unclear or is continually changing, people start to question what they are doing and why they are doing it, and they begin to disengage. It is the leader's responsibility to ensure that goals are clearly communicated to every member of the organization. Dave Patchell-Evans, the founder and CEO of GoodLife Fitness Clubs, never wavered from his vision of what success would look like for his company. Everyone in the company knew that success would be 100 clubs by the year 2005. Having achieved that milestone, he clearly communicated his new vision: 100 more clubs in the next 4 years. The second goal has since been achieved and surpassed. The new goal is 1,000 clubs.

## The Bottom Line

A challenge for any organization is continually communicating its goals and vision. This is easier with a young company, as employees know the owner, understand the organization, and buy into its cause. As a business grows, it becomes difficult to keep the message alive. The best leaders constantly focus on communicating goals and vision with their staff.

## Great Leaders Seek Great Mentors

Mentoring is a key part of becoming a great manager and leader. All great leaders can point to specific mentors they learned from. Look around you to find people in your industry or other industries you can learn from. There is no point in trying to reinvent the wheel when many others are doing what you want to do. Learn from their mistakes and get there quicker. All too often, I see owners and managers do their own thing and work in their own silo. If they had only reached out for some help or gone to a conference or workshop, they could have saved themselves a lot of heartache.

# Characteristics of Great Managers

This section discusses a few of the critical traits great managers must possess. You can be a good manager if you have only some of these qualities, but great managers have all of them.

## Great Managers Have a Nose for Talent

Great managers have a sixth sense about people. They are continually on the lookout for promising candidates outside of the organization and are continually assessing the talent they currently possess. There is a war for talent in North America—the workforce is shrinking, as is the birth rate, and the traditional sources of skilled workers are drying up. This has been predicted for years, but, in the words of Peter Drucker (1998), "the future has already happened," and most health club managers are struggling to adjust. How can you avoid the frightening prospect of having no talented candidates to fill the inevitable vacancies you will experience?

One obvious strategy is to keep the people you currently have, as I'll discuss later. Another is to constantly be scouting for people who have the right attitude and would be a good fit with your company culture and values. Prime scouting areas include the hotel, restaurant, and retail industries. These are the places you are most likely to find employees who are genuinely interested in people and who have the service mentality required to be successful in the health and fitness industry. Whenever you experience exceptional service, compliment the employees and present them with a low-key recruiting pitch. Recruitment is the highest form of flattery, and it is identical to selling. You may not lure prospective associates to your club immediately, but you will plant the seed so if they consider switching careers at some point, they will think of you.

## Great Managers Continually Assess Talent

Great managers need to constantly be evaluating and assessing their current talent. How can you ensure that you are consistently, fairly, and accurately assessing the merits of your people?

The former Chairman and CEO of GE Jack Welch was well known for getting rid of the bottom 10% of his employees. Welch would not settle for weak performers, and he knew that these people would bring down others in the organization. While his approach may seem aggressive and insensitive, it worked from the shareholders' standpoint. GE's stock skyrocketed during Welch's tenure, and to this day he is considered one of the great CEOs in recent memory.

The following are some basic tenets associated with evaluating talent:

- *Recognize and reward the top performers.* Everyone benefits from productivity, but not everyone deserves the same recognition. Never lose sight of your top performers and what their contributions are.
- *Don't settle for weak performance.* If some employees are not performing at the level they need to be, tell them and help them get there. If you have made every effort to help them and they are still not performing at the desired level, it is time to let them go.
- *Conduct formal evaluations on all staff.* This is the only way to let associates know where they stand and for you to know what type of staff you have. Evaluations are normally done once per year, but they can be done more often depending on the situation.
- *Always be on the lookout for new people to add to your team.* You never know when you will need to add someone due to unexpected growth or replace someone without notice. Great leaders and managers are known for finding and developing talent. The best time to look for

new people is before you need them rather than when you are on a tight timeline.

## The Bottom Line

One of the best ways to retain and motivate your staff is to ensure that associates have clear career paths mapped out for themselves. Once these paths are formulated, be sure you give employees the right opportunities to grow and prosper within the company.

## Great Managers Understand That Everyone Is Different

Great managers understand that they cannot treat everyone the same. Marcus Buckingham (2005) likens this to checkers versus chess: In the game of checkers, each piece moves the same way, but in chess, each piece moves in a different way and performs different roles. Different people are motivated by different things and respond differently to feedback and coaching. For example, some people love public recognition, whereas others are uncomfortable in the spotlight and prefer to receive their rewards privately. With some people you can be very direct when giving feedback but with others you will need to soften your approach. Great managers intuitively understand this and are constantly working on building great relationships with their team members so they can better understand how to help all members achieve their potential.

Some managers seem to build great relationships easily. They have that elusive sixth sense about people. They tend to be keenly observant and ask a lot of probing questions, and they are excellent listeners. They are genuinely interested and care deeply about the success and happiness of their charges. Daniel Goleman (1995) refers to this ability to build relationships and manage emotions as emotional intelligence (EI).

Using a worksheet such as that shown in figure 1.2 can provide structure for meaningful conversations with associates about their past accomplishments and future aspirations. These conversations provide the foundation for a great relationship. Once you understand what is important to your associates, you will be able to provide meaningful coaching and support as you assist them in moving toward their goals.

At GoodLife Fitness Clubs, managers and leaders use 12 questions as a primary form of feedback. The questions are from the book *First, Break All the Rules* (Buckingham and Coffman 1999). The first two questions—"Do you know what is expected of you?" and "Do you have the resources required to do your job?"— are the most relevant to this discussion and elicit the most important information from the manager's perspective. If people don't know what you expect of them or don't have the tools to do their jobs properly, then they don't have even a faint hope of being successful. Buckingham and Coffman use the analogy of climbing a mountain: You must spend the requisite amount of time acclimating at base camp before moving up to the summit; otherwise, you will die. Until your associates can strongly agree with both questions, any attempt you may make to motivate or empower them will ultimately fail. This is your foundation, and until it is solidly in place, you dare not move on.

Answers to the remaining 10 questions provide feedback about you as a leader or manager and indicate how well associates fit into the company culture and what they believe their futures in the organization look like; all of this is great information. It is not uncommon to have associates complete this evaluation on a quarterly basis. Building a history of responses from all associates will enable you to monitor their (and your) progress and will indicate potential sources of trouble or success. For example, if an associate answered the second question with a 5 (strongly agree) on one evaluation but dropped the response to a 2 (tend to disagree) on the next evaluation, you need to initiate a meaningful conversation with that person to ascertain what changed and how it might be rectified. This is a valuable method for scoring the effectiveness of managers and how engaged people are. It is short, easily understood, and quickly interpreted.

Another useful tool for determining how to best manage people is to use the StrengthsFinder profile (www.strengthsfinder.com). You will need to purchase one of the publications listed on the website to access the online questionnaires, but the information you receive will be well worth it. You will learn which situations and projects allow different people to thrive and which ones will cause them to become frustrated and disengaged. You will be able to define the top five strengths for each person who fills out

# LIFE AND WORK GOALS

Name: Thomas Johnson

## Mission

My mission is to make a positive difference for each person I come in contact with every day.

## Core Values That Guide Me

Care, trust, integrity

## Significant Life and Work Accomplishments

- Completed two marathons.
- Married for 16 years to the same person.
- Promoted to general manager (GM) in 2005.
- Graduated with an MA in exercise physiology.

## Work Goals

- Achieve all financial targets for my club.
- Improve member retention by 3%.
- Recruit and hire an excellent member-care manager.

## Professional Development Goals

- Win GM of the year award.
- Join Toastmasters.
- Present at canfitpro conference.

## Personal Goals

- Take a family vacation in Italy.
- Learn to speak Italian.
- Run two half marathons.

## How to Meet My Goals

### Work Goals

- Set up a monthly meeting with my divisional manager to review statements and correct variances.
- Beef up personal training revenue by 20%.
- To improve member retention, handle all cancellations myself whenever possible, focus on training front-desk staff for world-class meet and greet, and meet with member focus group once a month to invite feedback.
- To find a member-care manager, recruit from local restaurants and retail stores and post internally to see if there are any members who would be great candidates. Once the manager is hired, set up a rigorous training program. Develop an incentive program based on reducing member cancellations.

### Professional Development Goals

- Work out an action plan with my divisional manager to win GM of the year. Get clearly defined expectations and performance standards.
- Contact canfitpro and find out how presenters are selected. Join Toastmasters in November to improve presentation skills. Ask divisional manager to allow me to present at GM meetings.

### Personal Goals

- Book and pay for the holiday so we can't cancel.
- Buy Italian language CDs and commit to listening three times per week for 1 hour each.
- Join the half marathon running group in January.

**Figure 1.2** Goal-setting worksheet filled out by an associate. Managers can learn about their associates' motivations by asking them to fill out similar worksheets.

the questionnaire. More important, you will gain invaluable insight into how to effectively manage each associate.

## Great Managers Encourage Feedback

A climate in which feedback is encouraged is invaluable. If people feel safe giving you honest feedback about what works for them and what doesn't, you are well on your way to becoming a great manager. It sounds easy, doesn't it? Tell people what you really think about their behavior on a consistent and timely basis. What is so hard about that? Unfortunately, most people struggle with honest communication. You can create a feedback-positive climate in your organization by building relationships based on trust and caring. The adage "they don't care how much you know until they know how much you care" is highly applicable to managing. People will forgive you for many mistakes if you create an environment in which they understand you sincerely care about them and their success and they know you are prepared to invest in them.

A word of caution is warranted: There is a huge difference between caring and caretaking. Don't fall into the caretaking trap. Caretaking sounds something like this:

> Justin hasn't hit his sales goals in 6 months, and I told him if he didn't perform this month, he would be out. I know I should just go ahead and fire him, but he and his wife are expecting their first baby next month.
>
> I can't tell Kim what I really think of her performance, because she is so sensitive. I know if I'm totally honest with her, she will get really upset.

If you are unable to be honest with associates because you think they will be unable to handle the truth, then you have fallen into the caretaking trap. The highest form of caring is giving honest, timely feedback to people in a manner that allows their dignity and self-respect to remain intact. It may be challenging initially, but like anything else, it gets easier with practice. Eventually, you will be able to develop meaningful relationships because they are based on mutual trust and respect. Caring

is the most important implement in your managerial tool kit. Use it often and wisely.

## The Bottom Line

Giving feedback is one of the easiest ways to reward an employee, but studies show that managers do a poor job of this. The best way to motivate employees is to find them doing something correct and praise them for that action rather than trying to find them doing something wrong and disciplining them.

## Great Managers Understand the Importance of Systems

Strong managers understand that there is a formula for success. Once you understand the formula, you can teach it to the right person. Having systems in place essentially means that the business has a specific way of doing things, and they want everyone doing them the same way. High-performing fitness facilities have systems for every aspect of the business (e.g., a specific way to answer the phone, a specific way to handle member complaints, a specific way to sell and process memberships). A practice is considered a system only if it is written down and is regularly reviewed. A conversation is not enough, because things can be forgotten or misinterpreted, which leads to the desired outcome not being achieved. Great systems ensure a consistent client or member experience and ensure everyone knows exactly what is expected of them. The most successful fitness clubs in the world have achieved greatness by developing, borrowing, and changing their systems. Well-developed systems that are communicated to employees on a regular basis take the guesswork out of day-to-day decisions.

Systems are useless unless they are clearly defined and people are kept accountable to them. For example, all fitness facilities should have a clearly written script and a system for how they handle phone calls about membership inquiry. When a prospective member calls and the phone call is handled properly, that prospect should be booked for a tour and consultation at the gym.

When this call is not handled properly, a potential new client is lost. When people call a gym, their first question is normally related to costs or to a specific program. An important part of handling these calls properly is assessing the clients' goals and their exercise history. It is best to meet with prospects in person so they can see the facility and determine what programs are best for them. If prospects on the phone are simply given prices, the quoted prices may be for memberships or programs that are not right for them, and the prospects may be deterred or lose interest in the club. These are missed opportunities that cost the club money. Large facilities track their booking rates from incoming calls; when they start to get low, they address this to ensure everyone is following the specified system.

## Great Managers Provide Clear Expectations

Great managers are very clear about what they expect from their associates. After all, how can associates do a good job if they don't know exactly what is expected of them? This seems like a basic tenet, but you would be amazed to discover how few people in supervisory roles are able to state clear expectations for their direct reports. If in doubt how well you are doing in this area, use the 12 questions mentioned earlier, and pay specific attention to the responses to the first question.

When defining expectations for associates, be aware that a job profile is just the beginning. You need to have meaningful discussions about what it looks like to perform well. For instance, a job profile for people who work the front desk might state that the phone must be answered in a professional and courteous manner. Your definition of professional and courteous, however, may be quite different from someone else's. Thus, it is important to provide training that will clearly show what it looks and sounds like to answer the phone in a courteous and professional manner. Observe associates' performance so you can provide caring, honest feedback. As noted previously, the greatest gift you can give or receive is honest, timely feedback delivered in a manner that provides clarity on expectations and enhances the receiver's self-esteem.

Consider this example: You walk into your club earlier than usual one morning to find the person at the front desk reading the paper and paying no attention whatsoever to the members who are checking in. You have several choices:

- You can rant and rave like a deranged maniac, thereby scaring the associate and everyone else in earshot.
- You can ignore the behavior (more about the effectiveness of this strategy later).
- You can ask the associate to come to your office when the next person shows up to work the front desk.

Hopefully you chose the last option. Your mandate for giving feedback should always be to reward in public and reprimand in private. How can you deliver appropriate feedback that will leave no doubt about your future expectations but will also leave people feeling good about themselves? In the words of Stephen Covey (1989), great managers seek "first to understand." It is all too easy to jump to the wrong conclusion about the motivation for someone's behavior only to make an idiot out of yourself and damage the relationship. Take a deep breath, and find out why the associate felt compelled to read the paper when it was clearly not appropriate. You may be shocked to find out that she considers this to be appropriate behavior because no one told her it wasn't. Or you may find out that she was fulfilling a member's request that she look up the time and location of a movie. If, however, she understands that the behavior is inappropriate and simply made a bad decision, you need to take the appropriate action. Be sure to separate how you feel about her behavior from how you feel about her as a person so you don't damage her self-esteem.

For example, you might start by saying "Sarah, when I came into the club this morning, I observed that you were reading the paper. I am curious to know why you were doing that." This is an open-ended, nonjudgmental question (hopefully your body language and tone are neutral and nonthreatening). Now, let's assume Sarah knew and understood she had made an inappropriate choice, and she admits it to you. An effective response from you might be the following:

*I trust you to conduct yourself in a professional manner at all times when you are in the club, Sarah, even if I am not here. To our members, you are a walking, talking personification of our* **core values**. *I know I can count on you to make decisions about your behavior that are in the best interests of our members. Although I am disappointed in your behavior this morning, you need to understand that I think you are a fine individual, and I am proud to have you working here. In the future, please refrain from doing this type of thing at our front desk. If you have completed your list of daily tasks and need of things to do, please ask me. There are always things I can use your help with.*

## STRUGGLING AS A MANAGER: PITFALLS TO AVOID

The mistakes managers make are not usually easy to cover up, because they can affect many people. The following are 10 of the most common behaviors that will cause you to struggle and ways to avoid them:

1. *Hiring like-minded people with similar strengths.* It is no secret that most people like to be around others that are like them (e.g., similar interests, backgrounds, personalities). Although this might be great for a friendship, it is a disaster for a business. When managers hire people like themselves, they are loading up on certain skills and neglecting others. For example, you might be a great salesperson with a lot of enthusiasm and passion for people, but you might not be great at keeping yourself organized or understanding the financial effects of your decisions. Therefore, it is critical to have people with other skill sets around you.

The best managers try to hire people who are smarter than them or who at least have different strengths than they do, because they realize this will ultimately make the team and the organization stronger. Although some managers worry that an exceptional employee may eventually take their job, owners value managers who make good hiring decisions, which demonstrate the manager's value to the company rather than diminishing it.

2. *Undertraining.* This is one of the great weaknesses of many independent fitness clubs and small businesses in general. Managers get too busy with day-to-day business operations or don't understand the value in delegating, and they neglect to train their staff. Training is an ongoing function of a manager, and it is often the most important role. Most performance issues (when the right people are hired) boil down to training issues, and these fall on the manager's shoulders. New and experienced staff alike needs training to learn new tasks and to stay sharp on current ones. The best managers position their employees for success by developing or following training programs that will improve staff skills.

3. *Making quick hiring decisions.* This is a big one. Staff turnover is often unpredictable, and when an associate leaves unexpectedly, the manager is left scrambling to find a replacement. When this happens, proper hiring protocol is often thrown out the window, and bad decisions are made. Not spending the time upfront to get the right person on your team will always cost you in the long run. You will also lose credibility with staff and members because they see people come and go too often.

4. *Not setting a good example.* Weak managers ask staff to do things that they don't want to do (e.g., talking to a member about a strong body odor, which is not fun for anyone). Weak managers take shortcuts that go against company policies and procedures. Some managers do not maintain their own fitness levels and portray unhealthy images. The best managers willingly perform any job task, always follow policy, and practice good nutrition and exercise routines. They set the standard for the staff and the club members.

5. *Not making timely decisions.* Managers who put off important decisions can derail an organization. In addition, relationships suffer because people lose confidence in the manager's ability to make decisions. Weak managers ignore issues or rely on staff and others to solve problems. Although it is important to empower staff, there are decisions that must be made by managers. People may not always agree with the decisions, but they will respect managers who make them. To make the best decisions, strong managers should gather the relevant information, react without emotion, and consult with people around them as needed. The best managers also take ownership of their mistakes if they make the wrong decisions.

6. *Managing time inefficiently.* This is perhaps the challenge that new managers wrestle with more than any other. It takes great skill to create a flex-

ible schedule that allows for inevitable unanticipated events that will require your attention, and it takes great discipline to stick to this schedule. There are many books and courses on the best way to manage your time. Steven Covey, author of *The Seven Habits of Highly Effective People* (1989) and other books, is one of the authorities in this area. Virtually any system will work if you have the discipline to execute it. Managing your time well means prioritizing tasks and responsibilities and scheduling the most important tasks so you know they will get done with minimal interruption.

As a club manager, many people require your time and attention. If there is a secret to successfully managing your time, it is that you need to manage your interruptions. Train your team to respect your schedule. Create specific times during the day when they have access to you for asking questions. You should also apply **Pareto's Law** (also called the 80:20 rule) when creating your schedule: Focus on the 20% of your tasks that yield 80% of the results, and then schedule those tasks at the times you are most productive. Whenever possible, delegate tasks that do not meet the 80:20 criteria. This will help you focus on the most important items and will allow your people to assume more responsibility. No matter how well you plan and how disciplined you are, you will have days where nothing goes according to schedule, but as long as most of your days do not fall into that category, you will be winning the time management battle.

7. *Forgetting that members come first.* New managers are often so overwhelmed with the responsibilities of their position that they forget who is most important; this is a classic case of not being able to see the forest for the trees. In our industry, members always come first. This needs to be much more than rhetoric. This philosophy must be thoroughly woven into the operation of your club so members are never taken for granted or forgotten. Members put food on your table, clothes on your back, and a roof over your head. As such, they need to be treated like royalty. In addition, happy, satisfied members will become ambassadors for your club, which will ultimately bring you more members. Poor managers somehow forget this or overlook it. As the manager, you must always stay in touch with members and put them first.

A member of a club once complained that the manager was hard to find, and this complaint was corroborated by the low member retention in that club. The manager was transferred to a different position that was a better fit (he was enormously gifted in organization and administration and truly believed in the core values of the company) and replaced with a manager who went out of her way to create meaningful interactions with members. She scheduled time every day to walk the workout floor during busy times and inquire about members' concerns. It would be too simplistic to say that member retention improved due to this one act, but it certainly was a contributing factor. Perhaps more important, this manager's actions embodied the notion that members come first, and her team saw this and took a cue about how they should act with members.

8. *Micromanaging.* To the untrained eye, there is a fine line between coaching and telling, but to the trained eye and to those on the receiving end, there is a world of difference. The difference is that a good coach will act as a guide but will allow associates to find their own way, within reason. If you find yourself consistently telling people how they should act or fixing problems for them, then you have crossed into the realm of **micromanaging**. The net effect of micromanaging is that people never have to think for themselves, because you are always doing it for them. They will become incapable of finding workable solutions to problems. If you micromanage, associates will not grow and develop, and you will have to spend an inordinate amount of time at the club because things fall apart when you aren't there. In addition, people will never feel that you trust them. Ambitious people will leave, and the people who are content to have you do their thinking for them will stay; as a result, you will never experience the level of success that you are capable of.

9. *Trying to be everyone's friend.* Although it would be great to make new friends at work, it would be even better to challenge associates and develop them into stronger people and members of your team. Challenging staff often means causing some conflict and asking people to do things they do not want to do. This is hard for friends to do with one another, but it is easy for strong managers to do.

10. *Not fostering an atmosphere of fun.* All work and no play will make your club a very dull place to work. People spend a significant portion of their time working, and if they don't enjoy what they are doing, then they are not living their lives to their

full potential. We do important work that makes an incredible difference in peoples' lives, and we need to enjoy ourselves while we do it.

Enjoyment is apparent if people have fun while they work. This doesn't mean playing practical jokes or running around aimlessly. It means being able to laugh together and at yourself. Lighten up and see the humor in your job. It will allow you to keep everything in perspective and help you maintain your sanity. It will make your club a desirable place to work and to be a member. Read *Fish: A Remarkable Way to Boost Morale and Improve Results* by Stephen Lundin (2000) and watch "Fish!: A Proven Way to Boost Morale and Improve Results" on YouTube. Work with your team to brainstorm ways to have more fun at work. If a fish market can be that much fun, just imagine what can happen at your club!

## The Bottom Line

Great managers understand that to keep great people, you need to empower them. This can only happen when managers effectively delegate responsibilities to their staff. Once tasks have been delegated, managers need to allow associates to complete the tasks without scrutinizing their every move. If associates are only given mundane, repetitive tasks, they will become bored and eventually leave.

These 10 pitfalls will derail your success if you let them. The first step to mastering them is awareness. What you do with the information now is up to you.

## SUCCEEDING AS A MANAGER: A STRATEGY TO MANAGE TALENT

If you could choose only one component that would most affect your success as a club manager, what do you think it would be? If you guessed people, you are right. You need a **talent management strategy** to ensure your success. You may find it useful to use the alignment, capability, and engagement (ACE) model described in figure 1.3 to visualize your talent management strategy.

If your associates are aligned with the values, beliefs, and goals of the organization (**alignment**), if they are capable of good performance and are properly trained and equipped to do their jobs (**capability**), and if they are fully engaged in their work and give 100% (**engagement**), then they are operating in the sweet spot of performance. This is comparable to what athletes refer to as the *zone*—the state in which they are working at peak performance and loving what they are doing. People who are successful and love their jobs seldom leave.

Keeping good people is essential to the success of your club. You first need to measure associate retention just as you would measure member retention. What gets measured gets managed. Calculate

## Becoming a Better Manager

Continuous growth and education are critical elements to becoming a better manager. Networking with other people in your industry or with people outside your industry can facilitate this. Fitness industry conferences are a great way to learn and network. You can attend educational sessions lead by industry experts and meet other attendees that you can share ideas with. A few of the larger conferences that have strong management contents are the International Health, Racquet & Sportsclub Association (IHRSA), Club Industry, and canfitpro.

It is also a great idea to see what people are doing outside of your industry. Local chambers of commerce often hold networking and public speaking events that anyone can attend. Mastermind groups are another way to network and learn. These groups are normally made up of 5 to 10 people and are led by a coach or facilitator who walks the group through an issue. Members can provide feedback and ask questions.

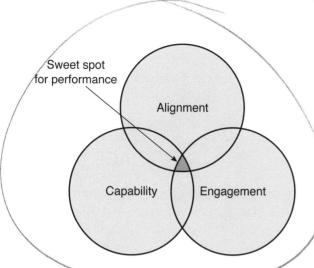

**Figure 1.3** The ACE model.

how much it costs to replace one associate, and you will understand how important it is to keep good people. To accurately calculate this, include the costs of recruitment, lost productivity during the hiring process, lost productivity due to not having the position filled, lost productivity during the associate's learning curve (the time it takes to get to full productivity), and training the new associate (including lost productivity by those training).

## *The Bottom Line*

The cost of replacing one membership coordinator (i.e., a sales associate) is approximately $17,500. In addition, when members see staff come and go on a regular basis, it can affect your brand and therefore your bottom line. When you gauge the cost of poor associate retention, it will quickly become apparent how much time and energy you need to invest in keeping good people.

You also need to closely monitor associate retention (or attrition). Those in the most important positions—that is, associates who have the most direct and significant effects on the financial performance of your club—should be of primary concern to you. You need to focus most of your time, attention, and resources on these positions, because these people are fundamental to your financial success. These positions are typically the club managers, membership coordinators, and front-desk associates. Whatever your own most important positions are, you need to be continually working to improve retention in them. Realistically, you will never reduce your turnover to zero. Picture writing a check for $17,500 each time a membership coordinator leaves the company to help you to stay focused on this critical goal.

In my experience, managers who have the lowest associate turnover (and who, not coincidentally, consistently deliver the best financial results) have these three traits in common:

1. They are extremely skilled in developing great relationships.
2. They give people the coaching and training they require to quickly become successful in their jobs and achieve their full potential.
3. They recognize and reward good performance and confront poor performance immediately and in a caring manner.

If you can develop these traits in yourself and apply them consistently, you will be in the enviable position of having experienced, productive, and engaged people working with you. When that piece of your success strategy is in place, your success and the success of your club will be guaranteed.

## Key Terms

| | | |
|---|---|---|
| alignment | emotional intelligence (EI) | sustainable competitive advantage |
| capability | engagement | |
| core values | micromanaging | systems |
| cultural heroes | Pareto's Law | talent management strategy |

# CHAPTER 2

# Understanding Organizational Design

## Learning Objectives

After studying this chapter, you will be able to

- understand the difference between vertical and horizontal aspects of a business;
- recognize key employees and their responsibilities;
- understand the importance of job descriptions in facility operations;
- discuss the differences between for-profit, not-for-profit, and corporate-based fitness facilities; and
- identify behaviors of successful leaders in the fitness industry.

Anjana was recently hired as the new front-desk person at the Lexington Athletic Club. She was excited because she has always wanted to work in the field. Anjana is a student and was told she would be working about 15 hours per week, including two evening shifts and one Saturday shift. She was interviewed by a general manager, but she was told she would be reporting to the front-desk manager, Marsha.

During the interview process, she was told that the job mainly involved meeting and greeting clients, answering phones, and doing some scheduling. She was also told it was a fast-paced job and she should expect to be busy the whole time. During her first week of training, she shadowed the other front-desk associates. She learned that there was a lot more to the job than she had originally envisioned. The front-desk software was very complex, and she was not looking forward to learning it. She also found out that she would occasionally be asked to give tours of the facilities and to go over prices with prospective new clients. This made her really nervous, because she is somewhat shy. At the end of her first week of training, Anjana felt overwhelmed and was starting to second guess her decision to take the position.

Anjana asked one of her coworkers if there were a job description for her position. Her coworker laughed and said "yes, it includes everything in the gym." Apparently, the other front-desk associates had asked for a concise job description on more than one occasion, but

The author acknowledges the significant contributions of Scott Lewandowski to this chapter.

they never got one. The lack of clarity about job responsibilities had often caused confusion and frustration, and it wasn't clear who the associates should talk to when problems arose.

Anjana decided to make it her personal mission to help the club create job descriptions for the front-desk positions. To help the workflow and overall communication, clubs should ensure that all positions have clear job descriptions.

───────────────────────●───────────────────────

Health and fitness clubs are fast paced. You must expect the unexpected, be prepared to maintain your composure, and execute superior service. Many employees, such as the front-desk staff, work part time, and they might not be as committed to the club as the full-time staff.

It is the manager's responsibility to provide a healthy, challenging, and rewarding work environment that encourages a greater commitment from and builds confidence in part-time and full-time employees. A clear and concise organizational chart that lists all job positions will help employees understand everyone's role in reaching the club's goals. Well-structured job descriptions are critical so employees know their responsibilities and management's expectations.

## The Bottom Line

Employees' job satisfaction is directly related to whether their skills are being used to the fullest potential. In addition, employee retention is directly related to member retention. If member numbers go down, the facility can no longer retain as many employees. So, it is important for employees to be vested in member retention to retain their own jobs, too. Create volunteer retention teams that focus on welcoming new members, retaining old members, retaining staff, providing social activities besides exercise, and getting members to participate in group exercise.

**Organizational design** is a critical part of any business. How an organization is set up will determine responsibilities, future career paths, and proper modes of communication when problems arise or when ideas need to be shared. When an organization is set up properly, communication and chain of command runs smoothly and staff members at all levels clearly understand their roles in the organization. The overall design of any organization is determined by the type of business, the number of employees, and the owners' philosophy.

When considering the type of business, you must look at the various departments and areas of responsibility. If the organization has numerous departments, then it will eventually need someone who is responsible for each one. For example, a large fitness facility might have a sales department, an administrative department, a personal training department, and a group exercise department. Each of these areas has a manager and 2 to 10 associates who report to that manager. There might also be subdepartments within each area. Within the group exercise department, for example, there could be an aquatics coordinator, a yoga coordinator, and a boot camp coordinator. In addition, as a business grows, there is a need to hire more people and expand specific departments. This is one way that a business becomes more complex.

The complexity of a business is determined by its vertical and horizontal aspects. The vertical aspects of a business are the various levels of management or responsibilities. You could see vertical growth due to the expansion of one department. For example, the sales staff may have originally reported directly to the club's general manager, as shown in figure 2.1a. As the business grows, however, the general manager's many responsibilities may make it difficult to manage the sales staff. In this situation, a sales manager or assistant manager may be brought in to oversee the sales staff (see figure 2.1b). This adds another position to the organizational chart.

## The Bottom Line

It is a good idea to project the organizational chart 3 to 5 years into the future so everyone can see the long-term plans and how their positions and departments might change. In a new small business, for example, everyone might initially report to the owner, but this will change as the business grows.

The horizontal aspects of the business are the various positions within the organization. When a business experiences horizontal growth in one area, the manager of that area will typically have increased responsibilities.

An organizational chart allows employees to see potential career paths within the organization, and it can be motivational for those seeking growth opportunities and promotions. The organizational chart reflects the current structure of an organization and shows the relative ranks of the positions therein. This framework is an efficient organizational structure because it provides a quick way to outline the roles, responsibilities, and relationships between individuals within an organization.

Communication is a critical part of any organization, and organizational design can help or hinder communication. The organizational chart should clearly lay out who is responsible for specific areas of the facility, and job descriptions should provide additional information on specific duties. For example, if a front-desk person receives a complaint about how a salesperson acted or receives a compliment about a specific group exercise instructor, he or she should know who is in charge of each of these areas so the information can be passed on to the appropriate person.

## GROWTH AND MANAGEMENT POSITIONS

As a business grows, it is inevitable that responsibilities will be shifted and new levels of management will be required. At the outset, a fitness club may be able to get by with one general manager who oversees everything. As the business grows, however, it may require new management posi-

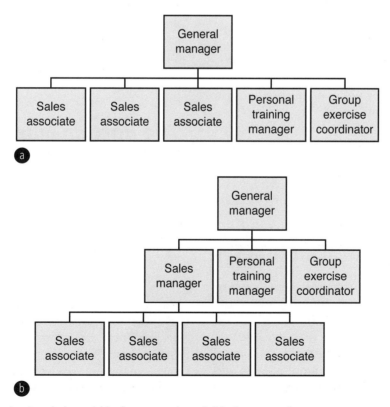

**Figure 2.1** Organizational chart *(a)* before growth and *(b)* after growth.

tions to oversee specific areas, such as sales, personal training, day care, group exercise, or the front desk. These positions will vary from club to club. The decision to restructure the organizational chart will rest in the hands of senior management as they seek to identify which facility needs require new positions due to growth.

## ROLES AND RESPONSIBILITIES

Regardless of the size of the facility, if the business does not have roles and responsibilities clearly defined in job descriptions and organizational charts, problems are bound to occur. The following are a few issues associated with not having formal job descriptions in place:

- Prospective new hires will not have a clear picture of the job duties, and this may lead to a poor impression of the business. If this candidate is highly sought after by other facilities, a business that provides a detailed job description will likely win the candidate.

- Without proper descriptions in place, evaluations can be vague and subjective. Evaluation processes should be largely based on the responsibilities laid out in job descriptions.

- Roles and responsibilities are not always clear, which can lead to some people taking on more duties and others taking on fewer. When this happens, staff inevitably develops animosity toward one another because it seems that some people are not carrying their weight.

- When people do not have clear expectations, they are not sure what they should be doing and they become unmotivated. This leads to complacency and doing meaningless jobs to look busy.

## WRITING JOB DESCRIPTIONS

The first step in developing a job description is to brainstorm the daily, weekly, monthly, quarterly, or yearly tasks for each position. Experienced staff members can create these lists, because it is unlikely you will know all the tasks completed at each level. Ideally, you will want at least one other person to review the brainstorming sheets for each position; this person should know the position relatively well. For key management and higher-level positions, the owner or general manager should review the lists.

Once the material has been reviewed, all items should be grouped and any redundancies should be eliminated so the job description is as concise as possible. It is a good idea to weight each task based on the time spent and its overall importance; then, list the tasks in order as follows:

1. Tasks that are essential to the position
2. Tasks that are important
3. Tasks that are not priorities

Therefore, using the rank ordering of tasks will identify and organize the tasks related to prioritization. This process should make it easier to identify those tasks in the job description, which are essential to the position.

Examine the lowest-priority tasks to see if they should be transferred to lower-level associates. For example, if the membership coordinator is spending a lot of time answering incoming calls that are unrelated to sales and dealing with customer complaints, perhaps these duties need to be transferred to the front-desk staff so the membership coordinator can spend more time on the essential tasks for that position (e.g., making outgoing calls, asking for referrals, conducting tours). In the final analysis, the goal of using the rank ordering is to align the essential tasks to the written job descriptions for the position. This alignment is key so a position does not include tasks that are not high priority or relevant to the position.

### *The Bottom Line*

Most businesses do not have job descriptions in place. There are various reasons for this, but the main one is often a lack of knowledge about their importance and the lack of urgency completing them. When you have sales targets to hit, customers to help, and machines that need to be fixed, writing staff job descriptions is oftentimes left on the back burner. As with any important task, time needs to be scheduled and things need to be delegated so the task gets done.

This chapter describes how various health and fitness organizations are set up and discusses the key positions in these organizations. Four types of organizations will be examined: for-profit organizations, not-for-profit organizations, hospital-based organizations, and corporate-based organizations. (Key components of job descriptions are discussed in chapter 3).

Although these types of organizations have different organizational designs to achieve their specific business goals, they do share common themes, positions, and processes. Their organizational designs and job descriptions for similar positions are different and meet the facilities' individual goals. I will compare a few different organizational designs.

# FOR-PROFIT ORGANIZATIONS

**For-profit (commercial) facilities** focus on membership, retention, and revenue. Earnings before interest, taxes, depreciation, and amortization (EBITDA) and revenue growth sales, membership retention, net membership growth, revenue per member, revenue per indoor square foot, and **nondues revenue** are tracked monthly and compared against the current budget, last year's budget, and industry standards.

Employees in facilities that are larger than 20,000 square feet (1,858 square meters) with more than 50 employees are very fast paced. Expectations at the beginning of the workday are seldom completed. These organizations have clearly defined roles and responsibilities. Key positions in a large commercial facility include the general manager, membership director, membership consultants (i.e., sales representatives), fitness director, and personal trainers (see figure 2.2). Sample job descriptions for some common positions in the health and fitness industry are outlined next.

For-profit facilities smaller than 10,000 square feet (929 square meters) differ from larger facilities in staffing and marketing. These facilities staff up to 15 employees. However, for businesses that employ 15 to 50 people, or businesses that are between 10k and 20k square feet, some staffing and marketing positions may include personnel with more specialized roles such as a social media specialist, marketing manager or membership sales, and membership sales manager or director. In other words, the "medium" size facility is a hybrid of a small or large facility with some positions written with a narrower scope. Most of these employees have titles such as member counselor and wellness coach (see figure 2.3). They have broader job duties, which include selling memberships, setting up exercise programs, and cleaning the facility.

The smaller for-profit commercial facilities must be adaptable and have attention-grabbing promotions unless they are part of a franchise that has their own standard operating procedures. A great way for smaller facilities to connect with their identified target markets is to offer health screenings at community events and corporate health fairs.

# General Manager

The primary roles of the **general manager** are to ensure the annual budget is met, develop a marketing plan with the membership director for continued membership growth, keep a high profile in the club, and work with department managers to achieve desired results. The general manager has the most difficult job when it comes to organization. When there is a problem, it is the general manager who is called upon. The general manager must be available to assist departments when needed and have a strong presence throughout the club, especially during peak times. The general manager can truly say there are not enough hours in a day.

## QUALIFICATIONS

- Have a bachelor's degree in business management/administration, fitness management, or related field. However, a master's degree is preferred.
- Have 2 to 4 years direct sales experience, preferably in a fitness related setting. Preference to those with at least 2 years of management experience, too.
- Be able to read and understand costs and budgets.
- Demonstrate ability to analyze information and situations to formulate logical and objective decisions.
- Work collaboratively with internal and external constituents; strong people skills.
- Have operating knowledge of Microsoft office.

## RESPONSIBILITIES

- Adhere to the core values and core purpose established by ownership.

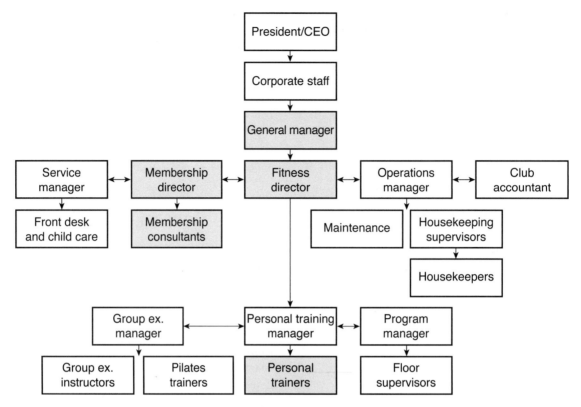

**Figure 2.2**   Organizational chart for a large for-profit organization (larger than 20,000 ft² [1,858 m²] and more than 50 employees). Shaded areas indicate positions described in the text.

Reprinted by permission.

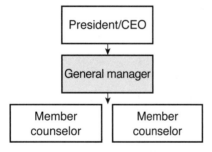

**Figure 2.3**   Organizational chart for a small for-profit organization (smaller than 10,000 ft² [929 m²] and fewer than 15 employees). Shaded area indicates position described in text.

- Improve the overall service level of the club based on the semiannual quantitative customer satisfaction survey.
- Increase the demand, usage, and net revenue capabilities of the club during off-peak hours. This is primarily accomplished through off-peak membership sales and

**subtenant** relationships established by the ownership. Subtenants (e.g., juice bar, pro shop) rent space from the fitness club and operate their businesses within the club.

- Nurture the existing subtenant relationships.
- Implement the strategic plan for the club.
- Hold quarterly staff meetings to reinforce the annual goals; work on team building; inform staff of new programs, services, and amenities; gather staff ideas; and train.
- Hold weekly meetings with the management team.
- Establish specific goals for each department manager and tie them directly to the manager's budget performance and compensation.
- Establish the annual club budget (to be approved by ownership).

- Meet budget profits by implementing the approved budget and adjusting the budget plan if the profit goal is not being met by midyear.
- Participate in the manager-on-duty (MOD) program on a regular basis.
- Produce a monthly variance report that documents differences in the budgeted versus actual income statements.
- Work diligently on the marketing efforts of the club, working closely with the membership director and the staff to ensure the marketing efforts are executed efficiently.
- Actively participate in the development of the yearly marketing plan. Work closely with the sales department to help sell memberships.
- Keep a high profile in the club and get acquainted with as many members as possible.
- Work with the operations manager and the director of human resources (corporate staff) to provide regular, thorough training of all employees.
- Conduct performance reviews at 90 days and then every 6 months for all department managers.
- Approve the hiring of all new employees and all changes of employment status.
- Submit assigned operating and retention reports.

## POSITION REQUIREMENTS

- Demonstrate a proven track record of success in fitness, retail, or customer service.
- Show effective and dynamic leadership skills with solid abilities in teamwork, decision making, problem solving, communication, and sales strategy.
- Excellent customer service skills, staff development, problem solving, and organizational skills.

## JOB SUMMARY

The general manager position is full time. The position reports to the regional operations director (corporate staff). The general manager oversees all sales, fitness, and operations functions within the fitness facility. Duties can include management of sales or fitness programs.

# Front-Desk Associate or Administrative Assistant

The primary role of the front-desk associate is to meet and greet clients and ensure that their experiences are tremendous. The front-desk associate is also responsible for controlling who comes into the club by ensuring all clients check in and all guests fill out a waiver or meet with their membership coordinator. The front-desk associate ensures all locker rooms are fully stocked and that the main reception area is clean and safe. The front-desk associate also assists various departments with projects that may be assigned on a daily, weekly, or monthly basis.

## QUALIFICATIONS

- Have high school diploma or GED equivalent required.
- Must be 18 years of age or older.
- Have a positive attitude and strong communication skills.
- Be able to multitask and work under pressure.
- Have strong organizational skills.
- Have a working knowledge of office software and computer skills.

## RESPONSIBILITIES

- Address all clients and guests as they enter and leave the facility.
- Handle all client or prospect inquiries in person or over the phone.
- Ensure adequate supplies are in place in all areas of the facility.
- Process all paperwork related to memberships and enter information into the club management software.
- Ensure the front-desk area is always kept neat and tidy.
- Convey any messages to staff in a timely fashion.
- Complete the front-desk checklist at the start and finish of each shift.
- Communicate any client issues with the appropriate staff.
- Answer any general questions about club programs.

- Ensure all paperwork is properly filed.
- Attend all individual and group meetings.

## POSITION REQUIREMENTS

- Have customer service background.
- Need basic computer proficiency.
- Demonstrate a passion for health and fitness.
- Possess a positive attitude.
- Must be punctual and reliable.
- Proven exceptional customer service skills.
- Show strong listening skills with the ability to empathize and problem solve.

## JOB SUMMARY

The front-desk position is often considered the most important position in a club. I think it is a grossly underestimated and underappreciated position in many clubs. A great front-desk person addresses guests in ways that make them want to come back, handles customers' complaints, sets the initial tone for prospects' first visits, and coordinates messages throughout the club. Anyone who thinks this is an easy job has never done it or has never worked at a club where the position was valued. Personal trainers and salespeople are notoriously bad with paperwork and staying organized. Often, the front-desk person keeps these positions focused and on track. As a manager, make sure all levels of staff are doing their part. If this is not happening, the front-desk staff will usually be able to tell you who is dropping the ball.

# Membership Director

Because 70 to 80% of total club revenue comes from dues, the primary role of the **membership director** is setting sales goals with membership consultants to maintain a constant stream of new members. The membership director organizes and leads a team of sales professionals and motivates them to achieve or exceed monthly and individual sales numbers and quotas.

## QUALIFICATIONS

- Demonstrate good communication skills.
- Demonstrate good leadership qualities.
- Demonstrate strong sales abilities and sales and promotional aptitude.
- Display good organizational skills.

- Have a minimum of 2 to 5 years of sales or sales management experience.
- Maintain regular attendance and punctuality.
- Have an outgoing personality.
- Have telephone sales skills.
- Effectively use one-on-one sales closing techniques.
- Effectively present and close corporate accounts.

## RESPONSIBILITIES

- Meet quotas as set forth in the membership director salary, commission, and quota agreement.
- Fulfill all assignments as requested by the general manager.
- Work within the approved guidelines of pay structure and follow proper procedures for hiring, disciplining, and firing.
- Train, coach, and manage membership consultants.
- Have monthly one-on-one meetings with each membership consultant.
- Chair weekly team meetings.
- Compile, publish, and maintain sales standards, including incoming and outgoing calls, number of tours, referrals, referral attempts, commissions, payroll, closing percentages, bonus records, and so on.
- Ensure the membership department meets its monthly goals.
- Set up and maintain standards of cleanliness and orderliness for the membership staff and membership consultant offices.
- Maintain professional dress and appearance.
- Set up and maintain staff standards of protocol with nonmembers.
- Set up systems to ensure consistent inventory of all membership and collateral materials.
- Ensure that membership staff promote and sell all club services and products.
- Stay up to date on sales and marketing information and disseminate this information to staff.
- Develop member referral programs with the regional membership director (corporate staff).
- Develop consultant recognition and reward programs.

- Lead by example, especially in the areas of appearance, punctuality, and professionalism.
- Be an active participant in club management meetings.
- Use training and quality-control techniques to ensure membership consultants are fulfilling the responsibilities set forth in their job descriptions.
- Create a membership budget.
- Write monthly variance reports as requested by the general manager.

### POSITION REQUIREMENTS
- Be proficient in scripted sales method (for which training will be provided).
- Be proficient in asking for the sale (for which training will be provided).
- Work during closeout (the last 3 days of each month).

### JOB SUMMARY
The membership director is a full-time position, and this person reports directly to the general manager.

## The Bottom Line

Job descriptions are constantly changing, so it is important to review them on a yearly basis. Staff evaluations are a great time to do this. As the business changes, so too should the job descriptions.

# Membership Consultants or Sales Representatives

**Membership consultants** reach individual quotas for monthly dues, annual dues, guest fees, seasonal memberships, and **I-fees** (enrollment fees charged when a member first joins) to ensure the membership team meets budgeted goals. They serve members on a daily basis, and they actively pursue inside and outside prospects. Prospecting outside the club can be achieved through mailings, participating in networking functions, and building relationships with local businesses. Prospects can be offered guest memberships to try out the facility. Prospecting within the club can be achieved by offering guest memberships for family and friends of current members. A member **referral program** rewards members who assist in recruiting new members.

### QUALIFICATIONS
- Have undergraduate degree in business, sales and marketing, or related field.
- Have prior sales experience.
- Possess excellent customer services skills, outgoing, motivational, and friendly.
- Be able to deal with pressure in meeting sales quota.
- Have excellent listening and verbal communication skills.
- Desire to build relationships with members.
- Be able to resolve conflicts in a professional, tactful manner.
- Be able to multitask and learn quickly.

### RESPONSIBILITIES
- Reach monthly quotas.
- Process all contracts and paperwork in a timely and accurate manner.
- Continually look for inside and outside prospects.
- Provide service that exceeds the expectations of all prospects and members.
- Complete all assignments given by the general manager or membership director.
- Adjust schedule as required to meet customer needs.
- Meet sales skill standards, build rapport, greet, identify customer needs, tour prospects around the facility, overcome objections, and close or ask for the sale).
- Schedule and confirm appointments with prospects.
- Track membership activity using daily, weekly, and monthly tracking sheets. Keep specialty mailing files up to date (e.g., past tours, guest passes, cancelled memberships).
- Obtain referrals from current and new members.
- Send thank-you notes to all new members.
- Attend all required membership meetings and training sessions.

- Research competition by touring and calling other clubs on a regular basis.
- Represent the club in an outside sales capacity at corporate events, chamber of commerce lunches, and after-hours special events.
- Contribute ideas to and help implement internal and external marketing campaigns.
- Meet and exceed individual and team goals.
- Organize and file all membership-related paperwork.

## POSITION REQUIREMENTS

- Be proficient in the scripted sales method (for which training will be provided).
- Be proficient in asking for the sale (for which training will be provided).
- Work during closeout (the last 3 days of each month).

## PHYSICAL REQUIREMENTS

- Be able to walk stairs repeatedly during your shift.
- Be able to spend extended time on the phone.
- Be able to lift 15 to 20 pounds (7-9 kilograms).

## JOB SUMMARY

The membership consultant **or sales representative** position is part of the revenue-generating membership department. Consultants work full time and report directly to the membership director.

## The Bottom Line

If the membership department does not have a structured follow-up plan with new members, the chances of retaining those members decreases. This is especially true with members who do not participate in their integration appointments or who sign up for fee-based fitness programs.

## Fitness Director

The primary responsibility of the **fitness director** is to retain members by offering a variety of programs that help them attain their health and fitness goals. The fitness director develops, evaluates, and grows programs to increase participation and revenue. Clubs offer a balance of free and fee-based programs that add value to the membership. Free programs include integration, group exercise classes, seminars, and motivational contests. Fee-based programs include personal training, Pilates training, weight management programs, sport-specific programming, leagues, and special events. To offer this variety in programming, the fitness director actively recruits, trains, and evaluates employees for continued success. Successful fitness departments produce 25 to 30% of the total revenue of a club (International Health, Racquet, and Sportsclub Association 2006).

The purpose of this position is to originate, coordinate, promote, supervise, implement, and evaluate quality fitness programs that will assist all members in achieving their fitness goals and to ensure that the fitness department is profitable and meets or exceeds the annual budget goals.

## QUALIFICATIONS

- Have a bachelor's degree in exercise physiology or exercise science. A master's degree in exercise physiology is preferred.
- Have one or two **third-party, nationally accredited certifications** and current cardiopulmonary resuscitation (CPR) and automated external defibrillator (AED) certifications.
- Have 3 to 5 years of experience in a health and fitness facility, 2 years of experience at a fitness facility or in program management, and 1 to 2 years of supervisory experience.
- Have experience conducting submaximal fitness assessments.
- Have experience in performance management and staff motivation.

## RESPONSIBILITIES

- Provide a clean, safe, and healthy environment for members, guests, and coworkers.
- Help retain current members and obtain new members through club promotion and **customer service** excellence.
- Acquire, maintain, and serve members by supporting their participation in programs and activities.
- Define performance standards and objectives for fitness staff.

- Develop, promote, grow, and evaluate fitness programs.
- Conduct all facets of fitness assessments.
- Maintain knowledge of all programs offered at the club.
- Conduct staff training sessions on fitness and service on a regular basis.
- Conduct performance evaluations for fitness managers.
- Track completion of managers' evaluations of fitness staff performance.
- Track fitness staff attendance, vacation, and sick days.
- Attend national industry trade shows and conferences.
- Instruct group exercise classes.
- Provide personal training for club members as necessary.
- Provide education and training for members on proper use of exercise equipment.
- Recruit, hire, train, and supervise fitness department managers (personal training, group exercise, and program managers).
- Contribute articles to company quarterly newsletters.
- Actively participate in all phases of major club functions and special events.
- Participate in the MOD rotation.
- Submit the annual fitness department budget per the instructions from the general manager.
- Help develop the fitness department operations manual.
- Oversee the maintenance, cleanliness, and upkeep of the facility and equipment.
- Inspect all fitness equipment to ensure the highest standards of maintenance and cleanliness.

## POSITION REQUIREMENTS

- Be proficient in scripted sales method (for which training will be provided).
- Be proficient in asking for the sale as role playing during training will be provided to assist in this process.
- Work during closeout (the last 3 days of each month).

## PHYSICAL REQUIREMENTS

- Be able to bend and stand.
- Be able to move fitness equipment and lift weight plates and dumbbells.

## JOB SUMMARY

The fitness director is part of the revenue-generating fitness department. It is a full-time position, and this person reports to the general manager.

# Personal Trainers

The entry-level position in the fitness department is the **personal trainer.** Personal trainers are responsible for integrating members into a facility and generating revenue by helping members reach their fitness goals. To maximize personal training sales and membership penetration, personal trainers should be hired as full-time employees. It is difficult for employees to build rapport with members, let alone a client base, if they spend little time interacting with members.

Members who spend additional money beyond their dues reinforce their commitment to the club. According to IHRSA's *Profiles of Success* (International Health, Racquet, and Sportsclub Association 2006), there is a direct correlation between clubs that have a high percentage of nondues revenue and clubs that have high retention rates. The trainers must be held accountable to monthly individual and team goals. Personal trainers sell personal training sessions and packages and establish, implement, monitor, and maintain individual exercise recommendations for clients in a professional manner to ensure member satisfaction and retention.

## QUALIFICATIONS

- Have a bachelor's degree in exercise physiology or an allied health field or a third-party nationally accredited personal trainer certification and 1 year of experience.
- Have current CPR and AED certifications.

## RESPONSIBILITIES

### Member service

- Provide a clean, safe, and healthy environment for members, guests, and coworkers.
- Help retain and attain new members through club promotion and customer service excellence.

- Conduct a fitness consultation orientation for all new members within the first month of joining. All members must be given a workout card upon completion.
- Assist members with specific fitness concerns on the fitness floor.
- Conduct 8-week reassessments on all members.
- Provide quality exercise recommendations for clients and ensure the attainment of their specific fitness goals.
- Wear appropriate attire while training clients.
- Maintain and update a 2-week schedule for appointments.

### Client file maintenance

- Physical Activity Readiness Questionnaire for Everyone (PAR-Q+)
- Medical health history
- Needs analysis
- Informed consent
- Fitness evaluation
- Copy of exercise program

### Education and training

- Maintain current involvement in professional organizations.
- Maintain current certification through continuing education.
- Attend all required department and continuing education meetings.
- Provide a free personal training session to all new sales staff.

### Equipment

- Spot members during exercise sessions.
- Restack all weights.
- Maintain supply of towels on the floor.
- Clean weight and cardiorespiratory equipment after client or personal use or when necessary.

### Special Events and Community Service

- Volunteer for special events and programs and various community events.
- Participate in member appreciation parties.

## POSITION REQUIREMENTS

- Be proficient in scripted sales method (for which training will be provided).
- Be proficient in asking for the sale (for which training will be provided).
- Hit quotas for personal training sales in the first month, second month, third month, and beyond.
- Work 36 to 40 hours in the club and maintain so many paid personal training sessions per week by the third month of employment.
- Complete a set number of complimentary sessions per month.
- Work certain fitness floor shifts to ensure proper service for and safety of all members and guests.
- Work during closeout depending on individual or department budgeted goals.

## PHYSICAL REQUIREMENTS

Have physical strength and manual dexterity.

## JOB SUMMARY

The personal trainer is a full-time position. This person reports directly to the personal training manager, fitness director, or general manager.

## *The Bottom Line*

Qualified, energetic, and well-organized personal trainers are successful whether they are full-time or part-time employees. For full-time personal trainers, however, you can control the schedules, establish higher revenue goals, and require a minimum number of paid sessions and integration appointments per month. You can accomplish some of these expectations with part-time personal trainers, but they are usually only present for their appointments, which limits their interaction with other members.

## NOT-FOR-PROFIT COMMUNITY FACILITIES

**Not-for-profit community facilities** are unique in that they receive tax-exempt status for providing affordable health and wellness programs for communities. Examples of these organizations include YMCAs; Jewish Community Centers (JCCs); and hospital-based, faith-based, and park and recreation centers. A board of directors made up of local business members governs each facility. The board members serve 2- to 4-year terms depending on the organization. Along with the president and CEO, the board develops the budget and plans major renovations and purchases. Revenue generated through memberships and programs pays the operating expenses, and the remaining revenue benefits the community.

Not-for-profit organizations also campaign for donations to provide scholarships that offset membership and program costs for families in need. The goal of these organizations is to provide programming that meets the needs of today's youth, families, adults, and seniors regardless of their financial situations. The programs offered focus on health and fitness, child care and development, education, arts, and summer and overnight camps. Key positions in these facilities include the directors of the various programs and the director of fund-raising. Unlike many for-profit centers, which focus on a niche market, not-for-profit facilities try to provide something for everyone. A sample organizational chart for a not-for-profit community facility is shown in figure 2.4. One key position in a not-for-profit

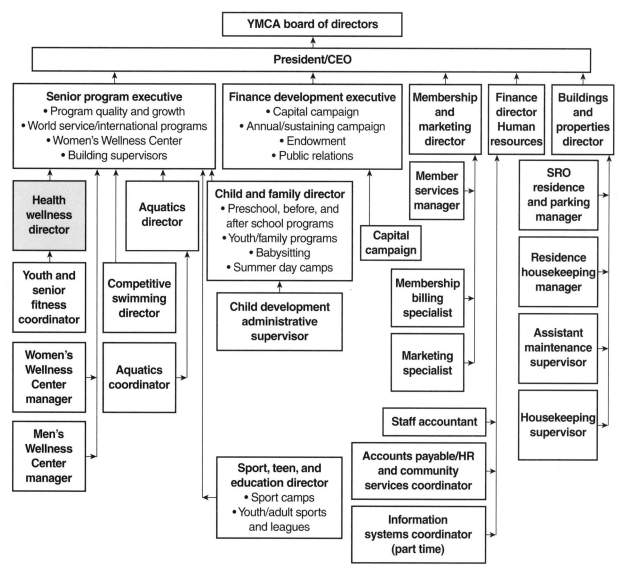

**Figure 2.4** Organizational chart for a not-for-profit community facility. Shaded area indicates position that is described in the text.

Reprinted by permission.

facility, the health and wellness director, is described next.

## *The Bottom Line*

Fund-raising is an important source of revenue for not-for-profit organizations. The finance development team and the staff continually conduct fund-raising competitions and events. Staff members also set fund-raising goals for themselves.

## Health and Wellness Director

The **health and wellness director** in a not-for-profit community center is responsible for the organization, delivery, and quality of all health, fitness, and wellness programs for all age groups. The director's emphasis is on offering high-quality programs, remaining up-to-date on fitness trends, increasing the number of participants served, and managing the budget.

### QUALIFICATIONS

- Be able to perform each essential duty satisfactorily. The requirements listed are representative of the knowledge, skills, and abilities required. Reasonable accommodations may be made to enable people with disabilities to perform the essential functions.

- Have a bachelor's degree in exercise physiology, physical education, or a related field. A master's degree is preferred.

- Have additional certification from a national organization.

- Show sensitivity to the needs of populations served and have strong organizational, communication, and fiscal skills.

- Have 1 to 2 years of experience and be able to provide leadership in developing program designs, fitness testing, exercise prescriptions, personal training, and programs for special populations.

- Be able to read, analyze, and interpret general business periodicals, professional journals, technical procedures, or government regulations. Be able to write reports, business correspondence, and procedure manuals. Be able to effectively present information and

respond to questions from supervisors, members, customers, participants, and the public.

- Be able to calculate figures and amounts such as discounts, proportions, percentages, area, circumference, and volume. Be able to apply concepts of basic algebra and geometry.

- Be able to solve practical problems, deal with a variety of concrete variables in various situations, and interpret a variety of instructions furnished in written, oral, diagrammatic, or schedule forms.

### RESPONSIBILITIES SPECIFIC TO HEALTH AND WELLNESS

- Perform all duties required for successful fitness, health and wellness, and related programs for all ages.

- Hire, manage, recruit, and supervise job performance of fitness staff.

- Commit to developing character in all participants, especially young people.

- Keep fitness staff informed of new programs, program time changes, special fitness events, and other fitness-, health-, and wellness-related events. Market the department programs to the community.

### RESPONSIBILITIES SPECIFIC TO DIRECTOR STATUS

#### Program related

- Promote and incorporate the core values and character development model in all programs and activities.

- Work with the marketing department to market and distribute program-specific information during each session.

- Compile program statistical reports as needed.

- Develop and maintain collaborative relationships with other community organizations.

- Assist in special events.

- Respond to all member and community inquiries and complaints in a timely manner.

- Assist with and attend department head meetings and other meetings as needed.

- Conduct informal or educational staff meetings at least once during each session to ensure that information flows through all levels of the organization.

- Secure the internal facilities needed for program implementation. Seek community areas outside the facility as programs grow.

- Maintain, monitor, inventory, and purchase equipment. Collaborate with all other departments regarding the status of facilities and equipment needs.

- Develop and monitor programs to meet fiscal objectives with the program executive and finance director.

- Facilitate fund-raising to meet budget goals. Collaborate with other directors regarding events and ideas.

### Member services

- Keep front-desk staff informed of all programs and special events and of any changes.

- Assist member services during busy registration times as needed.

### Relationship building

- Consider all interactions with members as opportunities to create relationships.

- Maintain an average of 10 to 12 contact hours with members per week (teaching, personal training, or other interactions).

### Teamwork

- Work in cooperation with all staff to ensure that safety and quality member services are the top priorities.

- Work within all established deadlines. Follow all procedures related to meeting communication and report expectations (e.g., purchase orders, new-employee documents, bulletin board messages, marketing requests, check requests, budgeting and operational goals, and brochure information).

- Assist in maintaining building cleanliness and repairs through service requests.

- Perform other duties as assigned by your supervisor.

### POSITION REQUIREMENTS

- Demonstrate the ability to motivate, engage, and be friendly.

- Show excellent customer service and relationship management skills.

- Be able to time manage, organize, and communicate.

### JOB SUMMARY

The health and wellness director is a full-time position. The position reports to the general manager. The health and wellness director oversees all aspects of recruitment of new members, retention of existing members, and supervises assigned staff, as well as the development and implementation of high quality program(s).

# HOSPITAL-BASED FITNESS CENTERS

**Hospital-based fitness centers** are more often not-for-profit organizations than for-profit businesses. Many of these centers have community members and physicians who serve on a health system board or board of directors and set standards of health care that integrate prevention, lifestyle changes, and rehabilitation of members and patients and that create a continuum of care for the community. Most patients have temporary access to the hospital fitness center.

Hospital fitness centers offer cardiorespiratory equipment, strength equipment, group exercises, and programs that are similar to those in for-profit centers. They also offer programs such as cardiac rehabilitation, arthritic programming, osteoporosis programming, smoking cessation, aging seminars, and cancer wellness. Most of the centers are located on a hospital campus, which facilitates easier blood cholesterol testing, bone density testing, and stress testing. The success of medical programming depends on enthusiastic physicians who firmly believe that exercise can assist in the prevention of and rehabilitation from many diseases. In some cases, a hospital may have a health promotions department that works closely with the program manager of the fitness center to run wellness programs.

Employees at a hospital-based facility work with a wide range of members. Some members will be healthy but will have complications or injuries they are recovering from at the hospital. Doctor involvement is not unusual in fitness programming. Employees need to be comfortable reading health history forms and be aware of exercise limitations for various conditions, such as cardiac rehabilitation, asthma, arthritis, and high blood pressure.

A sample organizational chart for a hospital-based fitness center is shown in figure 2.5, and two key positions are described in the following sections.

## The Bottom Line

There has been much discussion about medical referrals to fitness centers. A hospital-based center is more likely to be successful with medical referrals due to the wide array of professional network and resources available to treat those conditions identified because they are often owned by the hospital and some of the medical programming from the hospital occurs there.

## Group Exercise Supervisor

### QUALIFICATIONS

- Proven experience in fitness and group exercise (i.e., teaching classes, maintaining certifications, etc.).
- Have experience in management.
- Possess high school diploma or GED. College degree preferred.
- Must have a minimum of two years' work experience in a fitness-related field.
- Be able to spot, recruit, and hire talented group exercise instructors.
- Be able to work evening or weekend hours, as assigned.
- Organize class schedules.

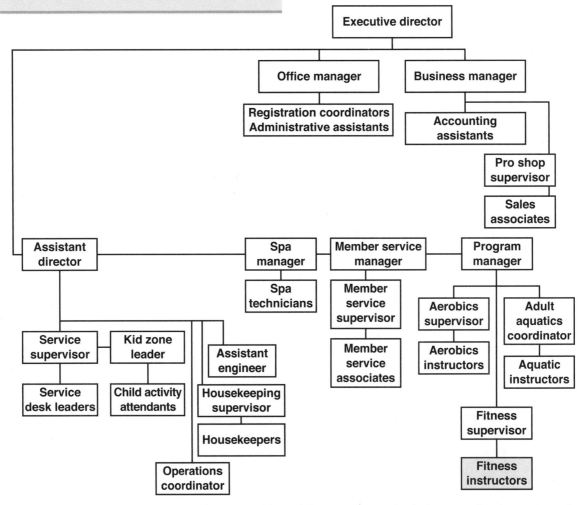

**Figure 2.5**   Organizational chart of a hospital-based fitness center. Shaded area indicates position that is described in the text.

Reprinted by permission.

- Attend all required staff meetings and any requested individual meetings.

## RESPONSIBILITIES

- Develop aerobic programs, establish exercise class contents and schedules, maintain supplies and equipment, and so forth.
- Prepare work schedules to ensure adequate coverage of classes. Monitor attendance at classes and recommend changes to the schedule to better meet the needs of members.
- Interview, hire, orient, train, and evaluate the performance of subordinate instructors. When necessary, discipline and discharge subordinate instructors. Work with the supervisor to resolve difficult problems in employee relations.
- Prepare and administer the annual operating budget for the assigned area, ensure adherence to this budget, and notify the supervisor of significant variances.
- Maintain the equipment and music system in proper working condition, order routine supplies, and recommend purchases of capital equipment.
- Act as a resource for assigned personnel in resolving complaints and problems. Evaluate suggestions for improving the exercise program, and implement new routines and classes to enhance it.
- Develop, recommend, and implement policies and procedures for the aerobic exercise program and ensure adherence to them. Modify procedures as necessary to improve services.
- Instruct aerobic and conditioning classes weekly.
- Prepare aerobic exercise classes, select music, lead classes, provide instruction in proper form and technique, and so forth.
- Perform related duties, such as conducting periodic staff meetings, presenting in-service sessions, maintaining logs and reports of incidents and activities, and so on.

## POSITION REQUIREMENTS

- Obtain CPR certification within the first 6 weeks of employment.

- Have a moderate level of analytical ability. Work is performed in accordance with standard procedures and requires basic technical knowledge or in-depth, experience-based knowledge to analyze and interpret information.
- Demonstrate adequate communication skills to explain policies or otherwise handle situations that require sensitivity and tact.
- Be able to complete work that is not completely standardized. Assignments are often received in the form of results expected, due dates, and general procedures.
- Be able to lead and instruct various levels of aerobics classes; walk or stand for an hour or more at a time; lift or carry objects that weigh 5 to 20 pounds (2-9 kilograms); and use a keyboard to enter, retrieve, or transform words or data.
- Exercise caution when working with equipment or performing activities; carelessness could result in minor cuts, bruises, or muscle strains.

## REPORTING RELATIONSHIPS

The group exercise supervisor reports to the program manager and is responsible for supervising approximately 10 to 20 employees.

## JOB SUMMARY

The group exercise supervisor is a full-time position and reports to the health and wellness director.

# Fitness Instructor

## QUALIFICATIONS

- Have a bachelor's degree in exercise science or a closely related field, or have a bachelor's degree in any field plus a nationally accredited certification. (Degree may be in process and completed within 2 years of employment.) A minimum of 1 year of previous fitness specialist experience is preferred.
- Have previous experience and knowledge of fitness equipment and principles of weight training necessary.
- Demonstrate strong communication skills.
- Must possess at least one national fitness or personal training certification.

## RESPONSIBILITIES

- Provide individualized fitness consultation to members and nonmembers to assess their overall fitness levels. Prescribe exercise programs in accordance with established fitness consultation protocols. Provide continual follow-up services.

- Proactively assist members with exercise programs and provide orientation to equipment.

- Instruct group exercise and wellness classes for all members and nonmembers.

- Develop, coordinate, and implement clinical, fitness, and member motivational programming and special events as directed by the supervisor.

- Contribute to the development and administration of the budget and to fitness program plans as directed by the supervisor.

- Monitor quality, progress, and success of members and nonmembers engaged in fitness programs.

- Develop educational lectures on wellness and present them to members at hospital locations and to the community.

- Contribute to the member service of the center by having daily face-to-face interactions with members.

## POSITION REQUIREMENTS

- Obtain CPR certification within the first 90 days of employment.

- Demonstrate excellent customer service skills.

- Have a moderate level of analytical ability. Work is performed in accordance with standard procedures and requires basic technical knowledge or in-depth, experience-based knowledge to analyze and interpret information.

- Demonstrate adequate communication skills required to lead, teach, and persuade others and to interact effectively with people in difficult situations.

- Be able to complete work that is not completely standardized. Assignments are often received in the form of results expected, due dates, and general procedures.

- Be able to walk or stand for an hour or more at a time, lift or carry objects that weigh more than 45 pounds (20 kilograms), and assist members with exercise workouts.

- Be comfortable working in an area that is somewhat unpleasant due to drafts, noise, temperature variations, and other factors.

- Exercise caution when working with equipment or performing activities; carelessness could result in minor cuts, bruises, or muscle strains.

## REPORTING RELATIONSHIPS

The fitness instructor reports to the fitness supervisor at the center and does not supervise any other employees.

## JOB SUMMARY

The fitness instructor can be a part- or full-time position and reports to the health and wellness director.

# CORPORATE-BASED FITNESS ORGANIZATIONS

**Corporate-based fitness organizations** provide convenient, cost-effective, customized, and flexible plans to meet the demands of a company. As health care costs continue to rise, companies are investing in their employees' health and well-being, which is increasing work productivity and decreasing physician visits. By offering health promotion and screening programs, employees can benefit from more balanced living, including exercise and improved self-monitoring of adverse health symptoms (e.g., stress, mild depression). Through well-organized programs and ongoing promotion of the facilities' activities, increased participation is realized. Heightened awareness results in increased membership enrollment, and the facility helps foster a positive workplace mindset. The facility becomes a healthy environment through which employees' health and well-being are nurtured and improved.

Corporate facilities consider all pertinent influences on the employees' health, such as family medical history, eating habits, and cholesterol levels as well as life satisfaction, stress, and work–life balance. An employee on the verge of a breakdown appears no more at risk on the outside than any other employee does. While companies are containing health care costs and reducing medical claims, their employees are addressing pertinent work and life issues and living healthier lives. Together, they make the everyday work experience more productive and positive, and the company becomes a progressive leader in healthy, effective change.

A wellness model

- targets healthy populations;
- improves exercise participation to relieve stress and increase self-esteem;
- provides a social structure outside the workplace, which lowers incidences of mild depression from job or life burnout;
- reports progress with systematic and accurate diagnostic measurements that result in greater motivation and sustained participation; and
- alerts chronically at-risk populations (e.g., those who smoke or are obese, depressed, or hypertensive) to seek medical care in conjunction with lifestyle programs.

Figure 2.6 is an organizational chart for a corporate-based facility. Two of the key positions are described in the following sections.

## The Bottom Line

A successful corporate-based facility needs a comprehensive wellness tracking system to report the overall health of its employees. Improving health conditions will increase productivity in the workplace, and this information can increase the likelihood of corporate memberships at the facility.

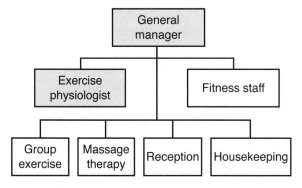

**Figure 2.6** Organizational chart for a corporate-based facility. Shaded areas indicate positions that are described in the text.

Reprinted by permission.

# General Manager

The general manager reports directly to the corporate management team and oversee all aspects of the club operation by working directly with manager and key staff on a day-to-day basis. The key responsibility of the general manger is developing and implementing the organization's strategic plan.

## QUALIFICATIONS

- Have at least 5 years hands-on general management experience with a proven track record of successfully leading multimillion dollar business operations.
- Possess a bachelor's degree in business administration, sports management, fitness management, or related fields.
- Have a minimum of 3 years of management experience and experience in teaching customer service techniques with a sensitivity to maintaining staff relations and cohesiveness.
- Understand the fundamentals of business including sales, operations, service, and profit and loss.
- Have prior history of reducing expenses, growing revenue, and increasing profits.
- Demonstrate sound judgment, effective decision making, and strong problem-solving skills.
- Have experience building productive teams and managing associate performance.
- Be able to effectively share skills and knowledge with others.
- Possess exceptional verbal and written communication skills. Listen to others and quickly build rapport.
- Have proficient computer skills.

## RESPONSIBILITIES

- Manage all aspects of the center's operations, marketing, and financial reporting.
- Know and understand all company and club policies and procedures and direct the operating affairs of the club within these parameters.
- Ensure the highest level of customer service and fiscal success.

- Provide an organized leadership role, including ongoing staff training, club programming, and new business development.

- Establish a staffing plan that efficiently achieves the operating standards of a first-class club operation, including appointing department heads, creating job descriptions for all positions, and developing work schedules to optimize successful club programs. Positions could include assistant manager, fitness staff, or housekeeping.

- Establish a personal schedule that provides high visibility at peak operating times, such as managing the club and walking the exercise areas at busy times to meet and greet members.

- Manage daily operations to achieve the financial and operational objectives as described in the annual operating budget.

- Create a cohesive and seamless delivery of services and operational standards to maintain a high level of member satisfaction.

- Establish and implement monthly marketing strategies, membership policies and procedures, and club programs to maximize club revenue.

- Become familiar with and direct personal efforts to monitor and participate in business, athletic, and cultural events that will result in new opportunities for business development.

- Learn and present the wellness programs and services offered by the company.

- Advise, guide, direct, and authorize staff to complete club events and to uphold housekeeping and member service standards that are consistent with established policies, ownership's expectations, and the annual club budget.

- Become familiar with and use the club operating, billing, collections, membership utilization, and other management systems necessary to achieve the operating standards and annual budget for the center.

- Review all financial reporting for accuracy, monitor all purchasing practices to ensure expense controls are sufficient to meet budget, and prepare staffing plans and pricing policies to achieve club operating budgets.

- Establish and maintain an effective system of communication throughout the organization, including among staff, members, and management. Respond to the needs, questions, suggestions, or complaints of members and staff.

- Conduct interviews and assist department managers with budgeting, interviewing, supervising, and staff training. Maintain all employee policies and procedures as defined in the employee handbook.

- Report any actions, rumors, allegations, or negative insinuations made by any employee, member, or other person that may detrimentally affect the operations of the club.

- Support and protect the interests and views of all employees as they pertain to enhancing the best interests of the company and their personal development.

- Maintain a facility standard of excellence and cleanliness. Ensure proper maintenance of all club equipment, furnishings, and fixtures, and make sure written diaries of all preventive maintenance and repairs are maintained.

- Continually review the operating results of the club, compare these with established budgets, and prepare and compile the month-end financial report and executive summary. Include an explanation of any variance in operations that exceeds 10%. Recommend steps to ensure appropriate measures are taken to correct any unsatisfactory results.

- Assist the marketing and sales staff with the implementation of corporate and individual membership campaigns and provide creative suggestions to continually improve these programs and membership enrollment.

- Monitor department managers and their staff for customer service and satisfaction levels.

- Conduct employee performance reviews on an annual basis and maintain current employee files.

- Ensure the completion of and contribute to the membership newsletter.

- Coordinate and conduct biweekly staff meetings.

- Approve and track club expenses and work cooperatively with the accounting department to facilitate purchase order processing.

- Process staff payroll.
- Perform other duties as assigned.

## POSITION REQUIREMENTS

- Have an outgoing personality and be able to effectively communicate, teach, and motivate a variety of people.
- Have a personal commitment to a fit and healthy lifestyle.
- Be a results-oriented leaders who can achieve organizational objectives in highly competitive markets.
- Dress professionally and maintain a well-groomed appearance.

## JOB SUMMARY

The general manager is a full-time position. The position usually reports to the owner(s) of a small-to-medium sized health club or vice president-level, depending on the organizational structure, at a large organization. The general manager oversees the financial targets of a club; provides leadership in areas of customer service, staff relations, sales, in-center business performance, and membership participation; and recruits, hires, and trains new staff.

# Exercise Physiologist

The **exercise physiologist** reports directly to the general manager and to the corporate management team on request. During MOD hours, the exercise physiologist is an extension of the authority of the general manager.

## QUALIFICATIONS

- Have master's degree in exercise science or related field and certification in cardiovascular clinical area or American College of Sports Medicine Clinical Track certification.
- Have prior ECG and exercise testing experience, which includes basic ECG interpretation skills. ACLS certified.
- Possess at least 3 to 6 months experience with cardiac rehabilitation or stress testing preferred.

## RESPONSIBILITIES

- Design and implement patient-specific therapeutic exercise programs, both individual and group programs.
- Treat and educate medically complex patients on disease management, symptom management, and appropriate behavioral modifications.
- Perform follow-up on all patient therapeutic interventions.
- Document and provide feedback on patient progress.
- Work closely with physicians and other healthcare professionals directly involved in patient care.
- Prepare and maintain required reports and statistics.

### Health profiles and heart risk assessments

- Supervise and ensure the safety and cleanliness of the fitness floor.
- Have a working knowledge of all aspects of the testing system and evaluation standards.
- Have knowledge and competency in exercise testing, including screening for potential contraindications.
- Assist members with exercise programs and provide clinical testing.
- Interpret results and design safe, appropriate, and enjoyable individualized exercise prescriptions.
- Monitor workouts and exercise routines, provide guidance on proper form and technique, and answer questions as necessary.
- Complete and maintain all member files in accordance with the fitness manual.
- Contact every member for a 6-month reevaluation.
- Compile and analyze data from the testing system for group reports and reports on specific groups with identified risk factors.
- Correspond with members after evaluations to facilitate continued education and awareness and to answer questions.

### Orientation

- Review the exercise prescription and data provided by the health profile and heart risk assessment and prepare a personalized exercise prescription for every member.
- Implement personalized cardiorespiratory and strength programs.

- Give each member a detailed orientation on how to properly use each piece of equipment.
- Encourage interaction between members and fitness staff, and encourage members to contact fitness staff for questions and concerns.

### Floor supervision

- Monitor equipment maintenance needs and immediately advise the general manager of any developing problems.
- Clean each piece of equipment daily according to the manufacturer's specifications.
- Assist, motivate, and educate all members on the use of machines and on personal fitness goals.
- Be proactive and approach every member to ensure proper training techniques are followed.
- Provide routine blood pressure and heart rate checks.
- Maintain a safe, productive, and inviting exercise environment for members and guests.

### Health promotions

- Assist in the implementation of all health promotion, medical screening, and educational programs.
- Contact special populations from previous member files about upcoming events.
- Develop creative strategies for encouraging participation.
- Assist in the development of specific interventions that serve the needs of members and subsidiaries.
- Work with the member services staff in implementing health fairs.

### Personal training

- Motivate and educate participants.
- Follow specified guidelines and personal training services as stated in the fitness manual.
- Conduct complimentary training sessions for new members.

- Assist in the development and implementation of marketing initiatives designed to generate awareness of personal training programs.

### Other

- Ensure that aerobics staff members are present and on time for all scheduled classes. Report any tardiness or missed classes to the general manager.
- Prepare all assignments and correspondence in a neat, timely, and professional manner.
- Keep all business-related interests, resources, and correspondence organized and neat.
- Maintain a high level of professionalism at all times.
- Remain active in industry associations and education.
- Work well with others and maintain professional working relationships with all employees.

### POSITION REQUIREMENTS

- Have a bachelor's degree in exercise physiology (or a related field).
- Have clinical exercise testing experience.
- Have current CPR certification and national training certification.

### JOB SUMMARY

The exercise physiologist is a full-time position and reports to the fitness director or health and wellness director.

## *The Bottom Line*

Creating or revising job descriptions might not be a top priority for a fitness professional who loves interacting with members. Who wants to sit behind a desk when you can be touching people's lives with education? However, if you want to start your own health club or become a manager for a health club, the probabilities of employee, facility, and overall success will be improved by having clear, concise, and comprehensive job descriptions.

## Key Terms

corporate-based fitness organizations

customer service

exercise physiologist

fitness director

fitness instructor

for-profit (commercial) facilities

general manager

health and wellness director

hospital-based fitness centers

I-fees

membership consultant

membership director

nondues revenue

not-for-profit community facilities

organizational design

personal trainer

referral program

subtenant

third-party, nationally accredited certifications

# CHAPTER 3

# Recruiting the Best Staff for Your Facility

## Learning Objectives

After studying this chapter, you will be able to

- identify and use critical industry and marketplace employment benchmarks to positively influence strategic planning for recruiting and hiring;

- identify essential internal review processes so appropriate personnel adjustments can be made by reorganizing, creating, or replacing positions;

- define the criteria for creating purpose-driven job descriptions to form the framework for successful personnel management;

- understand and implement efficient recruiting processes that identify qualified candidates and ensure the greatest possible buy-in from current employees;

- create organization-specific standards for screening and reviewing applications and résumés to ensure the best candidates move on to the interview stage;

- learn to apply a wide range of interviewing techniques to best bring out the talents, skills, experiences, and work styles of candidates for long-term retention and productivity; and

- ensure that the hiring process provides a solid foundation for the business and the new employee with regard to legal, operational, and cultural orientation.

Priya, who earned the recognition of master trainer at XYZ Club for the past 2 years, heard about an opening for the facility's fitness manager position and decided to apply. The fitness manager oversees the club's 15 to 20 personal trainers.

The first round of interviewing began the following week with a group interview. Ten people from within the club were competing for the position. Priya was told by her supervisor that one of the first questions of the group interview would be what the most important responsibility of a fitness manager is. During the group interview, Priya listened to the other candidates answer this question by talking about motivating the staff, training them, or teaching them how to sell the personal trainer packages. When it was Priya's turn

The author acknowledges the significant contributions of Kevin Hood to this chapter.

to answer the question, she said "The most important thing I can do as a fitness manager begins with my ability to spot, recruit, and hire talent, because as the manager, I can only be as successful as the talent I recruit to put on our gym floors to serve our clients." Suddenly, everyone in the room became very quiet. The interviewer asked Priya a follow-up question: "What is your strategy for accomplishing this task?" Priya replied, "Immediately look for people who have strong whys. *Why* do they want to be in this business of personal training? If they want to make a difference and serve the client's needs, then they may be good candidates." Based on that response, the interviewer invited Priya to a one-on-one interview with the club's management team the following week. After her second interview, she was offered the position.

---

As this story illustrates, a fitness manager must to able to spot, recruit, and hire talent. This is a key to success for most managers. People who are responsible for recruiting and hiring staff have some of the most important roles in any organization. In almost all circumstances, businesses are successful or fall short based on the performance of their employees. This chapter discusses a range of techniques and tactics for those who are charged with recruitment and hiring.

The first section of this chapter deals with analyzing staffing needs so the recruiting efforts match the needs of the organization. The next sections explain how to formalize and refine job descriptions in a practical way so they can be used in developing quality interview techniques. The latter sections provide information on positive profiling and the important interview questions that can come from the profiling exercise. Finally, strategies for selecting the best candidate for the job are discussed.

## ANALYZING STAFFING NEEDS

One of the most important jobs for any manager is understanding the personnel requirements necessary to get the job done. As discussed in the previous chapter, much of the knowledge about what it takes to get the job done will come from the **job description**. One goal of managing is ensuring that the right number of people are assigned to a given task and that those people produce the best work possible in the most efficient and effective way. Understanding the mission, vision, and culture of the organization; the appropriate

salary ranges based on selected **benchmarks** for the fitness industry; and the overall marketplace is necessary to achieve this goal.

Wage and salary benchmark categories are derived from comparing types of clubs (e.g., fitness, multipurpose, women's only, personal training) and jobs with similar responsibilities, hours, and benefits. Understanding the wages, benefits, and other forms of compensation competitive clubs provide helps shape an offer that motivates desirable candidates. This information also helps evaluate past, current, and predicted future trends so they can be put into perspective and necessary actions can be planned and undertaken.

Some important questions to answer before beginning the recruiting process include the following:

- How many people need to be hired to accomplish the job? Staff to member or supervisor to frontline employee ratios may need to be evaluated from productivity, customer service, or legal standpoints.
- What are the hourly wages for comparable positions?
- What is the availability of trained and untrained labor in a given market?
- What is the turnover rate for this position?
- How do the answers to the previous questions affect the **wage position** (i.e., toward the high, average, or low end of the market) for the job?

The IHRSA provides detailed information on salary ranges for a variety of positions in different club types (e.g., large multipurpose clubs, small studios). Professional associations such as the National Strength and Conditioning Association (NSCA), the American College of Sports Medicine (ACSM), and the American Council on Exercise (ACE) provide salary data for different types of positions in the fitness field. Your local economy and the level of competition will ultimately determine what you should pay to hire and retain great people.

The staffing needs of every organization evolve over time. Employees accept positions with other organizations or advance within your organization, or they might have to be terminated because of poor performance or personnel reorganization. The amount of turnover in specific positions that is ideal, acceptable, or damaging is hard to define. It is clear, however, that employee attrition is related to member attrition (International Health, Racquet, and Sportsclub Association 2006), so hiring and retaining high-performing people is critical to the success of any health or athletic club.

## *The Bottom Line*

High employee turnover is a drain on management's time and can be a reflection on the business. Taking the time to hire the right people who fully understand what they are in for is a critical step in managing employee turnover. In my business, I often try to talk people out of a position by emphasizing the challenging parts of the job. For example, when hiring for the front desk, I tell them how demanding it can be answering phones, scheduling appointments, greeting clients, and dealing with an overflowing toilet all while maintaining a smile and peak attitude. I tell prospective personal trainers how hard it is to get new clients and the wide range of hours they will be required to work to be successful. There is nothing worse than losing employees because they did not know what to expect going into their positions.

Employee turnover is not always a bad thing.

- New employees frequently approach business challenges in a refreshing way and bring new perspectives to solving old problems and new ideas to keep the business energized.

- The natural evolution of employees seeking more challenging opportunities in other organizations can be a healthy indication of a stable company in which upward movement may be limited because of long-tenured and productive employees.

- Turnover in organizations can simply mean the evolution of high-performing employees moving out of one position into another of more responsibility, thereby creating the need for additional personnel.

- Seasonal requirements can also contribute to the need for hiring new employees on a regular basis.

When hiring for a vacated position, you should examine whether the personnel organization chart can be redesigned to absorb the duties that were associated with the position. There are several methods for covering the responsibilities associated with the vacated position or changing the position, including the following:

- Change the supervisory **reporting structure** or move the position to a different department.

- Combine the responsibilities with those of one or more positions that are already filled. (This may mean there is an opportunity to advance or promote someone from within the organization or change compensation structures.)

- Hire contract or temporary employees to fill the position for the short, medium, or long term.

- Reorganize the position by changing it to full or part time, adding or removing job responsibilities, changing the pay rate, adding or removing benefit opportunities, and so on.

## UTILIZING JOB DESCRIPTIONS

Refer to the detailed job description when outlining desired skills and attributes in an advertisement or job availability notice. For example, the **performance expectations** portion of a job description for a front-desk position might include the following:

*Constant attention to proactive customer service is essential to creating a consummate member-*

*focused environment; this includes all aspects of service delivery, such as appropriate phone etiquette (greetings, transferring calls, voice tone, and grammar). The applicant must have a warm and friendly communication style that facilitates a personalized relationship with each member and must be respectful of members' preferences (e.g., being addressed by first or last name).*

In addition, the tasks addressed in a detailed job description should form the basis for interview questions. Questions designed to reveal a candidate's ability to deliver the kind of personalized service desired in a front-desk position might include the following:

- Describe situations in which you've experienced excellent customer service. What specific staff behaviors did you notice that contributed to this excellence?

- What businesses or organizations do you feel have reputations for providing great customer service? Why do you think they deserve or don't deserve these reputations?

- What books or articles have you read that deal with delivering great customer service?

- What do you think are the critical elements of answering the phone?

- How would you handle a situation in which a member is signing up for a program at the desk and the phone rings and no one else is available to answer it?

- What are some **defined behaviors** that front-desk personnel could display that would be consistent with the highest levels of customer service?

In addition to providing information for job announcements and interview questions, job descriptions form the framework for training, resource planning, wage and benefit decisions, and job performance criteria. The following sections discuss factors to consider in creating a job description.

# Key Elements of Job Descriptions

A good job description addresses the aspects of the position that are important to the organization and to the employee. In creating a job description, the organization should sufficiently address the following elements:

## QUALIFICATIONS

- *Importance to organization.* The organization needs to define the criteria used to choose the candidate who has the greatest chance of being successful.

- *Importance to employee.* Applicants can determine whether a job is appropriate for them and what training, experience, or education might be necessary to become eligible for the position.

### Issues to Address

- Education
- Experience (overall and specific to the industry)
- Special skills
- Commuting distance
- References

## WAGES

- *Importance to organization.* Positioning wages appropriately within the marketplace is also critical in determining the quality of employee candidates the company attracts. Organizations may decide to pay more than the average for some specialty positions and less than the average for others that it deems less critical to its success. This process of comparing pay rates to the marketplace is designed to position the company to compete for employee talent and is called **external equity**. It is also important to ensure that employees' salaries are positioned proportionately within the club based on levels of responsibility and accountability.

- *Importance to employee.* Defining pay guidelines helps employees understand the structure of the company and their current place within the hierarchy of the organizational structure. In addition, guidelines for pay advancement give workers clear pathways to increase their compensation.

### Issues to Address

- Compensation methods and wage classifications (hourly versus salaried; full versus part time; performance-based compensation with opportunities for commission and bonuses versus base wages; opportunities for overtime; 90-day, semiannual, or annual)

- Internal versus external equity

- Benefit status (vacation eligibility, accrual schedule, personal time, and sick days)

- Starting wages as low as possible without demotivating employees to provide room for increases
- Setting expectations for range and timing of wage increases

## PERFORMANCE EXPECTATIONS

- *Importance to organization.* Establishing performance expectations allows organizations to review how all jobs fit together to ensure the most efficient and effective personnel structure. Performance expectations provide a framework supervisors can use to structure performance coaching and goal setting for their employees.

- *Importance to employee.* Performance expectations make priorities clear and eliminate uncertainty during performance reviews.

### Issues to Address

- Performance review structure, including objective, subjective, results-based, and process-based performance criteria
- Time frames for achieving goals and objectives
- Appropriateness of tying performance goals to potential salary adjustments and bonus rewards (e.g., monetary compensation, vacation time)

## MANAGEMENT SUPPORT STRUCTURE

- *Importance to organization.* Managers and supervisors must understand that they are responsible for the development of workers. Their number one job is to support those they supervise by being accessible and providing necessary resources.

- *Importance to employee.* An established management support structure provides a framework so employees know who to turn to regarding critical aspects of the operation. Defining the chain of command allows all employees to understand the available resources and how their jobs fit into the organization.

### Issues to Address

- Internal and external training provided by the organization
- New-employee orientation or mentoring programs to help new workers acclimate to systems, people, and procedures

- Appropriate chain of command to facilitate effective and efficient communication
- Ensuring managers don't have too many subordinates (typically, it is best to have 5 to 10 direct reports)

## CAREER ADVANCEMENT WITHIN THE ORGANIZATION

- *Importance to organization.* Opportunities for advancement can make a position more attractive by adding future value to a job that may not meet the ideal requirements of candidates who are slightly overqualified. Supervisors can tailor training needs for workers who want to advance within the company.

- *Importance to employee.* Detailing these opportunities helps employees understand how they might advance within the organization.

### Issues to Address

- Potential timing of opportunities for career advancement
- Qualifications for next-step jobs

## PERSONAL APPEARANCE STANDARDS

- *Importance to organization.* These standards can be challenging to define, but once they are established, managers and supervisors can consistently enforce them for all employees. Personal appearance standards contribute to the culture of the organization and can attract certain types of employees.

- *Importance to employee.* Clear communication of company standards reduces unnecessary conflict and provides clear and concise guidelines about the type of attire that is acceptable or unacceptable.

### Issues to Address

- Jewelry, body piercings, and tattoos
- Clothing
- Posture and body language
- Makeup and hair styles

## PHYSICAL REQUIREMENTS

- *Importance to the organization.* Thoughtful consideration of the physical demands of the job helps companies recruit workers who are suited to the job and can increase employees' longevity and productivity.

- *Importance to the employee.* Potential employees must understand the physical nature of the job. Physical limitations that are unexpressed could lead to underperformance or injury. It's best to be up front about any limitations and determine whether there are ways to mitigate physical requirements of a job.

### Issues to Address

- Precise physical expectations (e.g., up to 2 hours of uninterrupted standing)
- Ability to lift heavy loads (e.g., for putting away weights)
- Ability to bend, twist, kneel, and lift throughout the day
- Ability to work outside in the heat or cold
- Potential exposure to chemicals (e.g., working in the maintenance department or around a pool)

## Refining Job Descriptions

Managers may find there are certain types of people that have proven to be good for certain types of positions; as a result, they can grow comfortable looking for a particular mixture of personal and professional assets in a candidate and overlook other qualified applicants. Outlining the most important qualifications in the job description results in guidelines managers can use to determine whether candidates meet experience, skill, and education criteria rather than simply being personable and having familiar behavior patterns.

**Positive profiling** can be helpful. Certain skill sets, educational backgrounds, or career stages might be desired in candidates applying for specific positions. For example, receptionists need to relate to members; therefore, life experience that mirrors the maturity level of the members can be helpful. Candidates in formal career transitions who have predictable commitments (e.g., part-time graduate school for the next 3 years) can be great assets in positions for which long-term employees are challenging to maintain, such as at the front desk, in housekeeping, or in food service.

Some forms of profiling, however, are illegal, immoral, and unfair. In the United States, the Civil Rights Act of 1964 and the Equal Employment Opportunity Act of 1972 cover the types of profiling that are illegal. These two pieces of legislation form the foundation of employment protection provided in the United States, and managers and owners of clubs should be familiar with the information and laws associated with them. The U.S. Equal Employment Opportunity Commission (EEOC) enforces federal laws against discrimination based on race, national origin, sex, age (between the ages of 40 and 70), disability, veteran status, handicap, and religion. Managers should review the preferred qualities listed in job descriptions to ensure they are appropriate, fair, and legal; this will contribute to further refinement of the job description.

## The Bottom Line

Do not overlook the people that are in front of you every day—your customers and staff. Clients can be great for positions in a fitness facility; they value fitness and already have a solid grasp of your culture. Your staff can also be a great way to generate new leads. If they have been with you for a while, you know they will be good promoters. Some words of caution about this: You do not want staff to become so friendly that they lose focus on their jobs, and you need to be aware of the dynamic that is created if a friend of a staff person is terminated. Neither of these, however, is a reason not to consider staff referrals.

## DESIGNING THE APPROPRIATE RECRUITING VEHICLE

It's important to make conscious recruiting choices that lead to choosing the candidate from a large group of less-qualified applicants or a small group of applicants whose qualifications are specifically matched to the predefined needs of the job. The following are five variables to consider in choosing the appropriate job applicant.

1. *Technical nature of the skill set required.* How likely is it that the target audience of the recruiting vehicle will have the technical skills and other requirements of the position? Are the skills relatively common or hard to find?
2. *Available recruitment budget.* Is there a large or small budget?
3. *Urgency of hiring need.* How soon does the position need to be filled?

4. *Geographic reach.* Is it important for employees to live close to work? Might the candidate relocate as a result of taking the job?

5. *Compensation range.* Do the pay parameters of the job vary depending on the applicant's qualifications?

Table 3.1 lists recruiting vehicles and their advantages, disadvantages, and costs.

The most effective position advertisement maximizes the number of highly qualified respondents and minimizes the responses of those who are less qualified. The recent shift

**Table 3.1**   Sources for Recruiting Candidates

| Recruiting vehicle | Pros | Cons | Cost |
|---|---|---|---|
| Web-based search engines; social media advertising | Attract people you would not normally reach | May be overkill; can result in many responses | $100-$6,000 |
| Job websites | Offers quick response call-to-action to access information and apply; provides data analytics reports | May take time to conduct initial screening based on the number of applications | |
| Newspaper ads | Reach large population (regional ads) or a more targeted population (local ads); may be free in university publications | May not reach qualified candidates | $200-$600 |
| Trade journals; association websites | Can be very effective for technical jobs | Journals with national distribution may attract applicants who have to relocate | $400 and up |
| Temporary labor companies; job fairs | Effective bridge during search for long-term candidate or for seasonal hiring | Efforts required to train short-term workers may outweigh advantages; best for basic manual labor tasks | 20%-30% more per hour than regular employees for temporary labor; varies for job fairs |
| Regional employment offices | Provide no-cost brokerage of applicants who have been screened based on work experience, education, and some psychological testing | Doesn't always produce the most qualified candidates | Free |
| Recruiters | Good investment for essential positions or those that require state- or nationwide searches | Can be very costly | 10%-50% of annual salary for the position |
| Staff referrals | Reliable method of finding trustworthy people; requires positive employee culture | Possible friction if referrals aren't hired | Monetary incentive (e.g., $50) |
| Member or customer referrals | Generally invested in the success of the business and understand needs | Possible friction if referral is mishandled | Referral gift (e.g., product or service) |
| Vendor referrals | Vendor may have abundance of qualified applicants or be downsizing | Poaching employees could jeopardize the relationship with the company | Complimentary service or product (can help build relationships) |
| Current employees | Can keep employees excited about their jobs and about learning new skills | Eliminates opportunity to get new ideas and perspective; may need to hire someone else to fill vacated position | Free or small gift |

toward communicating through a company's website and social media channels should be considered as an effective strategy to reach a global audience in real-time. In fact, it is easy to post a job advertisement and provide a direct call-to-action link for the applicant or job seeker to be directed to a specified landing page for capturing their information. Therefore, the key is to follow the recommendations in chapter 7 regarding the best days and times to make these postings on the various social media platforms. To ensure a high percentage of qualified respondents, a job advertisement should include the following:

• *Managing response.* In general, an advertisement should limit the number of respondents by tightly defining the parameters of the opportunity to encourage the largest possible response in the hopes of engaging candidates who might typically be screened out. Sometimes, through conversation or review of résumés, unlikely initial candidates become worthy of consideration.

• *Number of words.* The number of words is directly related to the cost of print ads; therefore, brevity means money saved. However, not adequately describing the job circumstances can lead to an inadequate response. Use active words to describe and clarify work responsibilities to inspire greater response.

• *Headline.* Headlines differentiate ads and help attract appropriate candidates, so keep them interesting.

• *Section.* If applicable, choose the appropriate section (e.g., service, housekeeping, reception) for your ad.

• *Contact method.* Giving candidates several ways to respond to ads can increase response. Be careful when using a phone number as a response option; being swamped by phone messages from unqualified candidates can result in wasted time. For jobs that require phone skills, it may be appropriate to get first impressions of candidates by phone, but be sure to include enough information to limit the calls.

• *Necessary skills.* It is essential to describe the required skills in detail. If degrees or certifications are required, be sure to include that information as well.

• *Required experience.* Ad response can be increased or decreased by simply using the words

preferred or required. If there are no other factors that trump that requirement, list it to affect response to the ad.

• *Wages and benefits.* Depending on the type of position, you can provide specific wage information in the ad. A phrase such as "compensation commensurate with experience and education" can broaden the response and allow for negotiation toward an appropriate compensation package. Providing a range of wage or salary options is also appropriate, as is using the phrase "to start" to indicate room to increase the wage as the employee increases tenure or value within the organization. If there is an absolute wage that the job pays (e.g., $8.50 per hour), be specific about it.

• *Work schedule.* Be specific about the required work days and hours to receive responses from people who can work at those times.

• *Number of days to run ad.* Pricing is usually based on the number of days the ad runs. The best value in terms of cost per day is typically an ad that runs 7 to 10 days. It is usually possible to stop the ad and recoup some of the cost if you receive enough résumés, calls, or applications.

• *Days to run the ad.* Many people look for job advertisements on Saturdays and Sundays, but these are also the most expensive days to run ads. Running the ad for a week beginning on Saturday provides the most exposure early in the run, which allows you to evaluate the response and make decisions about continuing the ad for the duration of the week.

• *Special touches.* Several techniques can make an ad more noticeable, such as bold lettering, an outline or frame around the ad, and a large font size. Each of these incurs an additional cost. Choosing the most compelling aspect of the ad to highlight can be effective in increasing qualified response. Table 3.2 offers examples of more effective and less effective print advertisements.

Another important part of the recruiting phase is to set clear expectations for the ways applications and résumés will be processed and for how you will respond to candidates. For example, if candidates are calling in response to an ad, you might want to leave a voice mail greeting such the following:

*Thank you for calling XYZ Company and expressing an interest in employment. Applications and résumés are being accepted by fax at 303-555-7720 and in person at 1234 Bellevue Drive. The deadline for receipt of applications is August 25. We are in the process of reviewing applications and will be responding to applicants by September 1. If you do not hear from a company representative by that date, you can assume that you were not selected for further evaluation in the hiring process for this position. Thank you for calling XYZ Company.*

If candidates respond in person, a written note similar to this message could be posted.

## The Bottom Line

In my experience, one of the best ways to hire new staff is to work closely with local colleges, universities, and certification instructors in your area. One of my best employees was hired as a result of a talk I did at our local university on the benefits of a career in fitness. He said my enthusiasm was one of the main things that came across to him, and prior to this he had never really considered the field as a career. Many years later, we are both glad he did.

## DEVELOPING INTERVIEW STRATEGIES

To prepare for the interview process, you must develop thoughtful questions that elicit information about the applicant's characteristics, skills, and experience as identified in the job description. Developing interview questions can be a team-building exercise with existing employees. In addition, current employees who have been involved in the hiring process are more committed to ensuring the success for a new employee. Oftentimes, current employees understand the position better than the person doing the hiring. One note of caution: If a group of coworkers is dysfunctional or the current culture of the organization is not representative of the ultimate direction of the company, it may not be appropriate to involve existing employees in developing interview questions. Employees who are at odds with the organization may seek to disrupt the hiring process or derail the well-intentioned efforts of other, more positive employees.

To conduct a brainstorming session for interview questions, begin by choosing the group of employees who will be involved in the project. You can ask for volunteers (if there is no concern about who might volunteer) or choose the employees best suited for the task. You can then involve the rest of the staff by asking for their

**Table 3.2** Sample Print Ads

| Less effective | More effective |
|---|---|
| General help wanted: Club seeks night custodian. Experience preferred. Applicants should call Jan @ 918-555-8926. | Janitorial: Prestigious ACME Health and Fitness Club hiring hardworking, self-motivated night housekeeper. Full time, Sun-Thurs 9 p.m.-5 a.m. shift. Min 2 yr professional cleaning experience pref. $10/hr to start; paid vacation & additional benefits provided. Qualified applicants apply in person at 1234 Broadway Ave., Cleveland, OH 97241, or mail résumé to Jan. |
| General help wanted: Front desk help needed—greeting customers & opening club, wage negotiable, several shifts available; send résumé to john@xyzathletic.com. | Customer service: XYZ Athletic Club is hiring friendly, fitness-focused, outgoing, people-oriented, energetic reception desk service specialists for Sat & Sun 6 a.m.-2 p.m. Benefits include use of club facilities, uniform, free parking, & shift meals. $8.50/hr with opportunities for advancement and wage increase with outstanding performance. Send résumé to john@xyzathletic.com or mailing or applying in person @ 3465 Cherry Lane, Denver, CO 80224. |

input, questions, or concerns about the resultant questions.

Involving employees in the review of job descriptions for their positions or related positions can help remind them of expectations for job performance. In addition, the employees can provide feedback about updates that should be made to the job descriptions.

According to Boydell, Deutsch, and Remillard (2006), there are two main reasons that interviews fail. This first is incompetent interviewers; most people have never been trained in interviewing, so it is no surprise that they are not very good at it. Learning to probe deeply into what interviewees are saying only comes with training. The second reason interviews fail is vague questions. When an interviewee does not fully understand the question, the answer is not likely to be in line with what the interviewer is looking for.

## Job Preview

A crucial task in developing a recruiting strategy is to identify the skills, attributes, and personal characteristics that provide the candidate with the greatest chance of success in the job. This helps ensure a good fit between the organization and the candidate. A **job preview** gives the candidate a snapshot of what it might be like to work at the company and allows you to observe the candidate's response to these conditions.

If there are some conditions that could be **deal breakers**, it's better to communicate these up front. For example, if nose rings are unacceptable, this should be stated at the outset; if a candidate is unwilling to give up his or her nose ring, that will be a deal breaker. If shifts are only available in the early morning and it is unlikely that will change, it is better to communicate that information up front so the candidate understands that going in. If the position is fast paced and there is little opportunity for downtime, such as working the front desk, you should clearly communicate this. Identifying job conditions can streamline conversations and reduce wasted time for you and the candidate.

## Types of Questions

There are several types of questions that can be used in an interview. These are discussed in the following sections.

## Closed Ended Versus Open Ended

**Closed-ended questions** can be answered with a simple *yes* or *no*. **Open-ended questions**, however, should require more than a single-word response and invite people to expand on their answers. The following are examples of open- and closed-ended questions:

- *Open ended:* In your last position, what level of input did you have in the design of the member use tracking system? What did you think were particularly effective components of the system, and what do you think could have been improved?
- *Closed ended:* Is your CPR certification current? Do you possess any national personal training certifications?

## Experiential Versus Situational

**Experiential questions** draw on people's experiences and ask them to relate how they handled some problem in the past. **Situational questions** create circumstances that candidates must react to and can give insight into the problem-solving abilities of candidates. Including both types of questions in an interview is most effective.

## General Questions

The following are questions that could be used when interviewing for different types of positions.

### EXPERIENCE

- Describe your professional experience. How does it apply to this position?
- What are some examples of jobs or experiences you've had that required you to successfully [insert task]?

### MOTIVATION

- What is it about this position that interests you?
- How do you see this position contributing to your career aspirations?

### WORK ETHIC

- What was the hardest job (physically, emotionally, or mentally) you've ever had? Why?
- Are you interested in overtime hours if they are available?

- What's the best job you've ever had? Why?

## CUSTOMER SERVICE

- Give an example of a situation in which you provided service that was significantly more than was expected by the customer.
- A member approaches the front desk and is upset because the whirlpool has been out of order for 5 days. She is aggressive and threatens to quit her membership. How do you handle this situation?
- What have been some of the biggest customer service mistakes you've made? What did you learn from them?

## PERSONALITY TYPE

- Would you say you are more outgoing or more reserved? Give an example of a time when this has been an asset and a time when it has been a liability.
- Give an example of a personal characteristic that you would like to be different. How are you working toward changing it? Or, are you comfortable not changing it? In what situations do you notice this characteristic, and how do you handle yourself?
- If we're chatting over coffee one year from now, what will I say surprised me most about you that I wouldn't have guessed from meeting you in this interview?

## TEAMWORK

- Give an example of a conflict you had with a coworker and how you contributed to resolving it. If it wasn't resolved, explain why.
- Give an example of a poor boss you've had. Explain why the person was not a good manager and what strategies you used to manage your relationship.
- Give some examples that demonstrate your ability to successfully contribute to a team project or effort.

## PROBLEM SOLVING

- You're the shift manager. The air conditioning is not working and it's 7 p.m. on a Sunday. It's getting very hot in the cardio room, and members are complaining. What do you do?
- After coming out of the whirlpool, a member complains that he feels lightheaded and nau-

seated. While talking to you, he collapses and is unconscious. What do you do?

## TIMELINESS AND AVAILABILITY

- What personal examples from jobs, activities, or hobbies can you offer to indicate you can consistently be on time for early-morning shifts?
- Why is the [late-night, early-morning, weekend] shift attractive to you?

## PASSION

- Give examples of things in your life that you're passionate about. If I watched you engage in these things, what sort of behaviors would I see that would convince me of your passion?
- Is there someone in history, sport, politics, or your personal life that you admire because of his or her passion for something? Explain why you admire this person.

## COMMITMENT TO PERSONAL GROWTH

- Have you recently done any professional reading or participated in any professional education programs? If so, please tell me about these.
- What accomplishments are you most proud of? Include at least one professional example, and include personal examples if you desire.

Always remember to ask whether the candidate has any questions. The type and depth of questions offered by the candidate can provide information on his or her level of preparation for the interview. In addition, when closing the interview, ask the candidate if there is anything that you haven't asked or that he or she would like you to know.

## *The Bottom Line*

The best way to determine whether someone is lying during an interview is to ask the person to elaborate on an answer. According to the *Complete Reference Checking Handbook* (1998), most people do not want to elaborate on their lies and will give brief answers or trip over their words.

# Questions Relevant to Specific Positions

Some of the questions you ask during a job interview are directly related to the performance criteria and skills needed to perform the job. In the following examples, job-related criteria and skills and a sample interview question are provided for each position.

### FRONT-DESK PERSONNEL

- *Job performance criteria.* Candidates must be able to multitask and must maintain a positive and upbeat customer-centered approach in an environment that requires a constant shifting of attention.
- *Skills and characteristics associated with these tasks.* Making appropriate eye contact, being unflappable, being patient but energetic, and having a quick mind are all important in these tasks.
- *Sample question.* What are some situations in which you've successfully dealt with multiple tasks in a time-intensive manner while maintaining a high level of customer service?

### FITNESS SPECIALIST

- *Job performance criterion.* Candidates must be able to administer a variety of health screenings and use the resultant information to determine participant goals and establish an appropriate exercise regimen.
- *Skills and characteristics associated with this task.* Knowledge of anatomy, kinesiology, physiology, and special health conditions and the ability to develop rapport are essential.
- *Sample question.* A new member wants to lose 20 pounds (9 kilograms) before he attends his high school reunion in 2 months. He is 40 years old, has diabetes and arthritic knees, and is 30 pounds (13.5 kilograms) overweight. How you would approach this situation and develop appropriate exercise recommendations?

### MEMBERSHIP SALESPERSON

- *Job performance criterion.* Candidates must be able to perform needs analyses as part of the sales process to determine prospects' motivation for considering club membership.
- *Skills and characteristics associated with this task.* This job requires an engaging personality, the ability to mirror a client's energy and personality style, and familiarity with specific techniques associated with needs analysis.
- *Sample question.* Explain the concept of needs analysis and its importance in selling club memberships.

### HOUSEKEEPER

- *Job performance criteria.* Candidates must be able to be on their feet for extended periods of time; lift up to 40 pounds (18 kilograms); travel up and down stairs; and bend, twist, and reach when vacuuming, dusting, collecting trash, and cleaning windows.
- *Skills and characteristics associated with these tasks.* Candidates must be in good physical condition and have good strength and flexibility.
- *Sample question.* What physically demanding jobs have you had in the past? Indicate the specific tasks associated with these jobs.

In many situations, you might want to test the candidate on a specific skill or task. For example, it would be difficult to hire a personal trainer without observing the person in action. In this situation, you could have the trainer conduct a workout with you or a staff member based on some predetermined guidelines (you would need to give the candidate time to prepare for the session). As another example, you might ask a candidate for a sales position to sell you a pen. Again, the candidate would need to know about this task ahead of time so he or she is prepared; the candidate will be representing your business, so you want this done in a professional way.

## Quality of Answers

You should spend as much or more time thinking about the right answers to questions as you do the questions themselves. Some general questions to evaluate the quality of the candidate's answers include the following:

- Did the candidate answer the questions succinctly?
- Did the candidate stay on track while answering questions?
- Did the candidate ask for additional information to improve the quality of his or her answer?
- If the candidate did not know the answer, did he or she admit it?

Take the time to answer the questions you plan to ask the candidate. This exercise can help you consider follow-up questions that better illustrate the kinds of qualities or expertise the ideal candidate should have. For example, say you are planning to ask the applicant to tell you about situations in which he or she had to deal with a disgruntled customer. Identify the ideal components associated with the answer. When dealing with an unhappy customer, you should do the following:

- Apologize for how the customer feels.
- Acknowledge the customer's perception of the problem.
- If there are several ways to solve the problem, ask for the customer's input.
- Proactively offer a reasonable range of solutions to the problem.
- If you are uncertain how to fix the problem, seek out an employee who might be able to help.
- If the problem is a condition of the business (e.g., the club doesn't open until 5:30 a.m. or no shaving is allowed in the steam room), state that the policy is a commitment the company has made to the members and that making occasional exceptions reduces the credibility and consistency of the company's overall image and product.

- Reflect the customer's feelings and specific concerns, and confirm how you will fix the problem (if possible) and how you will follow up with the customer.

Identifying these components ahead of time clarifies the ideal answer.

## SELECTING THE BEST CANDIDATE FOR THE POSITION

The procedure for assessing the applicants generally follows these steps:

1. Review of applications and résumés
2. Phone screening
3. In-person interviews
4. Background and reference checks
5. Comparison of candidates
6. Job offer

### Review of Applications and Résumés

All candidates should fill out a **job application** even if they provide formal résumés. The job application provides a standardized list of requested information and compels the applicant to tell the truth. Many applications explicitly state

## Questions to Avoid in Interviews

Hiring preferences related to age, religion, race, ethnicity, social condition (membership to clubs or organizations), and gender are unethical and illegal. The following interview questions (U.S. Small Business Administration 2004) are illegal in the United States because they seek to determine personal characteristics that cannot be used when making a hiring decision:

- How old are you?
- Are you married?
- Do you have any children?
- How old are your children?
- How will you care for your children during work hours?
- Do you receive alimony or child support?
- Are you pregnant?

- Where do you attend religious services?
- Are you [insert ethnicity]?
- Send a picture with your application.
- How much do you weigh?
- What is your maiden name?
- What is your father's surname?
- Where were you born?
- What clubs do you belong to?

that fabricated information on the application is cause for elimination from the applicant pool or immediate termination of employment. Consult with a reputable labor attorney to ensure that you comply with all federal and state regulations in developing an appropriate form. Many consulting firms work with small businesses to provide advice about applications, such as where to get them, what information should be included, why candidates have to fill them out, and legal protection for the company. Applications also allow the personnel manager or hiring supervisor to compare applicant content with résumé content to ensure the information is accurate and consistent.

It can be helpful to keep a checklist of qualifications to review with each application. You can also use this checklist for comments or questions about some aspect of the application (never take notes on the application; if the candidate is hired, it becomes part of the employee file). The notes can be helpful in managing a stack of résumés to ensure the pertinent information from each one is summarized for review later. The checklist is a great place to note where one candidate's experience may be more applicable to the position or where a graduate degree is more compelling than an undergraduate degree. This initial **paper screening** should sort applications into two or three categories such as excellent, possible, and disqualified.

## Phone Screening

Once the initial paper screening has been completed, the next phase is typically **phone screening** for the priority candidates. The chance to evaluate a candidate's phone etiquette and phone presence is valuable, and phone interviews save time compared with meeting all candidates in person.

In the phone interview, confirm the candidate's interest in the job and the information listed on the application. Discuss potential deal breakers that could sabotage the second interview, such as basic pay range, work hours, work environment, availability date, professional certifications or education, and ability to perform critical job tasks. By expanding on the information provided in the job advertisement, you can screen out a few candidates that look good on paper but are not worth interviewing in person.

Ask candidates a couple of questions from the list you developed from the job description. Ask each person the same questions so they have equal chances to demonstrate their competence. If you are inspired by the answers to questions, ask follow-up or clarifying questions. If it becomes apparent early in the conversation the candidate is not right for the position, don't feel the need to continue the interview. Thank these applicants for their time, let them know that this a preliminary phone screening for potential job candidates, and tell them if they are being considered they will receive a phone call within a certain time period (e.g., 1 to 2 weeks).

Once you've identified good candidates, find out whether they're involved in employment conversations with any other companies. If a candidate will have to decide on another opportunity before you're prepared to make an offer, try saying the following: "I understand you may be entertaining an attractive job offer soon. Given our brief conversation and the early stages of our interviewing process, I think you are a very good candidate for the position. Before you commit to another company, would you consider giving me a call so I can try to speed up our process to take advantage of your availability? That way, if we determine we'd like to make you an offer, you'd potentially have a choice of employers."

## In-Person Interviews

The first interview is not only a chance for the applicant to make a first impression but also the company's chance to define itself as a business-oriented organization that takes the hiring process seriously. Establish a professional environment and circumstances for the interview as follows:

- Select a private, quiet room that is tidy and well organized.
- Provide comfortable furnishings, including a table and at least two chairs.
- Offer the candidate a beverage (some will be nervous, which can lead to a dry mouth).
- Allow adequate time (a typical first interview could take 5 to 30 minutes).
- Avoid interruptions from phones or other personnel, if possible.

The in-person interview begins with the interviewer being prepared with appropriate interview questions, including why the candidates believes he or she is best person for the job. As they ask questions, interviewer should be paying attention to the interviewee's responses, vocal tonality, and nonverbal communication, which are key to conducting a great interview. The interview should also provide the interviewee with an opportunity to ask questions that will reveal important information regarding the applicant. Finally, conclude the interview by thanking the applicant and outlining the process going forward. Indicate how long it will be before you make a decision, and detail the additional steps and approximate time frame for completing the process if the candidate is offered the job.

Some companies conduct more than one in-person interview. Generally, the more opportunities you have to interview a candidate, the better. Take it as a good sign if the candidate continually demonstrates timeliness, appropriate appearance and body language, and consistent, targeted, and accurate responses to interview questions.

Using different types of in-person interviews can also be an effective strategy. Table 3.3 describes different interview types and their purposes.

# Reference Checks

Some companies require three professional references, and others require contact information for one or more former employers to confirm employment history. Defining the value of and obtaining meaningful **references** can be challenging. Most candidates select people for their references that they know will make favorable comments, so you might wonder whether references are truly important. References can confirm impressions and beliefs you developed during the interview process. They also confirm that information listed on the résumé is accurate. Candidates who play it loose with the facts when listing their employment dates, job titles, responsibilities, or pay rates may not be trustworthy employees.

You should also pay attention to references that are not listed. Candidates frequently don't list their current employers because the job search is confidential or they don't want to put their current jobs in jeopardy. Candidates should, however, list one or two previous employers. If they don't, it could indicate problems they would rather not expose. Don't be afraid to ask for references that have not been provided. Even if the people who worked with the applicant are no longer employed there, dates of employment and other information

**Table 3.3** Types of In-Person Interviews

| Type | Description | Purpose |
|------|-------------|---------|
| Supervisor-directed one-on-one interview | This is a typical interview scenario in which the supervisor meets with the candidate. | This allows the manager to control all aspects of the interview process. |
| Support personnel-directed one-on-one interview | This type of interview is conducted by a team member the applicant would work with or a manager who works in a closely related department. | This allows the team member or manager to see the degree to which the applicant fits in with other personalities. This style can also create buy-in and provide additional perspectives on the applicant. |
| Group- or committee-directed interview | This type of interview involves a group of the applicant's potential peers or a committee of current employees charged with vetting candidates. | This demonstrates a candidate's ability to be consistent and perform in a group environment. |
| Trial interview | This type of interview involves having the candidate perform some of the functions associated with the job. The trial could take the form of role-play with a supervisor or could involve part of an actual shift working directly with customers or existing employees. Paying applicants as contract labor may be necessary for interviews that use a several-hour trial in an actual work environment. | This interview provides a realistic picture of how a candidate will perform. Because of the time involvement, this technique is typically limited to the best candidates. |

can be confirmed, which lends credibility to the applicant's résumé and experience.

In these litigious times, companies are sometimes reluctant to provide detailed information other than whether the candidate was employed and the start and end dates. You should ask for detailed information if the company is willing to provide it. Questions can be general (e.g., about work ethic, timeliness, punctuality), but they should be related to the job for which the candidate is applying. For example, if a candidate is applying for a position performing pre-exercise health screenings and exercise prescriptions, you could ask about the candidate's technical skills or ability to perform accurate blood pressure readings. Keep in mind, though, that you might want to test a candidate's aptitudes on technical issues during the interview process rather than relying on someone else's judgment.

## Comparison of Candidates

One dimension of comparing candidates may include **scoring** their responses to questions or scoring them on standards related to the position. Scoring the candidate can be very helpful if you use several interviewers or have a committee-based process for candidate selection. Agreeing on the preferred employment criteria in advance (e.g., undergraduate degree preferred) is necessary if this method is employed.

You can also create a rating system for preferred characteristics and skills. This can be time consuming, but it can help address the areas that are critical to making the best hire. For example, a rating system could ask interviewers to rate the candidate on the following using a scale of 1 to 5 (1 = poor, 5 = excellent):

- Appearance
- Relevant experience
- Likelihood of long tenure
- Relevant education
- Technical skills
- Personality characteristics
- References

You can then total or average the scores to determine each candidate's rating. You can also rank the criteria (ensure all those involved in the interviewing process understand the hierarchy).

If candidates are close, you can reevaluate the scores and focus on the most important criteria.

Rating systems add a degree of objectiveness to a process that can be subjective. These systems can be particularly useful when you are having difficulty choosing among several qualified candidates. The scores can highlight the differences between candidates and facilitate helpful conversation, which can contribute to a better final decision.

## *The Bottom Line*

You must use the same questions and the same scoring systems for all candidates. This is the only way to fairly compare people. This is another reason having a group of predetermined interview questions are a critical part of the interview process.

## Job Offer

Some companies make job offers in writing. These offers usually stipulate certain conditions, such as the candidate's ability to successfully pass a background or drug and alcohol tests. A well-crafted job offer should contain the details of the employment offer, which may include the following elements: job description, job title, reporting structure, starting date of employment, salary and bonuses, benefits information and eligibility, acknowledgment of offer, and confirmation of acceptance.

## Background Checks

Many companies require **background checks** before employees can be hired. These range from criminal conduct reviews to credit checks to drug and alcohol screenings. Candidates must provide their consent for background checks. There are several companies that provide background checks as part of their payroll management services (e.g., Automatic Data Processing, Inc.; Paychex Payroll Services; Kelly Management Services). These companies use their websites "locations near you" by state or zip in the United States. to offer services. Other information checks include asking applicants to provide university transcripts and documentation for professional certifications.

## New Hires

Most companies have a **new-hire packet** to ensure the necessary paperwork is completed. In the United States, standard new-hire forms include the W-4 (tax-related information) and I-9 (confirmation of citizenship). Employers might also include documents such as payroll information, information about direct deposits to personal bank accounts, a welcome letter, and the general policies of the organization (e.g., sexual harassment, drugs and alcohol, safety, payroll, benefits, vacation, sick days, paid holidays, dependent care savings). Other processes that need to be dealt with at point of hire are time card assignment (for hourly positions), uniform and name badge distribution (as necessary), and formalization and agreement of a work schedule.

## Key Terms

background checks
benchmarks
closed-ended questions
deal breakers
defined behaviors
experiential questions
external equity

job application
job description
job preview
new-hire packet
open-ended questions
paper screening
performance expectations

phone screening
positive profiling
references
reporting structure
scoring
situational questions
wage position

# CHAPTER 4

# Training and Developing Staff

## Learning Objectives

After studying this chapter, you will be able to

- use training as a powerful management tool,
- perform a training needs assessment,
- choose training topics,
- develop a training strategy,
- deliver training material effectively, and
- justify training investment.

Roz Greenfield, director of sales and marketing for Sports and Fitness Ventures, which operates eight clubs on the East Coast of the United States, does the majority of the sales training for all eight clubs herself. For ideas and inspiration, she uses industry-specific books and magazine articles, attends conferences, and occasionally invites an expert to give her inspiration and material to work with.

"Training and development is the biggest focus of my job," says Roz. She gets the entire team together once a month for intensive training on a specific skill (like informational calls or follow-up calls). She also hosts a weekly conference call. For very little cost, each representative calls in on the toll-free line and the group addresses an issue or a skill together with Roz at the helm. "I might ask them how a certain promotion is going and see how we can maximize that opportunity," she explains.

Roz feels that the most important element of training is the individual follow-up with each rep. In addition to the monthly training and the weekly call, Roz does an intensive coaching session with each rep (usually with the club manager present) to focus on a specific skill. "We role-play in these small groups to make sure the rep has the skill down pat," she says. "Follow-up is the most important part. When you train with the group, it's in this perfect setting, but it is not always reality. You have to get with the person and see what they're really doing. I go through steps of the presentation while we are together and then meet one on one to fine-tune the details."

---

The author acknowledges the significant contributions of Brenda Abdilla to this chapter.

One way a fitness organization can gain a competitive advantage is to develop a staff training strategy. This begins with great leaders who share a compassionate and passionate vision with those they lead and show them how the work they do contributes to results. The training strategy also adds tremendous value to health club members, personal training clients, guests, and others.

Great training programs are no accident, and they should be used as powerful management tools. To put this in perspective, consider the extensive training Disney University has for its cast members: Every cast member learns Disney's traditions and their line of business and then receives on-the-job training. Translating this to the fitness industry, every fitness organization that believes their front-line employees are key to creating the magic within the club must perform a training needs assessment, choose the right topics, develop a training strategy, deliver training materials, and justify the training investment. Those leaders who develop and manage the training need to consider the idea of creating emotional connections with customers. As Maya Angelou once said, "People won't remember what you said, people won't remember what you did, but people will always remember how you made them feel" (Gallo 2014). Staff should embody this mindset and focus on the overall customer experience. This culture is created through training.

Excellent club managers learn quickly that the only way for clubs to succeed in this intensively customer-focused business is through the employees who interact with the members. People in management usually have reached that level by providing excellent customer service, using effective communication, and mastering the skills of their jobs, but managers can't be the only ones to possess these qualities. The desire to have others behave in a certain way drives most managers to invest time and resources in staff training and development. The ability to influence the behavior of others becomes a critical element of effective club management. Even the most skilled manager has only a limited number of ways to influence the behavior of others.

Developing the skills and changing the behaviors of the team can be one of the most interesting and rewarding duties of club managers. Training requires a tremendous amount of planning and work, but the outcome can be remarkable. There are few actions a manager can take that will be more effective than delivering training with the intent of changing the staff's approach to a skill. If handled properly, the manager will see increased confidence in the staff as well as a better appreciation for the aspects of their jobs covered in the training. Quality training can help attract and recruit excellent staff and help the club retain current staff. Although a warm personality and bright smile can be hired, nearly any other skill can be trained with the right effort.

Training and development can produce results and deliver consistent behaviors among staff in any department, including sales, hospitality, group exercise, housekeeping, and more. Used properly and over the long term, training and development can help staff develop a **career path,** which promotes employee retention and professional growth. Furthermore, training can benefit employees by providing additional job skills and intellectual stimulation. Finally, regular training provides a forum for ongoing communication of important information.

## *The Bottom Line*

The world's best managers maximize the effects of training by developing employees' strengths rather than trying to improve their weaknesses (Buckingham and Coffman 1999).

# FIVE STEPS TO CREATING INTERNAL TRAINING PROGRAMS

Successful internal training programs are created through a five-step process. The steps are committing to a **needs analysis,** choosing the topics for the training, picking a strategy, delivering the material, and creating accountability.

## Committing to a Needs Analysis

Starting a training program in the club setting is easier than most managers think. The best way to start the process is to commit to an observation period, such as 2 weeks. You can easily continue to perform regular management duties during this observation period. To start, label file folders with every department name and club topic that needs enhancement. Keep the files nearby, and develop the habit of filing anything that comes into view that applies to the analysis process.

Items to consider could be memos, articles, notes on thoughts that come to mind, notes from a speaker or program, advertisements from local seminars—anything. Later, when it is time to put together a training program or delegate training to someone else, you will have a collection of discussion items. It should be noted that completing the needs analysis and creating the topics list are more than just management processes. Having a clear idea of training needs (even if the list is long) can provide tremendous stress relief if you have been observing bothersome behaviors. Awareness of specific needs often stimulates thoughts, ideas, and connections in your mind that can lead to resources and strategies for getting the training done.

The following are examples of departments that could have files:

- Fitness
- Group exercise
- Hospitality desk
- Sales
- Housekeeping (cleaning)
- Maintenance (fixing and upkeep)
- Aquatics
- Child care
- Café or restaurant

Files for general topics that might affect more than one department include the following:

- Customer service
- Dealing with difficult situations
- Cross-training
- Member retention

- Leadership
- Selling
- Special populations (seniors, members in postrehabilitation)
- Grassroots marketing
- Technical skills (electronic cash register, computers, pool maintenance)

During the 2-week observation period, assess the current needs in each department. This process takes about an hour for each department. It is easiest to start with the four departments that have the greatest effect on customer satisfaction and the bottom line: sales, hospitality, housekeeping, and fitness. This assessment is best done after you have worked in the department or spent some time observing the department in action while answering the questions.

## Choosing the Topics for the Training

Once the needs analysis is complete, take some time to read the notes made during the process and sort training needs into three categories:

1. Urgent need
2. Short-term need
3. Long-term need

Urgent training needs should be met within 30 days of the needs analysis, short-term needs should be met within 90 days, and long-term needs should be met within 6 months to 1 year, if possible. Table 4.1 is a sample list of training topics that includes level of need. You should also determine whether there are elements of the

**Table 4.1**　Sample Topics and Level of Need

| Training topic | Level of need | Staff to receive this training |
|---|---|---|
| Customer service | Urgent | All staff |
| Point-of-sale system | Urgent | Hospitality desk staff, personal trainers |
| Team building | Short term | All staff |
| Sales training | Urgent | Sales team, personal trainers |
| Cross-selling skills | Long term | All staff |
| Telephone skills | Short term | Desk staff, sales staff, personal trainers |
| Personal training for special populations | Short term | Personal trainers |
| Pool supplies and chemical safety | Urgent | Housekeeping staff, maintenance staff |

training that would benefit the entire staff or the more urgent needs are department specific. For example, if poor communication or marginal customer service were problems in most of the departments analyzed, then the general topic of customer service excellence is an urgent need that must be addressed before specific training occurs within departments. If observations revealed impressive levels of staff communication and customer service, then more specific training might come first (e.g., point-of-sale training for the front desk, training in how to perform fitness evaluations for the fitness team). For a more complete list of topics, see the Club Training and Development Planner sidebar later in this chapter.

## The Bottom Line

Clubs often struggle to get their staff to do what is at the core of their business: exercise. When associates work odd hours and split shifts in a fast-paced environment, exercise is often the last thing they want to do. Ensure that staff exercise regularly and ensure that the work environment encourages this (e.g., managers set an example by working out regularly). I can attest that exercise is often put aside for other pressing matters; when this happens, I remind myself what I do for a living.

## Choosing a Strategy

After coming up with a clear idea of training needs, work on finding resources to help with the training process and decide on training strategies for each need (see figure 4.1). To choose a strategy, determine who will provide training and where it will take place.

## Who Will Provide the Training?

For each of the training topics, determine whether you will deliver the training, there is someone on staff who can deliver it (both of these are considered internal resources), or an external resource is necessary. For some topics, such as CPR, pool care, or even sales training, an outside resource may be necessary unless you also have teacher certifications or special expertise in these areas. For many of these topics, however, there are options. Sometimes the budget is so limited that

internal training is necessary. If the budget permits, the best strategy is a combination of internal and external training resources, because no one resource or person usually has all the answers. A list of outside resources to consider is presented later in the chapter.

## Where Will the Training Take Place?

Choosing a training venue is important in creating a productive learning environment. Seemingly nonessential factors, such as room temperature or outside noise, can have a negative effect on how the training is received.

Fitness facilities typically hold most of their staff training on site. Be sure to have comfortable seating and tables, appropriate materials, and lighting suitable for learning. The in-club training venue should be free of member traffic, and training should not be conducted within earshot of members, which is often difficult for busy clubs with limited space. The ideal times for training are when the club is not busy (i.e., early morning, middle of the day, weekend). Planning the training in advance is critical, because you will have to arrange it around people's schedules. Ideally, you should schedule weekly, monthly, or quarterly meetings so staff know ahead of time what to expect.

Budget constraints need not limit venue options for staff training if **trade-outs** (i.e., trading goods or services with another business) are an option. Many local hotels would gladly take free guest passes in exchange for a conference room, audiovisual materials, and even meal service.

**Staff retreats** take **off-site training** one step further. Retreats are increasing in popularity in the business world; an internet search for *corporate retreats* yields nearly 20 million results. Staff retreats can range from something as simple as taking the staff bowling to hiring a company to take the team on a ropes course or rafting. After, a consultant or guest speaker can begin to train formally or informally on a plethora of topics agreed upon by senior management. A retreat is a fresh approach for a group that has seen it all. Retreats can also be taken for the following reasons:

- To encourage staff to think differently and change their approach to solving a dilemma
- To establish team spirit where it is lacking
- To facilitate transitions such as new ownership, staff changes, and so on
- To try something new

# Club Training and Development Planner

Training programs should focus on specific areas of need. Here are some examples of general areas, suggestions for topics that can be covered, and ideas for delivering the training.

## Safety and Compliance

- *Topics to cover:* Occupational Safety and Health Administration (OSHA) regulations, sexual harassment, CPR and AED, bloodborne pathogens, facility safety, first aid, water safety, personal training certifications, and lifeguard certifications (check state laws for positions that require drug testing or background checks as part of the hiring process)
- *Ideas for training:* Consider outsourcing this training or purchasing an e-learning program. Make certain classes mandatory for all employees and schedule them quarterly or more often. Call the local fire or police department and schedule drills for fires, bomb threats, first aid, and safety.

## New-Associate Orientation

- *Topics to cover:* company standards, cross-training for all departments, benefits, service strategies, and policies for uniforms, grooming, benefits, and so on
- *Ideas for training:* If the club's orientation is outdated, schedule a half-day brainstorming session with all department heads to commit to a new agenda and method of delivery. The ideal orientation is concise, upbeat, and has a test for maximum effectiveness.

## Basic Management Skills

- *Topics to cover:* recruiting, interviewing, budget processes, goal setting, organization, schedules, uniforms, basic coaching skills for managers, and discipline approach and policy
- *Ideas for training:* This training should be given to anyone who manages other people. These skills are critical to the success of new managers. The general manager can perform training with the human resources and finance departments or bring in a trainer.

## Leadership Skills for Experienced Managers

- *Topics to cover:* building a team, time management, leadership versus management, crisis prevention, advanced coaching, forecasting and accountability systems, inspiring others to serve, influencing others, and how leaders think
- *Ideas for training:* If possible, bring in a professional speaker for this program once managers have mastered the basic skills. Consider enrolling everyone in a public seminar and having all participants present what they learned. See the Taking Training to New Heights sidebar later in the chapter.

## Team Building

- *Topics to cover:* structured or skill-focused topics, such as goal setting, mind mapping, wealth building, personal health and nutrition, and life balance
- *Ideas for training:* Unless the club has a team-building expert, it will likely have to pay someone to provide this training. Try to do some things that are completely unexpected by the team like unstructured or fun-focused events, such as bowling, outdoor activities, weekend getaways, theme parks, ropes courses, awards dinners, movies, theater performances, or trips. Be sure to block out the time so there are no interruptions. Be sure to avoid anything that is physically dangerous or that may be offensive to team members.

## Sales Training for New Reps

- *Topics to cover:* industry-specific topics, such as competition, selling intangibles versus tangibles, product knowledge, needs versus interests selling, informational calls, following up, lead tracking, tours, and referrals
- *Ideas for training:* Start a training file and fill it with articles, memos, and any relevant information a new rep will need. See what books, tapes, and materials industry experts have published and start a library. Schedule new reps for 30 minutes of training with each department.

*(continued)*

**Club Training and Development Planner** (continued)

### Sales Training for Experienced Reps

- *Topics to cover:* personal development topics, such as dressing for success, time management, organization, wealth building, nutrition, and life balance; advanced sales skills, such as prospecting strategies, grassroots marketing, business-to-business selling, and networking

- *Ideas for training:* Look for relevant books to read as a team. Register everyone for the next full-day business rally that comes to town, or invest in a speaker or trainer. Ask the group what they are interested in learning and teach it to them.

### Personal Trainers

- *Topics to cover:* safety training, updated information on exercise science, selling skills that focus on needs assessments of members and closing the sale, time management, communication skills, and referral generation

- *Ideas for training:* Try to hire trainers who can sell, because trying to teach this skill can be an exercise in futility. Credibility is critical; personal trainers need someone they can believe in to teach them new skills. A person with a background in exercise who has proven business skills is ideal.

### Customer Service

- *Topics to cover:* greetings, telephone etiquette, handling difficult clients, behavior toward coworkers, service expectations, technical training, and cross-selling

- *Ideas for training:* If the club doesn't currently have a solid program, put the department heads to the task and supplement the program with videos that reflect club expectations. Periodically take groups on field trips to local businesses that offer top-notch service, and then discuss the trip. If the club wants to go big, consider Disney University, a program that is available in several cities and has more than 500,000 graduates.

---

For some employees, a staff retreat or team-building event is exciting and is a welcome departure from the ordinary, but for others, it can be uncomfortable or perceived as a waste of time. Keep this in mind during planning, and decide in advance how much to tell the team about the upcoming event. It might help to involve several members of the team in the planning process. As with all training, begin with the end in mind. Determine the desired outcome, and then plan the special event. Consider the following key elements:

- How much social interaction is wanted?
- Is there a theme?
- Will internal or external facilitators be used?
- Does anyone in the group have physical limitations?
- Are there safety considerations?
- Are there any liability concerns?

- What is the duration of the retreat? Will there be an overnight stay?
- How will success be determined?
- What is the total budget for the event?

## *The Bottom Line*

When a team has a corporate retreat or off-site business meeting, the investment of time is significant. The question is how to make the most of this limited and extremely valuable time (Withrow 2007).

## Delivering the Material

The most critical element of effective training is likely the method of information delivery. Many different employees work in clubs, and they all receive and process information in different ways,

# DEPARTMENTAL TRAINING NEEDS ASSESSMENT

Date: _____

Evaluator name: _____

Department name: _____

1. List the three to five most critical tasks of this department._____

   _____

2. List the names of the people who perform these critical tasks with expertise, consistency, and professionalism (if any)._____

   _____

3. If you were working the department yourself, what would you do differently?_____

   _____

4. What efficiencies are present in this department?_____

   _____

5. What inefficiencies are present in this department?_____

   _____

6. On a scale of 1 to 10, how would you rate the overall success of this department, with 1 being poor and 10 being excellent?_____

   _____

7. If applicable, from a financial perspective, how does this department rate (over budget, under budget, understaffed, profitable)?_____

   _____

8. What elements could be added to this department to make it more financially viable or to save costs?

   _____

9. What are your general observations about the department's current condition?_____

   _____

**Figure 4.1** Sample form for assessment of department training needs.

From M. Bates, M.J. Spezzano, and G. Danhoff, *Health Fitness Management*, 3rd ed. (Champaign, IL: Human Kinetics, 2020).

have different levels of comfort with technology, and have different learning styles. Keep these differences in mind when updating training programs. Professionally prepared seminars or training classes typically accommodate a variety of learning modalities; with time and preparation, this can also be accomplished with in-house training programs.

## Developing Effective Training Programs

The following are keys to developing effective training programs:

- *Keep the focus narrow.* Peruse the notes and items filed to determine specific topics to cover in the upcoming training. When putting together a training program, keep the topic narrow and focus on skills rather than concepts. If time is limited, it is better to focus on a few aspects of a large topic than to try to lump the entire topic into one training session. For example, when preparing training sessions on delivering customer service, it is better to focus on a few related topics, such as handling member complaints and dealing with difficult situations, in one session than to also include telephone skills, scheduling, and snack bar sales in the same session. It is better to cover narrow topics deeply than to cover wide topics broadly.

• *Begin with the end in mind.* Think about the desired outcome. Answer the following three questions:

1. What specific skills should the group come away with?
2. How will their knowledge be apparent?
3. What words, body language, or results will be present after the training that are not consistently present now?

• *Break it down.* Virtually any skill can be broken down into steps or important concepts. Come up with at least five steps or concepts that will help the group absorb the material. For example, if the topic is dealing with difficult member situations, come up with the steps necessary to handle the situation.

1. Listen carefully to the member (using both eyes and ears).
2. Remove distractions and pause before reacting to the member's words.
3. Calmly repeat the member's words back to the member for clarification.
4. Decide how to respond. Call reinforcements if needed, but keep the member informed of pending actions.
5. Take responsibility to resolve the situation.

Once the steps are in place, determine the best approach to teaching each step.

• *Bring training material to life.* Many people think the most difficult part of training is public speaking (see the Tips for Delivering Training Material sidebar later in this chapter). Anyone who has ever developed a training program knows the most difficult part is making ideas and training goals come to life. It is difficult to change

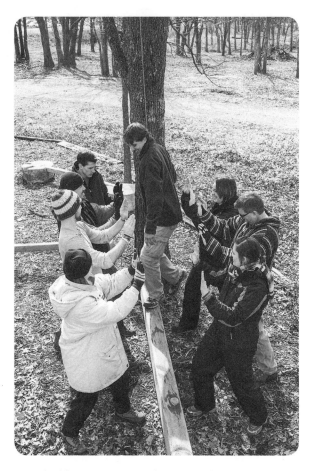

Team-building activities, such as a challenge course, can establish a team spirit among staff members and prompt a change in their usual approach to solving problems.

iStockphoto/Mark Rose

human behavior and habits, but getting people to change is the crux of training and development. The only measure of effective training is whether it changes the way people act and think. The goal of change requires a combination of good material and an effective teaching method.

## The Bottom Line

A common issue with experienced staff is the perception that they already know how to do everything. In my experience, they don't actually know how to do everything and have often developed bad habits over time. If you set a precedent that some form of training and review of procedures is always done at staff meetings, then you will ensure that staff are always sharp and meet your expectations.

## Tips for Delivering Training Material

It is perfectly normal to feel nervous or self-conscious when delivering training material. Focus on the material and the desired result instead of on personal appearance or nervousness. Immerse yourself in the material you are presenting, and the rest will fall into place. Keep these seven tips in mind:

1. *Never start with a joke unless you are a professional comedian.* Starting with a joke is common advice for nervous speakers, but this can be a mistake for several reasons: You might not be able to pull off a joke if you are nervous, you could offend someone, or you might repeat a joke the audience has already heard.

2. *Practice.* Rehearse until the message is committed to memory; that way, the material won't be lost to nerves. Practice makes perfect.

3. *Be positive.* Your thoughts about the upcoming training program will affect your performance, so make them positive. Also, do something positive before speaking (e.g., exercise, meditate) and avoid anything that might be upsetting to you (e.g., watching the news, checking voicemail).

4. *Focus on the material.* Focus on the material rather than how you will be perceived by others. If the material is good and the delivery is decent, you will be well perceived.

5. *Ignore insignificant distractions.* People sneeze, cough, move around, talk, and even fall asleep in training sessions. If someone requires disciplinary action, take care of it later. While presenting, focus on the material and ignore distractions.

6. *Plan each moment.* Take time to write down everything you will say and proceed in a step-by-step fashion. This will help with delivery, and it can also help if you get sidetracked. It can also help keep the program on a time schedule.

7. *Always start on time and end on time.* Begin as close to the starting time as possible (this often requires reminding staff of the starting time in advance). If given the choice, go short rather than long and leave the audience wanting more. Never exceed the time allotted. There is nothing worse than people looking at their watches and wondering when it is going to end.

## Selecting Interactive Exercises

Now that the training steps have been outlined, it is time to come up with a teaching method for each step. **Interactive exercises** keep the group interested in the material and can have a dramatic effect on information retention. Myriad interactive exercises and training games are available; the most effective training programs include a combination of these. Ensure that the exercises are related to the training topic (icebreakers are the only exception). The following are few types of exercises:

• *Icebreakers.* Icebreakers set the mood for the training and help the attendees get to know each other. The most common icebreaker is having attendees go around the room and introduce themselves. The possibilities for breaking the ice are endless.

A fun icebreaker is to have everyone fill out a name tag when they come in that includes their first name and their favorite color, food, or hobby. Another idea is to have everyone stand up and tell the person next to them something nobody would ever guess about them and later this information can be shared with the group for team building. Keep the icebreaker brief, and make sure everyone feels included.

• *Role-playing.* This is one exercise that new staff members typically dislike, but it can be the most effective way to train certain skills. It involves putting staff members into hypothetical situations and having them act out how they would handle them. For example, once staff have been trained on how to properly answer an incoming call, the best way to see if they have retained this information is to have them practice calls with management or other staff. This exercise can also be used for topics such as dealing with unhappy customers or selling memberships. Ensure that trainees have time to review the training material so they are fully prepared for the role-play.

- *Fill-in-the-blank handout.* This is perfect when the training topic is something the trainees do not know or understand. The fill-in-the-blank element keeps the group guessing until the answers are addressed in the training. For example, if training covers CPR, one item on the handout might be: The number of compressions for an adult victim is _____ to every _____ breaths.

- *Reading aloud.* Having group members read aloud can help emphasize a certain part of the training, such as the company mission statement or a case study. Reading aloud can keep attendees on their best behavior because they have empathy for the person reading and feel trepidation about being selected next.

- *Case studies.* A **case study** can be a powerful tool, especially when there is more than one way to handle a situation. A case study should be designed to get participants to think through a problem, and it should have a lasting effect on the group. The Sample Interactive Exercise Using a Case Study sidebar later in this chapter is designed to help the group develop empathy for difficult club members, but this goal should not be immediately apparent to the participants.

- *Team brainstorming.* The team brainstorming session involves the entire group and has no guaranteed outcome. Many topics are good candidates for brainstorming. The basic rule is that all ideas are good ideas. The leader typically records the group's ideas and distributes them later. Only a portion of the session should be devoted to brainstorming, because it can wear on the group after a while.

- *Demonstration or skit.* This can be a fun, serious, or poignant part of a training session, and there are many ways to incorporate it. One idea is to choose some people in the group who have already mastered the step that is being taught (e.g., overcoming an objection in sales) and asking them to act it out for the group. Another strategy is to improvise the skill for the group (e.g., ask attendees to give their worst member complaints and demonstrate how you would respond). Another

entertaining open is to plan and rehearse a skit with some key staff members. With some exaggerated behaviors and a bit of humor, you can address a whole host of awkward and frustrating subjects (e.g., associates on the internet during work, cell phone usage, lax attitude, lack of attention to detail).

Ideas for other types of interactive exercises can be found in the following recommended books:

- *Games Trainers Play* by Edward E. Scannel and John W. Newstrom
- *The Complete Games Trainers Play* by Edward E. Scannel and John W. Newstrom
- *The Big Book of Team Building Games: Trust-Building Activities, Team Spirit Exercises, and Other Fun Things to Do* by John W. Newstrom and Edward E. Scannel
- *The Big Book of Humorous Training Games* by Doni Tamblyn and Sharyn Weiss
- *The Big Book of Customer Service Training Games* by Peggy Carlaw and Vasudha K. Deming
- *The Big Book of Motivation Games* by Robert Epstein and Jessica Rodgers
- *Team-Building Activities for Every Group* by Alanna Jones

Be aware of copyright laws when using published materials. Copyright is a form of protection provided by the laws of the United States to the authors of original works, including literary, dramatic, musical, artistic, and certain other intellectual works. This protection applies to published and unpublished works. Most copyright laws apply internationally. Using copyrighted material without permission may be a violation of copyright law, and you can be sued by the copyright owner. More information is available at www.copyright.gov.

## Creating Accountability

The final step in this process is to create elements that test the effectiveness of the training and provide information or data to help justify future training expenditures. Sometimes, knowing they will be tested in some way makes people pay more attention during training and therefore makes the training more effective. Training effectiveness can be measured in the following ways:

## Sample Interactive Exercise Using a Case Study

Lucy Blankenship has been a club member for about 15 years. Her husband died suddenly in a car accident last year. When Mrs. Blankenship tried to remove her husband's name from the membership statement, the accounting department had an internal miscommunication, and it took 3 months to correct the error.

Last fall, Mrs. Blankenship's personal trainer of 6 years left the club to move to another state. The other trainers on staff have had trouble meeting Mrs. Blankenship's special needs.

Mrs. Blankenship has lost her temper with our desk staff several times in the past few months. Seemingly small mistakes, such as not having change for a dollar or the club opening a few minutes late, are causing her to complain loudly about the club, the service, and the staff.

### Discussion Questions

- What, if anything, should be done about Mrs. Blankenship?
- How long is a club expected to pay for its mistakes?
- Is Mrs. Blankenship's anger justified in any way?
- Is there ever a time when a club should ask a person to quit? When?

### Debriefing the Case Study

Divide participants into small groups and allow time for them to read the case study and discuss the questions listed. It is best if a group leader is assigned the task of making sure all group members get a chance to express their thoughts and opinions. Once everyone has had a chance to speak, ask for feedback from each group leader. When one a group has a response that shows empathy, expand on it and involve the entire group in the discussion. This exercise also allows you to note those who have open minds for solutions and those who have deeply entrenched negative views of members.

- *Testing.* The most common strategy for measuring the effectiveness of a training program is to test participants after each section of material is presented. The test can be written or verbal and formal or informal.

- *Role-playing.* A more intensive form of testing is to ask participants to explain what they have learned and use it in a simulated situation. This **role-playing** can be done privately after the training is complete or in the group setting.

- *Written follow-up.* After the session is complete, ask trainees to summarize what they learned and how they plan to apply it. This assignment should have a due date, and trainees should receive some feedback based on what they wrote.

- *Impromptu testing.* After the session, approach staff members in an impromptu fashion and ask them to explain or demonstrate the new skill taught in the training.

- *Financial tracking.* If the training was designed to increase profits or save on expenses, do a simple analysis by measuring the same line item before and after training.

Be sure to include a feedback mechanism after presenting or hosting a training program. It can be as simple as a short form that asks participants what they learned and what they would change about the program (see figure 4.2). You could also ask each participant to write a synopsis of the program and return it to you.

### *The Bottom Line*

The half-life of newly learned material is 3 days. If learners don't use it immediately, they lose it (Cross and O'Driscoll 2005).

# FEEDBACK FORM

1. Which program did you attend? _____

2. What was your favorite part of the program?_____

3. What was your least favorite part of the program? _____

4. What was the best thing you learned in the program? _____

5. Is there anything you would change about the program?_____

6. Do you have any comments about the speaker? _____

Thank you for your time!

**Figure 4.2**   Sample form for training feedback.

From M. Bates, M.J. Spezzano, and G. Danhoff, *Health Fitness Management*, 3rd ed. (Champaign, IL: Human Kinetics, 2020).

# OUTSIDE RESOURCES FOR TRAINING AND DEVELOPMENT

Combining do-it-yourself programs with proven, professional programs is an ideal approach for any business. The resources to select from are endless. Here is a partial list:

- *Industry-specific expert.* This person has a specific area of expertise that can benefit the team. Some of the topics include sales, service, and personal training. If you have not heard of the expert, be sure to check references from past clients and take the time to work out the details of the program far in advance of the training date. Check industry resource manuals and associations for recommended speakers. An ideal place to preview industry experts is at conferences and trade shows, which are held worldwide. Many industry experts also have recordings and books that you can purchase and add to the club library.

- *Professional speaker.* This person has either a general area of expertise (e.g., life balance, motivation) or a distinct one that is not specific to a particular industry (e.g., sales, service, and finance). A professional speaker should be polished and prepared and can be a wonderful adjunct to the annual staff get-together or special event. Be sure to clarify all fees, including travel, with a speaking professional. One great resource for finding speakers is the National Speakers Association (NSA) (www.nsaspeaker.org).

- *Professional training company.* There are several training organizations that can handle club training on a large scale. Ideally, the company would be local to save on travel costs. This is generally a big investment, so be thorough in your research and in outlining your expectations. Usually professional training companies sign on for at least 1 year.

- *Public seminar.* A public seminar is any training program or speech that is made available to the public for a per-person fee. The quality can range from poor to awe inspiring, so be sure to do research in advance. Sometimes the speaker is well known, but often you will register based on the topic or title (e.g., coaching tips for new managers) and will not know the quality of the material or the speaker ahead of time. Public seminars can be wonderful, low-cost ways to add training to the club; one downside, however, is the sometimes shameless focus on selling additional training materials. Most professionals subtly mention their materials during their presentations, but hawking materials throughout the program is considered in bad taste and is a waste of audience time.

- *Local networking event.* Many local networking groups invite local businesspeople to present topics at their regular events. These can be excellent sources of information and can also serve as networking events for the club. Call your local chamber of commerce and ask about networking events and local speakers.

- *Compliance and special certification.* Laws on CPR and AED requirements vary by state and country, so check to see if your club complies. Check with the local chapter of the Red Cross to see what programs they offer. In addition, check

## Instant Staff Training Idea

Training does not always have to happen in a class setting. An excellent way to get started with team training and development when time is short is to have all members of the team read the same book. Reading a book together opens the lines of communication, creates a forum for discussion, and gives everyone common knowledge on a subject. Another benefit of reading a book together is that it takes pressure off managers who have not led training sessions before. Choose a book that has universal appeal and a clear message. Self-help books are a great place to start; team members are more likely to read them because they may help with their personal lives as well. Read the book before buying it for the group to be sure it is appropriate. These following timeless self-help books are recommended for staff reading:

- *Think and Grow Rich* by Napoleon Hill (wealth, positive thinking)
- *How to Win Friends and Influence People* by Dale Carnegie (kindness, good deeds)
- *The Seven Habits of Highly Effective People* by Steven Covey (life balance, life mission, time management, relationships with others)
- *The Power of Your Subconscious Mind* by Joseph Murphy (positive thinking, affirmations applied to work and everyday life)
- *The Alchemist* by Paulo Coelho (inspiring parable of a boy in ancient time who goes on an adventure and finds his true value)
- *The Monk Who Sold His Ferrari* by Robin Sharma (fable about fulfilling your dreams and reaching your destiny)

with industry associations for lists of specific certification providers (e.g., personal training, lifeguarding, whirlpool maintenance, water safety, Pilates).

- *Online learning.* Online learning (also known as **e-learning**) encompasses any type of training done via computer. According to eLogic Learning (2017), numerous statistics triggered the e-learning industry to grow and prosper. For example, in 2017, 67 percent of organizations offered mobile learning. Also, eLogic Learning reported that by 2019, videos will be responsible for 80 percent of internet traffic globally.

The primary reason for adding e-learning to training programs is increased penetration of information. It does not require an instructor, and more people can access the information because they can view it on their own schedules. Experts advise that e-learning be one part of a program instead rather the only part, because only so much can be communicated via computer screens and talking heads. Mark LeBlanc, vice president of the NSA and president of Small Business Success, says "Do not underestimate the value of e-learning. Successful organizations are already taking advantage of this important medium. It is the ideal complement to regular training vehicles, supports the learning process, and helps put ideas into action" (personal communication).

## ASSESSMENT OF TRAINING COSTS

Many managers are reluctant to invest in training because it can be costly, and there is always the risk that the club will invest in training and then employees will take the newfound knowledge and find better work. This belief is contrary to the position of many experts who agree that training and development help retain employees. Also, as mentioned, employee retention has been tied to customer retention. When people grow personally and professionally through training and development programs, they often become more loyal to the employer and feel more competent in their work. They are more able to plot their own advancement within the larger framework of the company's growth. These factors help justify the costs involved in staff training and development.

When budgeting for training and development costs, be sure to consider the following:

## Taking Training to New Heights

Anne Nolen, training manager for the Houstonian Hotel, Club, and Spa, believes staff training is the answer to every problem and the key to achieving nearly any goal. Many top-rated employees join the enormously successful Houstonian Club based on its commitment to training and development. Training and education are used not only for improving critical skills toward profitability, such as sales and customer service, but also for recruiting and for saving money through safety compliance (litigation avoidance) and reduced turnover.

The first step in training at the Houstonian is to make sure new associates understand and absorb the club values, which they refer to as their *compass*. Even though the values may seem simple, the Houstonian takes them seriously and incorporates them into every training session, staff interaction, decision-making process, and disciplinary action. There are six Houstonian compass values:

1. Dignity
2. Trustworthiness
3. Accountability
4. Continual improvement
5. Personal and professional balance
6. Friendliness

### The Ultimate Commitment

In 1996, the Houstonian sent three of its managers to be certified by Franklin Covey in the famous program called the Seven Habits of Highly Effective People. "This process requires that the Covey people approve your organization for licensing and comes with a high-priced ticket and a commitment to the people you send since they cannot, by law, teach the training at any company other than yours," explains Nolen. The managers spent about a week learning the program. After the managers attended the program, they were required to teach segments to the group.

"The reason we are committed to this body of work is that it outlines a remarkable way of managing relationships. You must take care of your relationships. If you are trustworthy, then you have people's trust. To share that information and have that common language and connection with our entire staff is priceless. It infiltrates everything we do here," says Nolen. The Houstonian runs the Franklin Covey program approximately five times per year and encourages all staff to attend. They offer the program in English and Spanish and encourage all employees, including part-time and substitute employees, to attend as many times as they like.

### Training Programs Offered at the Houstonian

- *Customer service training.* All associates attend this required course once per year. "It is critical that you get together and talk about service and about relationships—why we are really here," explains Nolen.

- *Management development.* The Houstonian uses a Dallas-based training group to teach cutting-edge management strategies to their busy management team. Topics focus on the latest research in learning styles and effectiveness.

- *New-manager training.* This is an orientation-style training facilitated internally by the senior manager in each discipline. Hiring, corrective action, financials, and so on are covered.

- *New-hire orientation.* This program covers the compass values in detail. After orientation, each new hire is assigned to a peer partner (a coworker) who is not in a position of authority but can help the new associate. "It's like the buddy system," says Nolen. "They help them get oriented and have a friend, and the peer partners take pride in having been selected. Peer partners get some special attention, too, and it helps develop their careers. They do it voluntarily."

- *Specialized department training.* This is often taught by an outside expert and covers the needed legal compliance for that department (e.g., CPR and AED certification, bartender certification, sexual harassment training) or continuing education needs (e.g., bringing in a special yoga instructor to teach a master class).
- *Speaker track.* Outside experts are brought in to inspire and teach management-level employees.
- *Tuition reimbursement.* The Houstonian reimburses outside education expenses for its employees.

- Learner's time away from the job
- Cost of job coverage during training
- Training materials (e.g., books, handouts)
- Electronic equipment (e.g., computers)
- Audiovisual aids (e.g., flip chart, overhead projector)
- Licensing fees, where applicable
- Training venue or facility costs
- Fees and expenses of instructor, including travel expenses
- Support materials for follow-up
- Meals and refreshments

Untrained staff can have many negative effects on a club. One of the most significant is the impression that untrained staff can make on club members. Other costs of not training staff include the following:

- Potential liability from mistakes can be costly.
- Untrained employees can take up to six times longer to perform their tasks.

- Coworkers may spend extra time helping with routine tasks that could have been trained.
- Employee retention is not as high as it could be.

The following are some additional statistics that relate to staff training:

- A 4-year study by the American Society of Training and Development (ASTD) showed that firms that spent $1,500 per employee on training compared with those that spent $125 per employee experienced, on average, 24% higher gross profit margins and 218% higher incomes per employee (Avatech Solutions 2007).
- A 2% increase in productivity has been shown to net a 100% return on investment in outsourced, instructor-led training (Avatech Solutions 2007).
- A person who is paid $50,000 per year who is wasting just 1 hour per day costs the organization $6,250 per year (Wetmore 1999).

# Key Terms

| | | |
|---|---|---|
| career path | interactive exercises | role-playing |
| case study | needs analysis | staff retreats |
| e-learning | off-site training | trade-outs |

# CHAPTER 5

# Managing Staff Performance

## Learning Objectives

After studying this chapter, you will be able to

- identify the role of the manager in influencing staff performance;
- clarify job expectations;
- recognize the importance of the job description;
- provide performance feedback;
- address performance problems; and
- understand the importance of recognition, rewards, and incentives in influencing job performance.

Bob, the front-desk manager at XYZ Club, was desperate to get someone to cover the front desk in the middle of the busy season. Two of his best people had resigned, and he was covering the desk himself for a large part of the day. He placed an advertisement in the newspaper and received many messages about the job. After several days of phone tag with a few candidates and extensive phone conversations with people who turned out to want more money than the club was able to offer, he had a good conversation with a young nursing student and made a hurried appointment with her for the next day. Bob's schedule was so tight that he decided to interview her during a slow time while he was covering the front desk.

The candidate showed up a little late but was well dressed and seemed articulate and energetic. After a short conversation, during which Bob was distracted several times by member questions at the desk, he decided she was worth a try. He figured if he could just get someone in the position, he might be able to get caught up. Two weeks later, after Bob had spent considerable time training the new employee, she turned in her resignation because she had been accepted to a nursing school in another state. Bob thought she was already in nursing school, but she had just been applying. He had not thoroughly looked at her application or checked her references because he was so busy. Bob called the newspaper and restarted the ad, and he wondered when he would be able to get off this merry-go-round.

---

The author acknowledges the significant contributions of Bud Rockhill to this chapter.

Those who are responsible for recruiting and hiring staff have important roles in any organization. Think about it: In almost all circumstances, businesses are successful or fall short based on the performance of their employees. The recruiting and hiring process is the foundation that ensures organizations have the greatest chance of success. Therefore, it is imperative that managers master the art and science of managing performance.

Managing performance is the ultimate test of a manager's skill and the reason the manager's job exists in the first place. **Performance management** is the process of achieving business goals by building and working with staff. It is not simply a matter of conducting annual performance appraisals; it encompasses virtually everything in this textbook, from hiring to business strategy development to financial management, and it requires the manager to integrate staff, strategy, and business objectives.

Performance management is not separate from the other managerial areas; it is the outcome of being effective in these different areas and integrating them smoothly. The ultimate measures of a manager's skill in performance management are financial results and the more qualitative and subjective staff satisfaction.

Just as a successful new product, program, or service generates buzz—that sense of excitement that attracts customers—a successful organization has an intangible feeling of excitement and energy. It is the kind of environment that makes people want to go to work every day, where new ideas are valued, and where people take responsibility for their own job performance. This isn't a theoretical utopia or limited to textbook narrative. It's possible to achieve it in virtually any organization, but it takes a willingness to embrace the building blocks of performance management and use them consistently. As with most aspects of business, it requires a willingness to do the small things well and consistently, and it requires the manager to focus on the achievement of organizational goals rather than personal glory. When the team is winning, the spirit is contagious; success breeds success.

## ROLE OF THE MANAGER IN STAFF PERFORMANCE

In traditional management classes, the role of the manager has often been defined as planning, organizing, directing, and controlling. Although these are usually part of what a manager does, they don't provide a particularly instructive or insightful understanding of the job.

The management role could also be defined as organizing and directing resources to achieve the goals of the organization. This definition is more focused on results than the specific tasks and addresses the need to manage resources, including people, money, and time, but it isn't specific to performance management. To help make the topic as understandable and usable as possible, it may be more instructional to use sport analogies and terminology, given that most people involved in fitness management have some degree of experience in organized sport.

Therefore, the reference point for the effective performance manager is that the manager is the coach. A performance-oriented manager needs to address the same things a coach would:

- What's the game plan and does everyone understand it?
- Are the right players on the team and in the right positions?
- Do the players know what is expected of them and how their performance will be measured?
- Is their performance measured in a formal way (e.g., an evaluation or appraisal)?
- Are players given feedback during the game so they know how they're doing and what they could do better?
- If they're doing things well, let them know.
- If they need to make changes, let them know.

## The Bottom Line

The main driver behind performance management is ensuring everyone in the organization is working toward the goal and that each person understands how his or her role contributes to that of the greater team.

## Performance Management Today

Recent studies tell us we are failing at giving employees feedback. The latest Employee Outlook

Survey done by the Chartered Institute of Personnel and Development (2012) indicated the following:

- Only 46% of people received feedback on their performance from their manager.
- Only 39% had conversations with their managers about training and development needs.
- Only 30% of employees received on-the-job coaching from their immediate supervisors.

There is no question there is value in giving employees feedback both informally, through ongoing feedback, and formally, through evaluations once or twice a year. The challenge is ensuring that the process is as streamlined and efficient as possible.

## Managing With an Open-Book Philosophy

Most people are sincerely interested in contributing and doing a good job, and the more they understand how their positions contribute to the goals of the organization, the more effort they're willing to make. One way to create this type of work environment is to share information from corporate meetings, reports, and new developments. In addition to providing specific feedback on people's job performance, it is helpful and motivating to share information about business performance.

An article about last night's soccer game in today's newspaper most likely would not say "It was a beautiful, warm night; the grass was green; and the players looked crisp in their uniforms." Instead, it would mention the final score, describe the key activities that affected the outcome, and discuss highlights of the scoring or particularly brilliant defensive plays. After reading the article,

everyone would know what happened.

In some businesses, including clubs, managers often do not want to share performance results such as sales revenue from profit centers, customer service surveys, and company profit margins; therefore, the outcome is unknown. Maintaining company confidentiality is understandable, but several key numbers that impact results should provide some level of transparency with staff. For example, sales, termination rate, and performance results of profit centers could be shared with virtually all staff using a simple scorecard format (see figure 5.1), and that information could be reinforced with explanations about how each position in the club affects the key numbers.

At the level of department manager, there should be a level of transparency in sharing more in-depth information. This business practice of sharing information is an example of **open-book management**, but it can also be considered common sense.

## Succeeding Through the Success of Others

It may be helpful to visualize the role of performance management as removing barriers that prevent others from doing their jobs. As the manager, it is your job is to ensure the achievement of club goals through the most effective and efficient use of resources, including people, money, and time. It's not about you; it's about the organization.

If there are obstacles that prevent people from doing their jobs well, you must remove those barriers to allow the staff to be successful. This perspective and the willingness to derive satisfaction from the successes of others and to share the credit are the most critical factors to your success. Some people want to be stars, but the most successful

## CLUB SCORECARD

| | Month actual | Month budget | Variance | YTD actual | YTD budget | Variance |
|---|---|---|---|---|---|---|
| Sales | 125 | 115 | 10 | 560 | 540 | 20 |
| Termination rate | 3.2% | 3.0% | −0.2% | 3.5% | 3.0% | −0.5% |
| Average dues | $83 | $85 | $2 | $82 | $85 | $3 |
| Personal training | $4,356 | $4,000 | $356 | $34,578 | $35,000 | $422 |

**Figure 5.1**  Key performance numbers that can be shared with staff.

organizations are built on the **servant leadership model**. Servant leaders base their success on the success of others and share the credit. A book that elaborates on this perspective and supports the theory with quantitative research is *Built to Last* (Collins and Porras 1994).

## Determining the Identity of the Facility

In sport, everyone on the team knows the objective: to put the puck in the net, to score runs, to get the ball across the goal line. Players on the team understand the purpose of their respective positions and how they relate to the objective. Each team has a specific style of play based on its strengths (e.g., a running team, a passing team, a defensive team); thus, everyone knows the type of play that's expected.

The first task for the performance-oriented manager is to establish the club's competitive strategy and business goals so everyone knows what the purpose is and what the club is trying to accomplish. Every club has several things that it does (or should do) better than the competition. These things may relate to programming (e.g., tennis, kids' fitness, group fitness), or they may relate to the target market (e.g., families, seniors, singles). In business school, these strengths might be called the *unique selling propositions*. The performance-oriented manager who is focused on simplicity and results simply asks, "What are we famous for?"

Once it is determined what the club should be famous for, it must be constantly communicated to staff so everyone is clear about the club's identity. In many businesses, people often come to work with an understanding of the specific tasks they must do, but they don't understand the club identity or its competition and how their jobs support identity and positioning. For example, front-desk associates who work in an upscale club with an affluent membership base may think of their jobs as checking membership cards, answering the phone, and making sure guests fill out guest registers. They don't realize that they are the club's first impression on potential members, guests, and current members and that their enthusiasm and energy help make the club a club instead of a building with facilities and equipment.

Most people want to do a good job and contribute, but they need to know what the rules of the game are and what their position is expected to contribute. According to human resources

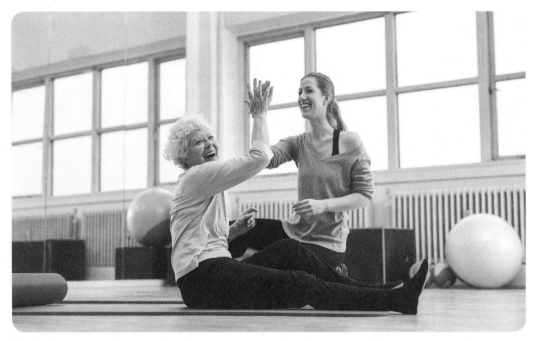

If a club's target market is seniors, the performance-oriented manager will make sure that all employees are aware of that objective so they can work toward building a unique identity for the club.

Jacob Ammentorp Lund/iStockphoto/Getty Images

## What Are We Famous For?

A general manager candidate was interviewing for a large, multipurpose club. He asked the interviewer, "What are you famous for?" When she looked puzzled, he explained that his club had a restaurant that had not been successful, and he and his management team decided they needed a clear identity. Given the many choices for fine dining in the city, they decided that they were going to be known for the best burger in the downtown area. He and his food and beverage director spent a month eating at different restaurants and trying different hamburgers. At the end of the month, they developed a recipe for what they thought would be the best hamburger and relaunched the restaurant appropriately. It was what they were going to be famous for.

Motivated by this, the interviewer told the story to the staff at one of the underperforming clubs and asked them what their club was famous for. Everyone looked at each other, and someone finally raised a hand and said, "We're really big." So much for differentiation! Over time, they clarified their market position and became famous for tennis and kids' programs. They found that focusing on what they were famous for helped get staff involved and enabled everyone to develop an effective competitive position.

consultant Denise Hartley-Wilkins, the overall goals of performance management should be

- *Effective.* They should ensure that people have the knowledge and ability to perform.
- *Strategic.* They should address broader issues and longer-term goals.
- *Integrated.* They should link various aspects of the business, people, management, and teams.

## STEPS IN MANAGING PERFORMANCE

Performance management can be the most challenging and the most rewarding of all the responsibilities undertaken by a manager, and it is one of the most critical in ensuring the continued financial and strategic success of the organization. Performance management integrates all the different facets of supervising people, including defining the job, interviewing to find the best candidate, orienting the new hire, setting goals, providing performance feedback, offering recognition and incentive compensation, and building a team committed to achieving the goals of the club.

### Clarifying Job Expectations

The first step for a manager to help an employee become successful is to clarify the expectations for the specific job in terms of expected results and the ongoing responsibilities and tasks.

Depending on the size of the club and whether it's part of a larger organization, many job descriptions are written in somewhat formal language or so-called corporate speak that makes it difficult to understand how the job fits into the business and what its overall purpose is. Alternatively, other job descriptions are overly task oriented and present a laundry list of daily responsibilities, which provides a checklist approach to the job but again neglects to demonstrate how the job fits into the overall organization and what results are desired.

As discussed in chapter 2, the job description is the perfect opportunity to define why the job exists, how it fits into the rest of the organization, and its primary objectives. Job tasks, although important, can be covered during the training process. Ideally, job descriptions make up the foundation on which the organization is built, and they must all fit together to provide a solid base on which the club can stand.

In addition to defining why the job exists and what the expected results are, a well-written job description identifies the experience and skills needed for someone to fulfill the job. It provides the basis for job postings or advertisements and for the types of questions asked during the interview process (as described in chapter 3). It also is the foundation for training new hires, establishing performance goals, and providing performance feedback.

For these reasons, the performance-oriented manager must look at the job description as the first step in building an organization that's focused on results rather than the administrative tasks of the job. If the job is not properly defined, employees will never be able to see beyond the tasks and understand how their jobs contribute to the purpose of the company.

Look at the two job descriptions in the sidebars. Controller job description A is for a club that is 60,000 square feet (5,574 square meters) and has 3,000 memberships. It is a fairly standard job description. Controller job description B is for

the same position, but it places greater emphasis on how the position fits within the company and the expected results.

# Hiring

Hiring the right person for the right job is the second step in managing performance. As discussed in chapter 3, this process begins with the job description and by determining the skills, experience, and personality characteristics that are necessary to ensure the greatest likelihood of success in the position. Once these have been

---

## Controller Job Description A

### Primary Focus

- Ensure the development of annual budgets and periodic forecasts that support the achievement of company growth objectives.
- Ensure that accurate financial and management data are provided to club managers on a timely basis.
- Ensure the development and maintenance of company financial policies and procedures to ensure integrity and accuracy of data.

### Detailed Listing of Controller Duties

- Prepare annual budgets; aid in period forecasting process; manage, train, and develop accounting and office management staff; and assist club personnel with accounting.
- Consolidate and prepare monthly financial statements for all operations.
- Create monthly financial package that consists of profits and losses, balance sheet, cash flow statement, financial analysis of operational results, variance reporting, and key business indicators.
- Provide owner, bank, and investors with required financial information.
- Perform internal audits for fitness clubs.
- Handle all preparation for and daily interaction with corporate auditors.
- Prepare reports required by regulatory agencies, including tax compliance and estimates.
- Maintain compliance list to ensure filing of all tax returns, corporate reports, and so on.
- Oversee human resource and insurance (employee and commercial) concerns and payroll.
- Manage all bank accounts and signature cards, including reconciliations, accounting system, credit and collections, accounts payable, and fixed assets.
- Manage cash on weekly basis and sweep excess into investment accounts as needed and records retention.
- Sign checks as necessary.
- Continually evaluate practices for improvement opportunities.
- Execute, review, and revise accounting policies and procedures as necessary.
- Assist club managers with return-on-investment and benefit–risk analyses.

defined, specific questions should be developed that will enable you to determine whether candidates meet the job requirements. For some positions, such as accountant, maintenance director, or personal trainer, there are specific mandatory technical skills or educational requirements, but for other positions, attitude and enthusiasm may be more important than specific experience.

In the U.S. National Football League (NFL), one of the most important activities each year

## Controller Job Description B

Great Lakes Fitness, Inc., based in Centerville, is looking for a controller whose experience includes work with multisite operations and who enjoys a small-company environment.

Great Lakes operate six commercial fitness clubs in suburban locations of Centerville. The company is focused on a well-rounded approach to fitness, sport, and wellness and targets the family market.

The controller position is an integral part of the senior management team and will participate in all major planning and reporting activities, including financial reporting, forecasting, budgeting, and business performance analysis. The controller will lead a small accounting staff that is responsible for generating the financial statements for each club, consolidating the reporting, and working with club managers on an ongoing basis to review financial performance and identify opportunities for improvement. The position reports to the CFO of the ownership group and has frequent contact with the owner.

In addition to accounting and financial expertise, the person in this position must have a management mindset and enjoy working with club managers in a support role to ensure that they continually receive the reports, data, and analyses that enable them to improve business performance. The position requires excellent communication skills, the ability to work effectively with club managers not located in the same building, and a hands-on approach.

### Key Responsibilities

- Oversight of and responsibility for preparation of monthly financial statements, including income statements and balance sheets, preparation of variance analysis, completion of account reconciliations for balance sheets, and participation in management review of performance
- Leadership responsibility for preparation of the annual budget for each club and consolidated clubs, which involves a hands-on role and frequent discussions with club managers to develop the detailed operating assumptions needed to support the line-item budget
- Responsibility for preparation of a detailed business forecast on a quarterly basis
- Management of credit, collections, cash, and payroll
- Preparation of tax returns and oversight of auditors

### Position Requirements

- 10 to 15 years of experience in accounting supervisory and management positions, including as a controller
- Certified public accountant (CPA)
- Preferably experience working with businesses that have multisite operations, such as hotels, restaurants, fitness clubs, or retail; service business or nonmanufacturing experience desirable
- Good analytical skills and a demonstrated ability to proactively identify problems and opportunities for improvement supported by clear analysis and recommendations
- Temperament to enjoy and succeed in small-company work environment with only five people in the office
- Excellent communication skills and the ability to establish productive rapport with managers in different locations

is the draft, in which teams select new players. There are two different approaches: drafting to fill a specific position or drafting the best athlete and then finding a position for him. Likewise, larger clubs or multiclub organizations can hire the best people and then find places for them, but smaller organizations that have limited payrolls must hire the people with the necessary skills, experience, and attitudes to fill the required positions. Clubs are hospitality and service businesses as much as fitness and health businesses, so hiring people with the right attitudes and enthusiasm will make it more possible to achieve the desired results.

## The Bottom Line

No amount of training and feedback will make up for hiring the wrong person. Learn from past hiring mistakes and get the right people on board the first time. It is always helpful to evaluate what went wrong with any employee who leaves. This can be an opportunity to learn and make a better hiring decision next time.

## Training

Even if the right person is hired for the right job, it is your responsibility to create the opportunity for that person to be successful. This goes back to the core definition of a manager as a person who is willing to succeed through others. Some managers because they are so focused on the day-to-day operations or responding to the crisis of the moment often adopt a sink-or-swim attitude toward new staff. This approach, however, will only result in having to spend more time in the reactive mode later either hiring a replacement when the new hire gets frustrated and leaves or correcting performance problems that result from a lack of clear direction.

New employees provide you with a fresh opportunity to instill the values of the club, share its strategy and vision, and ensure that staff understand the basic purpose of the club, its target market, its competition, what it does well, and how this job fits into the whole. If employees understand these things, they are much more likely to do a good job. It can't be said enough: People want to feel like they're contributing and

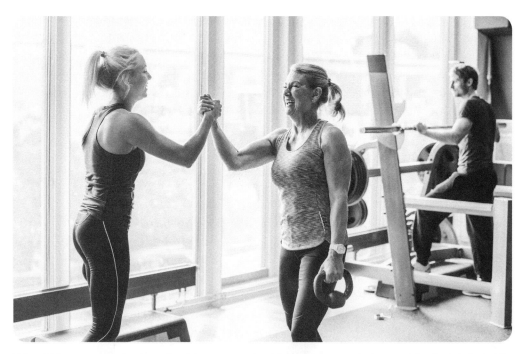

When hiring a personal trainer, the club manager should consider not only the candidate's technical skills but also his or her attitude, enthusiasm, and ability to get along with clients. Enthusiasm and attitude are difficult traits to train. If the person being interviewed does not wow you with these things at the interview, how do you think he or she will act with customers when you are not around?

Getty Images/Maskot

using their skills while fitting into the whole, but they cannot do so if their jobs are part of an assembly line of strictly emphasized tasks or if they have no sense of how they contribute to the whole organization. For more information on new-associate training, please refer to chapter 3.

# Measuring Job Performance

The expectations for each position should be reflected in measurement standards. The intent is not to micromanage or patronize the staff but to help everyone understand what is expected and how performance will be measured. It would be unfortunate to find out in an evaluation that your expectations were entirely different from what the employee thought was important. For example, a front-desk associate might think the most important part of his or her job is checking membership cards, handing out towels, and collecting guest fees, and thus, the associate might adopt a policing demeanor to ensure members do not sneak in with a guest or forget their cards. The manager, however, might think the front-desk associate is crucial in creating a good first impression with members, guests, and potential members and therefore would expect the associate to have an entirely different demeanor. This situation can be avoided with a clear job description that explicitly states the importance of the position in creating a sense of hospitality and welcome and outlines some simple goals that explain how job performance will be measured.

## Set Goals With Employees

It is your responsibility to try to ensure employees will be successful and the club will achieve its financial, strategic, and service goals. To keep people focused on the priorities that advance the overall goals of the club rather than maintaining the status quo, an effective performance manager works with employees to establish individual goals. **Goal setting** is generally most effective when you use the club's goals to provide an organizational framework and then address how the employee's position can contribute to these goals. Most people find it motivating to understand how their performance can affect the direction and results of the organization, and this understanding helps create more teamwork and integration across departments.

There is a difference between the ongoing tasks that people must perform on a daily or weekly basis and the goals that help improve overall business performance. For example, daily cleanliness inspections of the club are important, but they are part of someone's ongoing responsibilities. A goal for a supervisor responsible for club housekeeping might be to improve member satisfaction, as measured in the annual member survey, from a score of 8.3 to higher than 9.0.

Goals (as opposed to ongoing job responsibilities) should be

- specific,
- measurable,
- achievable,
- relevant, and
- time based.

You can remember this using the acronym SMART.

To identify goals that are effective for the employee and the organization, follow these steps and remember to write the actual goals using the SMART goal format.

- Focus on the three to five primary responsibilities listed in the job description. For each area of responsibility, list the ongoing accountabilities and tasks. (This list can also be used when training new employees.) The purpose of this step is to identify what the employee must do on an ongoing basis and clearly separate these tasks from any performance goals on which incentive compensation or recognition will be based.

- Develop performance goals that move the business forward and are not part of the ongoing responsibilities or tasks. They are most commonly used as the basis for salary increases, promotion, or incentive compensation.

## The Bottom Line

It is usually a good idea to have employees play a role in setting their own goals. This ensures their buy in and shows they are motivated to achieve the goals.

## Provide Performance Feedback

Once the right person has been hired and provided with orientation and training, you must monitor performance and provide ongoing feedback to ensure the person is successful. The emphasis is on helping staff members succeed, not on catching them doing something wrong. Positive feedback is just as important as corrective feedback.

Many organizations and managers believe that **performance feedback** is an annual event conducted in a formal setting (e.g., performance appraisal, performance evaluation). Although formal evaluations once or twice a year are necessary, you should also provide staff with ongoing, frequent feedback. To return to the sport analogy, if one player in the game was out of position, making errors, and not executing the appropriate tasks, the coach would provide corrective feedback on the fly or immediately after the game. Coaches certainly don't wait until the end of the season to give feedback, and managers can take a lesson from this.

Many managers, especially those who fear confrontation or negative experiences, quietly accumulate ammunition and unload it on the employee during the performance appraisal. This can catch the employee off guard because the manager has not provided any previous feedback about performance behaviors that needed to be addressed. Feedback in a formal review that comes as a surprise is an indicator of poor management. Anything discussed in the formal evaluation should have been addressed when it first occurred.

## *The Bottom Line*

Anxiety associated with performance appraisals can be reduced by setting clear and measurable goals for employees and ensuring they know how they are doing with respect to these goals throughout the year.

Providing staff with feedback is an important and challenging manager responsibility. It can be difficult for any manager, from the new supervisor to the experienced senior executive, to provide feedback that is likely to be interpreted as criticism. If you do not provide feedback, you are not fulfilling a basic job responsibility to the company and to the employee, who may not be aware of certain needs to improve performance. Feedback should be as specific as possible.

Most organizations have formal performance evaluation processes. It is good to have these systems in place to impose some discipline on the organization and force managers who might otherwise be reluctant to provide in-depth feedback to do so. In most cases, an organization will use specific forms that can be used guidelines to drive the process. There are many types of forms; see figure 5.2 for one example.

The following are the three components of a typical **performance evaluation form**.

1. The first section often consists of discussion items or questions intended to help the manager and employee talk about different qualitative aspects of job performance, the company, and the work environment. Typical items in this section include the following:
   - Overview of employee strengths
   - Areas in which the employee needs to improve or needs training
   - Employee's ability to work as an effective team member
   - Employee's problem-solving ability
   - Employee's willingness to take initiative

2. Next, overall skills and attributes that relate directly to the job description are addressed. These might include the following:
   - Technical knowledge for the job
   - Customer service
   - Meeting deadlines

3. The final section usually focuses on performance results for specific goals that were assigned for the measurement period. These should specifically relate to the job and the job description. These goals should form the basis for decisions regarding salary increases or promotions and should link to the overall strategic and financial goals of the club. Goals should, wherever possible, include measurement standards and target completion dates, as in the following examples:
   - Ensure achievement of annual sales budget of 980 memberships for the year.

- Ensure front-desk staff are trained on hospitality, emergency procedures, and problem resolution.
- Ensure that 80% of new members receive a fitness orientation and personally meet with at least one member of the fitness staff within 2 weeks of joining the club.

There is no doubt that evaluation forms are important; they are highly valued by many employees as tangible indications of their value to the club and to the manager. The most important aspect of the process, however, is the discussion between the manager and the employee.

The most effective way to start the performance evaluation is to schedule a meeting with the employee to discuss performance, obtain feedback on how the employee is liking the job, and look ahead to the club's goals for the next year and the employee's goals. Provide the employee with an evaluation form in advance, and ask the employee to fill it out and bring it to the meeting. The employee must play a legitimate role in the evaluation and feel that the self-evaluation is taken seriously. This is a two-way conversation. Ask the employee to come prepared to discuss major accomplishments, strengths, areas that need improvement, goals for the next year, and assistance you can provide, including specific training. During the meeting, you should use the form as the basis of discussion; this gives you the opportunity to provide feedback so the employee has the opportunity to make any necessary changes moving forward with their position based on the discussion. Many organizations supplement manager feedback informally or formally with feedback from customers, coworkers, or suppliers. This is referred to as a *360-degree evaluation*. This feedback can be extremely valuable, because managers are not always able to evaluate all aspects of employees' performance.

The meeting should end with a brief review. This is another opportunity to reinforce the employee's strengths and value to the club, to discuss areas that need improvement and what you and the employee can do to address these, and to outline the employee's specific role in contributing to the goals of the organization. You and the employee should sign the performance evaluation. Give one copy to the employee and keep another copy in the employee's records.

## The Bottom Line

The importance of ongoing feedback throughout the year cannot be overstated. It is critical that you give examples of good and bad performance during the formal evaluation. It is not useful to provide specific feedback (e.g., that the employee needs to improve his or her level of enthusiasm or needs to be more diligent answering the phone before the third ring) if this has not been previously discussed and there are not examples of this behavior in the employee's file.

## Addressing Performance Problems

Despite following the appropriate steps for defining the job, hiring a person, and providing feedback, there will inevitably be employees who have performance problems and do not achieve the expectations for the position. Your first reaction in this situation should not be to assign blame to the employee but to look at the situation objectively and examine how you might be contributing to the problem.

Questions to ask include the following:

- Have the expectations for the position been made clear?
- Can the performance problems be solved by training or coaching?
- Could this person be more successful in another position?
- If not, is it necessary to make a change?

## Providing Effective Feedback

Your goal is to help employees succeed in their jobs and achieve their performance goals. If employees are not doing this, you must provide feedback. To provide effective feedback, focus on the following:

- *Start with positive feedback.* Look for opportunities to compliment employees and make this part of your ongoing management style. If positive comments are not provided on

# NONEXEMPT PERFORMANCE REVIEW

Name: _____ Today's date: _____

Club: _____ Date of hire: _____

Reviewing manager: _____ Date of last review: _____

Job title 1: _____ Job title 2: _____

## Definition of Ratings

D = Distinguished (4 points): consistently exceeds standard expectations

E = Exceeds expectations (3 points): frequently exceeds standard expectations

M = Meets expectations (2 points): regularly meets or occasionally exceeds standard expectations

R = Requires improvement (1 point): occasionally meets expectations but frequently performs below standard expectations

U = Unacceptable (0 points): rarely meets standard expectations; improvement essential

N/A = not applicable

## Job Performance

| | | Comments |
|---|---|---|
| Displays thorough knowledge of job | 4 3 2 1 0 | _____ |
| Completes expected quantity of work | 4 3 2 1 0 | _____ |
| Completes expected quality of work | 4 3 2 1 0 | _____ |
| Performs work efficiently | 4 3 2 1 0 | _____ |
| Works well without close supervision | 4 3 2 1 0 | _____ |
| Works well under pressure | 4 3 2 1 0 | _____ |
| Offers practical suggestions to management | 4 3 2 1 0 | _____ |
| Shows initiative; solves problems that arise | 4 3 2 1 0 | _____ |
| Team player | 4 3 2 1 0 | _____ |
| **Total points** | _____ | |

## Job Skills

| | | Comments |
|---|---|---|
| Administrative | 4 3 2 1 0 | _____ |
| Communicative | 4 3 2 1 0 | _____ |
| Organizational | 4 3 2 1 0 | _____ |
| Technical | 4 3 2 1 0 | _____ |
| **Total points** | _____ | |

## Service and Attitude

| | | Comments |
|---|---|---|
| Complies with customer service standards | 4 3 2 1 0 | _____ |
| Always pleasant to members | 4 3 2 1 0 | _____ |
| Works well with other associates | 4 3 2 1 0 | _____ |
| Shows interest and enthusiasm for job | 4 3 2 1 0 | _____ |
| Shows respect for supervisor | 4 3 2 1 0 | _____ |
| Reacts well to feedback | 4 3 2 1 0 | _____ |
| Demonstrates pride in company | 4 3 2 1 0 | _____ |
| **Total points** | _____ | |

**Figure 5.2**  Sample nonexempt performance review.

(continued)

## Work Habits

| | | Comments |
|---|---|---|
| Maintains a clean and organized work area | 4 3 2 1 0 | _____ |
| Respects company property | 4 3 2 1 0 | _____ |
| Adheres to company dress code for position | 4 3 2 1 0 | _____ |
| Complies with company policies | 4 3 2 1 0 | _____ |
| Accurately logs work hours | 4 3 2 1 0 | _____ |
| **Total points** | _____ | |

## Job Development

Place a checkmark next to each training class required and completed (based on position)

Required training*                                    Additional training

_____ Team                                    _____ _____

_____ Bloodborne pathogens (exp. date _____)     _____ _____

_____ CPR/AED (exp. date _____)         _____ _____

_____ Sexual harassment (exp. date _____)     _____ _____

*All four classes are required for a rating of 2.

PT/group exercise required training and certifications*

_____ Personal training certification 1     Exp. date: _____

_____ Personal training certification 2     Exp. date: _____

_____ Group exercise certification 1     Exp. date: _____

_____ Group exercise certification 2     Exp. date: _____

*Current certification is required for a rating of 2 (in addition to required training sessions).

### Definition of Ratings

Distinguished (4)—All four required training sessions have been completed and additional outside and WU training or certifications.

Exceeds (3)— All four required training sessions have been completed and additional outside and WU certifications.

Meets (2)—All four required training sessions have been completed and all certifications are current.

Requires improvement (1)—Fewer than four of the required trainings have been completed or certifications are expired.

Unsatisfactory (0)—Fewer than three of the required trainings have been completed and certifications are expired.

**Job Development Score:** _____

## Overall Score

| | Total points | | Number of indicators | | Individual section score | | Weight | | Points |
|---|---|---|---|---|---|---|---|---|---|
| Job performance | _____ | / | 9 | = | _____ | × | .30 (30%) | = | _____ |
| Job skills | _____ | / | 4 | = | _____ | × | .15 (15%) | = | _____ |
| Service and attitude | _____ | / | 7 | = | _____ | × | .30 (30%) | = | _____ |
| Work habits | _____ | / | 5 | = | _____ | × | .15 (15%) | = | _____ |
| Job development | N/A | / | Varies | = | _____ | × | .10 (10%) | = | _____ |
| | | | | | | | **Total points** | | _____ |

(continued)

**Figure 5.2**    (continued)

*(continued)*

## Overall Performance

Score: _____

Letter rating: _____

Areas for improvement:


Strengths:


## Overall Performance Summary



## Signatures

Reviewing manager: _____   Date: _____

Next level supervisor: _____   Date: _____

Human resources: _____   Date: _____

Associate: _____   Date: _____

**Figure 5.2**   *(continued)*

From M. Bates, M.J. Spezzano, and G. Danhoff, *Health Fitness Management,* 3rd ed. (Champaign, IL: Human Kinetics, 2020). Reprinted by permission of Wellbridge Fitness-Wellness-Sports-Fun. Wellbridge is one of the leading health club chains in the USA today

an ongoing basis, suddenly doing so in a performance discussion will seem insincere or forced.

- *Provide frequent, informal feedback.* This is not a shooting gallery. Don't store up ammunition and then unload. More frequent, informal feedback is far more helpful and much less threatening.

- *Remember, less is more.* For corrective feedback or behaviors that require performance improvements, limit the criticism to one or two items. Don't attack; the employee will not be able to process the criticism, and it will feel personal. The goal is to correct the problem and improve performance, not to have the employee feel bad.

- *Be specific.* Generalities are not helpful (e.g., "You really annoy the other people in the office.").

- *Remember that recent history is more helpful.* Use recent examples rather than situations that are months old. Memory fades, and the situation being used as an example may no longer be relevant.

- *Have an open dialogue.* Ask whether the employee agrees that the specific result or behavior is a problem. If the person doesn't agree, bring the discussion back to the result or behavior, try to link it to the job description, and continue until there is agreement or you elicit some underlying explanation. Open dialogue is helpful for everyone.

- *Define specific corrective actions.* Define the actions to be taken to improve performance, how the results will be measured, and when there will be another conversation. Don't leave these actions vague or up in the air.

- *Offer to help.* You're in this together. Offer to provide assistance and support as needed (and as appropriate).

- *End on a positive note.* Provide encouragement and reinforce that you want the person to be successful.

## *The Bottom Line*

When giving an employee feedback about a performance that needs to be improved, you must give some level of coaching and support. For example, simply telling a salesperson to increase his or her closing percentage without helping is a recipe for failure. As the manager, it is your responsibility to put your staff in a position to be successful.

## Offering Recognition

Some managers, especially those who are new to supervisory positions, may think their job is to correct performance problems or identify things that associates are doing incorrectly. Many effective managers, however, operate under the opposite philosophy and look for associates' strengths and examples of positive performance and recognizing these to provide positive reinforcement.

When training a puppy, for example, the most important thing to remember is to use positive reinforcement. Dogs want to do the right thing; they just need to know what that is. The use of positive reinforcement is conveyed through simple gestures and words (e.g., *good boy*), an enthusiastic tone, a treat, or a hug. Unbelievably, managing effectively includes many of the same elements; a little bit of recognition and praise pays off in better performance and a more civilized and fun workplace.

Many managers think it's unprofessional, inappropriate, or a poor use of time to go out of their way to thank people for their work. But if people don't receive some type of recognition or acknowledgment for jobs well done, why should they bother? Some managers think employees are simply doing what they are being paid to do. But in a free country, people can vote with their feet. Thus, effective managers use recognition (and bonuses, as discussed next) as part of their ongoing management. Make it fun, recognize performance, and add a little competition to the workplace.

There are many ways to let staff know how much they're appreciated and to recognize good performance. Guidelines for effective recognition are similar to some of the guidelines for performance feedback:

- Make it specific to an individual achievement or action.
- Make it timely.
- Personalize it.
- Make it meaningful.

There are endless ways to let employees know how much they're appreciated. Examples include the following:

- Say thank you.
- Send a card or note.
- Remember birthdays or work anniversaries.
- Provide tickets to a ball game or movie.
- Buy lunch for an employee and a few coworkers.
- Give a book that relates to work.
- Offer longevity awards (for 1 year, 3 years, 5 years, 10 years, and so on).
- Give a gift certificate for a local restaurant or a favorite store.
- Provide a staff lunch, and let a different person pick the location each month.

Most of these cost less than $50, but they can have amazing payoffs, and they demonstrate that employees' work is appreciated and that management cares. A club with 1,000 members and $40 average dues could allocate $250 per month for little thank-yous, which is less than half of 1% of revenues.

The delivery is as important as the item. Don't just hand someone tickets and say "I have these leftover tickets and thought you might be able to use them." Instead, use the opportunity to reinforce your appreciation for specific work results, and mention how valuable the person is to the team and to the club. Depending on the achievement or circumstance, this can be done on a one-on-one basis, in front of the person's department, or in front of the whole club. Recognition can also be used for an entire team or department and can be an effective team builder. An excellent book on this topic is *Managing With Carrots* (Gostick and Elton 2001).

## The Bottom Line

Any time a client gives positive feedback about an employee, it should be celebrated so everyone on the team is aware of it. A very simple way to do this is to regularly follow up with clients and ask about their experiences with a particular staff person. Clients love the extra attention and will typically give you information that can be shared with all staff. Occasionally, a client's feedback may be negative; in this situation, provide constructive feedback to the employee in private.

## Providing Incentives and Compensation

Like it or not, money is a powerful motivator. For years, it has been the most successful motivator for sales staff. Monetary reward, even in small amounts, makes the game more fun, more competitive, and more rewarding.

**Incentive compensation plans** tied directly to the club's financial performance can be a powerful motivator and engage people in the results; this approach treats them more like owners. People want to make a difference, they want to do a good job, and they like to be rewarded. Ideally, an incentive plan is in sync with employees' individual goals, and it supports the company or business unit goals. The targets should be structured so if all team members do their jobs and the company or club does well, all team members are rewarded.

At the level of department manager, there is often some type of annual bonus plan that pays a percentage of the salary (typically 5 to 20%) if the club achieves a certain level of profitability. General manager bonuses tied to annual profitability may range from 10 to 25% of the base salary. Although these bonuses are appropriate and can be effective, these compensation plans can fail to motivate on an ongoing basis because the payout is so far in the future.

When structuring an incentive plan, consider the following:

• *Determine the approximate amount to be paid.* For example, a club may have an annual budget of $1 million in revenues and $150,000 in operating profit. When setting the budget, the general manager or club owner may determine that an operations manager who earns a salary of $30,000 is eligible for a $3,000 bonus (10% of base salary) if the club achieves its operating profit. This $3,000 would be included as an expense in the budget and must be covered for the club to achieve its operating profit goal.

With additional analysis and calculations, the general manager or club owner may determine that if membership sales at the beginning of the year exceed the plan, the termination rate can be improved by 0.5%, and the personal training business can be improved, it may be possible to earn $180,000 in operating profit. This would be a $30,000 improvement, which is 20% more than the budget. How much of that $30,000 is the owner willing to share with the key staff members who made it happen? There is no defined formula, but in many businesses, the owner would share between 10 and 30% of the upside. This would mean an extra $3,000 to $9,000 could be allocated to key staff. In the case of the operations manager, an additional $1,000 to $2,000 might be available if the club exceeds its goals by 20%. In this way, managers are motivated and compensated to think like owners and push beyond the budget target.

• *Determine the timing of the payment.* The shorter the time frame for the target, the more focused the staff remain. This is a fundamental principle of sales compensation, and it is why many salespeople are compensated on monthly or weekly targets in addition to being paid on each sale. The risk of shorter time frames is that bonuses or incentive payments could be made, but the club might not hit its annual target.

• *Make it simple.* The bonus calculation should not rely on a complicated formula or calculation. If it is too complicated, people will not be able to determine whether they are on track to receive the bonus.

- *Make it within the participant's control.* An incentive plan is only motivating if participants feel they can influence the results. For example, a bonus based on total club financial performance may not be especially motivating to a front-desk supervisor. Although the bonus will be appreciated, the employee will most likely be unable to determine which job performance behaviors or outcomes he or she should change to influence the bonus. It would be more effective to link specific compensation criteria to each position, even if part of the bonus depends on total club financial performance or the club must hit its goal for everyone to be eligible for a bonus.

- *Make it self-funding.* Incentives should be self-funding, especially if they're based on profitability. This means that a dollar amount for incentives should be included in the budget so achievement of the profit goal covers the cost of the incentive. For example, if a club aims for $100,000 in revenue and $80,000 in expenses for a certain period, the operating profit for that period would be $20,000. If club ownership decides they are willing to pay total incentive compensation of $2,000 for achieving the $20,000 target, that $2,000 expense should be added to the original expenses. Now expenses are $82,000, which means revenue must be $102,000 to achieve the $20,000 profit.

In setting the budget, the expected expenses for the incentive compensation are included as operating expenses under payroll, which means additional revenue must be generated to cover the expenses and still hit the operating income goal. The result is a **self-funding incentive program**, and everyone wins.

## Incentives for Nonmanagement Staff

Many companies provide annual or quarterly bonus plans to management staff, but the rest of the employees are sometimes overlooked even though the power of incentives may be greater for part-time or lesser-paid employees. The effects of daily, weekly, or monthly incentives with sales staff are well documented, and such incentives are used in many clubs. In most cases, salespeople are paid relatively low base salaries and relatively high commissions or bonuses.

Successful managers offset the challenges of being in sales—making 20 to 30 calls per day, lots of rejection, uncertainty while potential members make up their minds—by using incentives. Examples might include $50 for anyone who makes five sales in a week or $20 for the first sale of the day. From the outside, it looks like it's just about the money, but it also brings an element of fun and competition.

Nonsales staff sometimes resent the compensation sales staff receive. Rather than creating resentment, it would be more effective and useful to learn from what works and apply it elsewhere. Consider offering incentive compensation, rewards, or contests to other positions in the club.

## Examples of Incentive Compensation

Following are some examples of incentive plans and contests for staff. Regardless of the department or the specific criteria, the act of setting aside additional money for incentive compensation and taking the time to recognize the efforts of staff members can be a powerful management tool that has long-lasting results.

### Retention-Based Incentives for Fitness Staff

This type of incentive plan or contest focuses fitness staff on the ultimate measure of success for their job: the ability to help members integrate exercise into their lifestyles and to achieve results. This will result in member retention, which is the most profitable business outcome for a club; keeping an existing member is much less expensive and more profitable than obtaining a new member.

One way to create a self-funding incentive program is to develop an annual budget based on the expected member termination rate. After calculating the operating profit for the expected budget, try some different assumptions for termination rate and note the improvement in operating profit. For example, in a club with 2,400 memberships, $75 average monthly dues, and a 3.2% monthly termination rate, reducing the termination rate to 2.7% per month yields an improvement in operating profit of approximately $50,000.

Knowing this, a club might be willing to allocate some of this potential profit to the fitness staff (and any other staff members who focus on member retention) for incentive compensation. If the club is willing to share 15% of the incremental profits (but only if the member termination rate decreases and the club generates the additional $50,000 in operating profit before the payment of any bonuses), then $7,500 would be available; $3,000 might be allocated as a bonus for the fitness director and the remainder divided among full-time and part-time staff in a fair manner.

### Contest for Staff Who Answer the Phone

The purpose of this contest is to encourage front-desk staff to focus on answering the phone in a friendly, welcoming manner. Sometimes staff members think answering the phone is an interruption, but potential members usually call before they come in, and the person who answers the phone is responsible for the all-important first impression. In addition, members want to feel that they belong to a club, not to a building, and a friendly, welcoming voice on the other end of the telephone can help reinforce this club atmosphere.

This contest can work with a multiclub operation or a single club that has different employees who answer the phone. Criteria should be established in advance, such as answering the phone in three rings or less, speaking in a friendly tone, answering the phone according to club standard and exhibiting knowledge about questions. Judges can be management staff, family members of management staff, or members based upon the criteria of evaluating the performance. Prizes of $500 or $300 are usually enough to get the staff focused on telephone etiquette.

### Contest for Housekeeping Staff

In most industry surveys, current and potential club members rank cleanliness as the most important club attribute, but housekeeping staff members do not usually receive as much management attention and positive reinforcement as staff in other departments. One way to include them in the incentive compensation plan or recognition program is to create a contest.

It is important to establish evaluation criteria. Most clubs have a detailed inspection list the manager uses when walking through the club. First, the club could be evaluated by doing a walk-through and comparing it to other clubs in the market, or a baseline ranking could be established based on a walk-through completed on a specific day (possibly before the contest is announced). Then, the rating is given by conducting evaluations of other clubs in the market (by the general manager accompanied by the housekeeping supervisor) or evaluating the club on a date designated in advance to give everyone time to focus. The contest is won using quantitative predetermined criteria through improvement by a designated amount or having a higher score than the other clubs in the market.

For this type of contest, it might be most effective to ask the supervisor responsible for housekeeping or some of the housekeeping staff members what would be most motivating, such as a bonus, gift certificate, party, or dinner. Money is always welcome, but an activity that makes a lasting impression can also be effective; staff members will remember the great time they had and that they were appreciated and recognized by the club management.

## EMPLOYEE TERMINATION

There will undoubtedly be times when it is necessary to terminate an employee. Reasons for termination may include a business downturn that requires staff reductions, an employee's failure to meet performance expectations, or employee behavior problems on the job.

How the process is handled depends on the circumstances of the termination. The purpose of this section is to provide an overview of handling the termination process; it is not intended to be specific to any particular situation. Each situation will have its own circumstances and will require consideration of the factors outlined here. Employment laws vary by country and state, so check with a human resources expert or legal counsel before terminating an employee to ensure compliance with legal requirements.

## Recognizing the Importance of Ongoing Feedback

As mentioned previously, performance-oriented managers provide formal and informal ongoing feedback to all associates. Feedback is particularly important when an employee is not meeting the expectations for the job. If the employee is surprised when a discussion about termination takes place, this usually means you have not been providing appropriate feedback.

When providing feedback, make it clear to the employee that termination is a likely or possible outcome if specific changes in performance or behaviors are not made. Employees must know what behaviors will result in termination; failure to provide this type of feedback is a sign of poor management and could be a cause for legal action, which is expensive, time consuming, and demoralizing.

## Preparing for Termination

Terminating an employee should be a last resort, not a knee-jerk reaction to a performance problem. When you first identify a performance problem with an employee, ask the following questions:

- Have I made the expectations for this position clear?
- Have I provided the training necessary for the person to do the job?
- Is this person in the right position? Might the person be more successful in a different job?

If these questions have been addressed, review your prior communication with the employee about the issue. Whenever there is a performance or behavior problem, keep written summaries of all conversations (preferably signed by the employee) to prove that the employee was given prior notice about the issue and that termination was not the first line of defense. This helps ensure you have made every effort to let the employee succeed and reduces the chances of legal action.

Before proceeding with the decision to terminate, ask the following questions:

- Did I make the expectation regarding the performance, standard, or policy clear to the employee?
- Is the expectation, standard, or policy reasonably related to the employee's job?
- Did I have discussions with the employee about the problem, and did I provide any warning or notice?
- Did I make it clear that the consequences of a failure to meet the performance or behavior expectation could result in termination?
- Did the employee have a chance to explain?

- Are the same expectations in place for other employees in the same position, and are similar performance problems handled the same way?
- Is there anything in the employee handbook that contradicts the performance or behavior standard or that could be used by the employee to argue against the decision to terminate?

## Meeting With the Employee

Termination can be an emotional event for both participants, so it is critical to prepare a script and anticipate possible reactions. Now is not the time for a casual or improvised meeting. Possible employee reactions could include the following:

- The employee expects to be terminated and is relieved.
- The employee gets emotional and cries or refuses to talk.
- The employee gets upset and leaves the room.
- The employee gets angry, makes threats, or becomes violent.

Do not begin with small talk or do anything that avoids the main purpose of the meeting. Begin by stating that the employee is being terminated, and then explain the reasons as clearly and briefly as possible. Even if the employee does not agree with the decision, he or she must understand the reasons for termination and that they are for business rather than personal reasons.

Out of respect for the employee, hold the meeting in a private space where the conversation cannot be heard by others. Depending on the situation and the level of the person being terminated, it may be prudent to have one other person present as a witness, in case the dismissed employee later takes legal action. Schedule the meeting so the employee can quietly leave afterward without upsetting other employees; late afternoon is often an effective time. If possible, avoid terminating an employee late on Friday; terminating early in the week allows the employee to be proactive and begin a job search right away.

In the meeting, follow these eight guidelines:

1. Keep it brief (less than 10 minutes). It is not a discussion.

2. Get to the point. Avoid preambles and the temptation to recount history and previous discussions.

3. Speak decisively but calmly and without anger or frustration.

4. Accept responsibility for the decision. Don't blame it on a higher-level manager or the club owner. That will simply worsen the situation.

5. Be respectful and empathetic without signaling that there is any chance the decision will be reversed.

6. Be willing to listen, but do not get into a discussion or debate.

7. Provide any final paperwork (depending on company, state, or country legal requirements) and any compensation due.

8. After the meeting, document what was said and add it to the employee's file.

Termination is never a desirable outcome, but it is sometimes inevitable. Handling the situation appropriately reflects on you and the organization and may have legal and economic implications.

## Key Terms

goal setting

incentive compensation plan

open-book management

performance evaluation form

performance feedback

performance management

self-funding incentive program

servant leadership model

# CHAPTER 6

# Developing a Compensation Program

## Learning Objectives

After studying this chapter, you will be able to

- understand the importance of compensation policies and staff accountability,
- identify compensation needs,
- construct and implement a compensation plan, and
- understand the different forms of compensation and when to use each.

Mel was hired as the general manager of a large health club that recently merged with one of its smaller competitors and absorbed the club's staff and members. One of the first management tasks to tackle was a review of the compensation policy, because staff from both clubs were grumbling about the pay structure. Mel quickly realized that there was no direct connection between performance and compensation, which resulted in some productive employees not being adequately compensated.

After discussing the compensation issue with the club owners, Mel hired a consulting firm to conduct a compensation study and devise a new policy based on the following principles:

- Reduce the compensation entitlement mentality within the company to produce a lean, top-performing company.
- Pay should be tied to how well the company and the individual employee performed.
- The company should provide a competitive base pay and have performance-based pay increases.

After reviewing compensation history, pay structure, and competitor pay rates, the consultants proposed the following compensation strategies:

- Target salaries at top quartile of the industry to provide a strong incentive for employees to stay in their jobs and put forth greater effort, thereby enhancing productivity and lowering supervision costs (with the incentive to be more productive, fewer supervisors are needed to monitor performance).
- Reduce job turnover with above-market pay. This discourages workers from voluntarily leaving jobs. The lower turnover rate reduces the costs of hiring and training workers and results in a more experienced and more productive workforce. Above-market pay can contribute to employees feeling like they work for an elite organization with competent people, and it can make them feel fortunate to be there.

- Hire quality workers and demand above-market performance. Five people can be hired to do the work of 10 and can be paid like seven. The above-market pay practice is closely tied to demanding performance standards.

- Develop a culture that supports the compensation philosophy, and realize that negative culture cannot be overcome with higher salaries. Ensure that job descriptions and performance expectations are communicated throughout the organization.

These new strategies were enthusiastically received by Mel and the club owners. To make sure the compensation system was fair, Mel decided to get input from various sources, including select employees and various operating units. The input process helped get buy-in and agreement from employees and ensured management concerns were addressed and market trends were not ignored. Successful implementation depends on communication up and down the organization and rigorous follow through by management.

———————————————————————●———————————————————————

Even though the health and fitness industry has undergone major changes over the last decade, some clubs are still compensating employees the same way they did 25 years ago. Standard pay raises based on length of service and organizational rank and minimal or nonexistent benefits packages are still found in many clubs. Some creative managers are attempting to modify existing pay systems for top personnel to stay competitive and fit their changing environments. For some organizations, these changes include performance-based pay, insurance and retirement benefits, and bonuses or other incentive plans. Whatever the situation, the challenge with pay systems is keeping them flexible and focused on meeting the needs of the employees and the business.

In this chapter, I address the basics of compensation programs and discuss how to develop one to fit your organization. Further discussion centers on the various elements of compensation, surveys and job pricing, job evaluation, and pay-for-performance issues. Finally, I discuss the most common pay practices in the industry.

The health and fitness business is a customer service–driven industry. Continually meeting the needs and expectations of members and guests requires a skilled and knowledgeable staff. Personnel is the most important resource a club has in today's competitive market, and managers should consider it an asset. Successful managers realize that regardless of their state-of-the-art facilities, sophisticated equipment, or extensive services, their clubs cannot survive without skilled, helpful, and highly motivated employees.

To attract and retain the caliber of people needed in the health and fitness field, you need a well-designed and properly implemented compensation plan. An up-to-date plan will show the value of all employees and reward their contributions to the organization. An all-too-common complaint of fitness employees is that they feel a lack of recognition for the work they perform. For this reason, every owner and manager must ensure that the compensation package is fair for the employees and the employer.

## The Bottom Line

If left unattended by management, employees' feelings of underappreciation can have a negative effect on employee morale.

## FORMS OF COMPENSATION

Employees in the health and fitness industry receive their pay in various ways. Each form of compensation reflects an organization's philosophy, managerial style, and commitment to its employees. Some elements of compensation include wages or salaries, overtime pay, commissions, bonuses or profit sharing, pay for time not worked, insurance and retirement benefits, fringe benefits, and compensatory time off.

As a manager, you should identify the specific elements of compensation that best fit your organization. Once identified, determine a value or cost for each item. Although this is sometimes difficult to do, it is the only way to fully understand and manage a compensation program.

# Wages and Salaries

The term **wages** usually applies to payment for employee services rendered on an hourly or daily basis. Depending on the setting, front-desk attendants, maintenance personnel, fitness center instructors, and child-care attendants typically receive this form of payment. The term **salary** refers to compensation paid weekly, biweekly, or monthly to the owners, managers, and directors of major departments, such as personal training, sports, sales, and group fitness. Each form of compensation represents a fixed cost and the basis for administering other forms of compensation.

# Overtime Pay

Hourly workers, such as front-desk attendants, fitness center personnel, child-care workers, and most other nonsupervisory employees, are eligible for overtime. By law, these employees must be paid one-and-a-half times their regular base pay for each hour worked in excess of 40 during a week (this number can vary from country to country and possibly region to region). You cannot combine or average work weeks beyond 1 week, and you cannot give compensatory time off (details follow) outside of a work week in lieu of overtime pay.

Most health and fitness organizations pay either time and a half or double time for work on holidays or scheduled vacations. For those employees who occasionally work overtime, the additional pay they receive increases their overall rate of pay. The economics of overtime pay are important business considerations that need to be closely planned and scrutinized.

## *The Bottom Line*

Regularly monitor employee overtime and instigate a procedure for obtaining overtime approval from supervisors. Without these safeguards in place, an annual payroll budget can erode quickly.

# Commissions

**Commission-based pay** has become a popular method for compensating specialty employees in the industry. Sales personnel, massage and spa therapists, personal trainers, tennis pros, and sports program personnel are some of the employees who might receive commissions. A straight commission plan pays employees a percentage of what they obtain in total sales. The rate of commission pay depends on industry standards and the estimated volume of sales generated. For example, a massage therapist could start at a commission rate of 60% to the therapist and 40% to the club. As the volume of massage sales increases, management could increase the commission to 70–30 to reward the massage therapist for an increased client base, thereby allowing the therapist to earn more money and the club to receive additional revenue through increased sales.

Survey results (IDEA 2015) for 1,300 health and fitness staff showed that

- 64% of all full-time employees were eligible for commissions or other cash incentives,
- 40% of all part-time employees were eligible for commissions or other cash incentives,
- 37% of personal trainers received commissions or other cash incentives,
- 7% of group fitness instructors received commissions or other cash incentives, and
- 21% of Pilates and yoga instructors received commissions or other cash incentives.

Although commission-based pay can motivate employees, commission-only plans may cause employees to sell too aggressively, which can sometimes generate unfavorable member reactions. Another factor to consider is that organizations sometimes find it more difficult to get commission-based personnel to perform other necessary duties.

Another plan with wide industry acceptance is the salary plus commission combination. Employees earn a basic salary and can earn a percentage of sales as a commission. This combination guarantees employees a base level of pay and provides an extra incentive to sell their services.

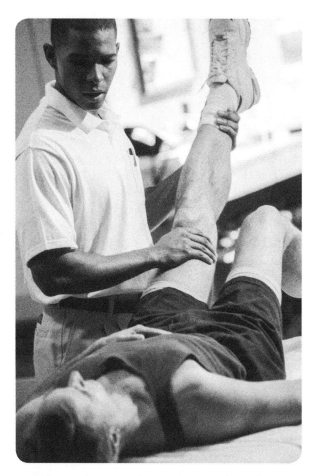

Specialty employees, such as massage and spa therapists or sales personnel, are increasingly compensated through commission-based pay.

Eyewire

## Bonuses and Profit Sharing

Bonuses and profit sharing are periodic lump-sum payments, such as annual or quarterly payments for meeting predetermined financial goals or monthly bonuses to sales personnel for reaching pre-established new-member goals. Bonuses may also provide an incentive for achievements such as cost savings; for example, some clubs may structure the bonus plan entirely on quarterly net profits. With this approach, employees can influence their quarterly bonuses by being constantly watchful of all expenses associated with their divisions.

For an employer, all such payments represent a variable cost. More important, many organizations believe that some type of bonus plan contributes significantly to improving overall operations and member services by providing financial motivation to employees. An example of a club-sponsored bonus program is explained in the Ojai Valley Racquet Club Employee Profit-Sharing and Point System sidebar later in this chapter.

## Pay for Time Not Worked

Pay for time not worked includes vacation time, holidays, sick-leave days, maternity leave, and personal days for such things as jury duty, religious holidays, a death in the family, and military service. There is also pay for time not worked during working hours, such as scheduled rest breaks. Sick-leave days provide employees with continued income in the event of a short-term illness. Vacation and holiday payments allow for paid rest from work. Being paid for nonworking periods allows employees to have more time for families, travel, recreation, and, most important, a needed break from the daily demands of the customer service business.

## Benefits

Employee **benefits** include retirement plans and protection against economic risks, including death, disability, and illness. Many of these are insured benefits, and the employer pays some or all of the insurance premium.

### The Bottom Line

In some cases, employer-sponsored benefits provide coverage at a level the employee could not obtain alone.

Offering benefits to employees provides needed protection at a lower cost than would be available individually. Providing benefits can also assist in meeting the needs of the organization by helping organizations attract new employees and retain existing employees. For example, a 401(k) match or other retirement plan incentive can help employees save for the future, which can provide financial security for current and future employees. Awarding a designated number of paid vacation days for each year worked rewards employees for their years of service, which is a great way to both incentivize and attract employees. In today's

# Ojai Valley Racquet Club Employee Profit-Sharing and Point System

Each quarter, the accounting department computes the net profit (after all expenses) during the previous 3 months. Twenty percent of that profit is designated for employee distribution as cash bonuses. For the first three quarters, 50% of the profit-sharing bonus is paid to employees directly and 50% is held back to offset possible quarterly losses. At year-end, the remaining 50% is paid in addition to normal quarterly bonuses.

## Who Is Eligible?

All hourly and some salaried employees are eligible.

## What Determines the Bonus?

- Quarterly mini review results
- Overall productivity with respect to others in the same department
- The number of hours worked per week
- Employees' attitudes toward each other
- Length of employment
- The degree to which the department meets its expense budget

## What's the Purpose of the Profit-Sharing Plan?

The plan sends an important message about performance that is spelled out in the bonus amount as follows:

- A check for a large percentage means you are meeting or exceeding your job requirements.
- A check for a smaller percentage means that you are a valuable person but could use improvement in some areas.
- A check for a small percentage means that your performance is not always what it should be.
- No bonus means you should consider seeking employment elsewhere.

The overall objective of the plan is to help create a higher performing team and to tangibly reward those employees who are doing the best job for the club.

## What Are the Criteria for the Best Job?

- Meeting department expense budgets (exceeding these goals will result in a larger share of the total profit allocated to each department)
- Meeting member needs within each department
- Supporting company policies, rules, and regulations

## Point System

The profit-sharing plan is based on a point system that has positive and negative points. Positive points can be accrued by attending a club event, performing a special act for a member, suggesting an idea to improve the club, and other actions that benefit the club. Negative points are recorded for tardiness, complaints, failure to attend mandatory meetings, and other actions that fail to meet job requirements.

Each item counts for a certain number of points, which are logged in workbooks and totaled each quarter. Any negative net is used as a percentage, which is multiplied by the profit-sharing amount to decrease the profit bonus paid to the employee (e.g., an employee who has −50 points receives 50% of the profit-sharing amount). Being even would result in an employee receiving 100% of the profit-sharing amount. Positive net is carried into the next quarter and to year-end when employees may exchange positive points for vacation days or additional bonuses beyond the profit-sharing amount.

market, providing a sound benefits package is necessary to attract and retain employees.

Each form of compensation can represent a significant portion of an employee's overall remuneration. However, usually only the financial elements of compensation are expressed in monetary terms; therefore, all employees see is the paycheck amount. They give little thought to the added benefits the employer pays for. Consequently, benefits are often viewed as soft costs. Employers should calculate a hard cost for items such as taxes (i.e., unemployment, workers' compensation, and disability); health, dental, vision, and life insurance; holiday and vacation pay; sick leave; retirement plans; bonuses; training and education; staff uniforms; and club memberships. This is the only way to show employees the total value of wages and benefits. Figure 6.1 provides a sample employee benefits worksheet that any organization can adapt to reflect an employee's complete compensation and benefits package.

In the figure, an additional 32% was added to the base pay because of the benefits package. Understandably, most managers would view this figure as excessively high. However, a consideration when creating a similar model for employees is turnover. Sometimes people do not stay long enough to earn all their vacation, sick, or holiday pay. Others decide against taking health or life insurance. Consequently, depending on turnover rates, a correction factor could be included to adequately represent payroll taxes and benefits. A worksheet similar to figure 6.1 can also assist employees in understanding that if the organization incurs an increase in the cost of health care, employees might have to share some of the additional cost.

Although for most employees money is the primary driving force to work, there are some noncash elements of remuneration. In the health and fitness industry, working in a fitness environment is a perceived value to the employee. This value can relate to the social merits of helping people become physically fit or improving self-image.

The job itself can be another area of great worth to the employee. Those entering the fitness field consider the opportunity to have a job that combines physical and social skills an added benefit. The opportunity to use club facilities for personal workouts is also of value. Thus, the work itself not only determines direct pay but also has psychological value.

Other forms of fringe benefits may include club discounts for programs, services, and pro shop merchandise; continuing education assistance; tuition reimbursement; flexible medical or child-care spending accounts; or other child-care benefits. It is the responsibility of an owner or manager to identify these areas for the organization and include them in the personnel manual as added benefits.

# COMPENSATION AND MANAGEMENT

A compensation plan is a vital component of management. It contributes to the success of any health and fitness operation and provides the mechanism to compensate employees for their productivity. Management style must be reflected in the method of compensation. Does the compensation plan consist of only salaries and hourly wages, or are performance-based incentives, commissions, benefits packages, or bonus plans included? Addressing these issues reflects management's commitment to employees.

## Five Compensation Suggestions

A well-developed compensation program can affect the success of a health and fitness organization in a number of ways: It can set you apart from the competition, assist in recruiting candidates for employment, help retain existing personnel, and contribute significantly to employee morale. To create a compensation plan that contributes to the success of the operation and is supported by employees, consider these five suggestions:

1. *Ensure pay is competitive with similar positions in the field.* With the increasing number of health and fitness facilities and the decreasing number of hourly wage employees, more attention has been directed to the competitiveness of pay. Use available industry surveys that list national salaries and wage scales to compare similar positions in the field. You should also monitor comparable facilities within the community to maintain a competitive pay scale. As the industry has matured, the price paid for labor has increased along with the demand for additional services and facilities.

2. *Recognize that employees are income-producing assets.* View each employee as a major contributor

# ABC ATHLETIC CLUB EMPLOYEE COMPENSATION AND BENEFITS WORKSHEET

Position: Assistant fitness manager, full time

| | Hourly rate | Annual hours | Base annual earnings (BAE) | |
|---|---|---|---|---|
| | $10.00 | 2,080 | $20,800 | |
| Taxes | BAE | Factor | Total | % of base |
| Federal unemployment | $20,800 | 0.008 | $166 | 0.80% |
| State unemployment | $20,800 | 0.016 | $333 | 1.60% |
| FICA (Social Security) | $20,800 | 0.0765 | $1,591 | 7.65% |
| Worker's comp insurance | $20,800 | 0.024 | $499 | 2.40% |
| **Total** | | | $2,589 | 12.45% |
| | | | | |
| Medical insurance | Monthly | Annual | 50% paid by employer | |
| Health advantage HMO employee | N/A | N/A | N/A | |
| Health source HMO employee | $128.00 | $1,536.00 | $768.00 | |
| **Total** | | | $768.00 | 3.69% |
| | | | | |
| Dental insurance employee | $14.64 | $175.68 | | |
| Dental insurance employer | $7.32 | $87.84 | $87.84 | 0.42% |
| Paid holidays* | | | | |
| Salaried (daily rate × 7) | | | $560.00 | 2.69% |
| Paid vacation* | | | | |
| Salaried (hourly rate × 13 days) | | | $1,040.00 | 5.00% |
| Paid sick leave* | | | | |
|   (hourly rate × hr taken) up to 32 hr | | | $320.00 | 1.54% |
| Employee staff shirts | | | | |
|   ($8.00/shirt at 4 shirts/employee/yr) | | | $32.00 | 0.15% |
| Training and educational courses* | | | | |
|   ($12,000/yr for qualified staff) | | | $1,000.00 | 4.81% |
| Total benefits | | | $3,807.84 | 18.31% |
|   (less benefits included in base earnings) | | $2,920.00 | Salaried | 14.04% |
| | | | | |
|   Net benefits | | $887.84 | | 4.27% |
|   Bonus plan | | $3,200.00 | | 15.38% |
| | | | | |
| Total compensation and benefits paid by employer | | | $27,477.44 | 132.10% |

**Figure 6.1**  Sample employee compensation and benefits worksheet.

*Represents cost for nonproductive time.

to the overall success of the organization. Because health and fitness programs and services are not considered tangible products, every employee must assist in creating the overall value or image associated with belonging to the facility. For this reason, managers in all settings must recognize that compensation has to do with acquiring and using a club's most important asset: the people who work there.

3. *Balance payroll costs with employee productivity.* Unfortunately, traditional accounting practices have impeded the way most managers view personnel. On balance statements, employees are considered liabilities; on income statements, they are listed as expenses. Rarely do you hear managers talk about the income-producing potential of employees; instead, they emphasize wage cost containment. With this view, there is inevitably an overemphasis on cutting payroll and little emphasis on increasing the output per payroll dollar.

4. *Manage payroll costs in addition to pay rates.* The single largest expense in the health and fitness industry is payroll. According to the IHRSA *Profiles of Success* report (International Health, Racquet, and Sportsclub Association 2017), salaries and wages, benefits, and payroll taxes make up the largest expense category for all health clubs at 44.5% of the total revenue. For this reason, you should manage payroll costs like any other expense, even though payroll costs are not like other expenses. For example, if a successful member-retention program is the result of trained and enthusiastic employees, you should seriously consider the negative effects of reducing payroll or eliminating training and development programs. In this scenario, if you reduce payroll costs, then the overall business will likely suffer. Payroll management involves weighing the effects of payroll cost against the financial results of the business.

5. *Consider payroll costs to be an investment in the future.* An accountant views every dollar of payroll as an expense. Although this is sound accounting, a good manager considers other factors when determining appropriate compensation. For example, if a club compensates employees by paying a straight wage, this is considered a direct expense: pay for time worked regardless of the output of the work. However, if the club decides to incorporate profit sharing as an incentive for employees to receive higher pay while contributing to the increased profits of the business, this is considered an investment opportunity for the business as well as the employees. Although both options are recognized compensation plans, one is considered an expense and the other is an investment.

## *The Bottom Line*

Controlling compensation means optimizing the margin between output and payroll costs.

## Compensation Policies

Once you have developed views and strategies on compensation, establish policies that reflect the values of the organization. Identify and address compensation concerns to ensure all personnel are treated fairly and consistently during their employment. Basic policy issues that you should address include the following:

- What should the pay for jobs be compared with similar positions in the field?
- What is the policy with respect to pay for performance?
- Is there a standard policy for performance-review pay adjustments?
- Will the organization provide health, dental, vision, and life insurance; an employee assistance program; and a 401(k) or other retirement plan? If so, what will the employee contribute?
- What will be the compensation policy differences for full-time employees, part-time employees, and independent contractors?
- Are employees provided a club membership at no cost as a form of compensation? If so, are there any restrictions on membership usage? Are family members included on the membership?
- Which positions will be designated salaried, hourly, commissioned, or paid per class or session?

Although in every setting there are additional compensation issues you must address, these items represent the major policy concerns for most health and fitness organizations. The compensation policies that evolve from answering these questions should meet certain requirements.

When an employee makes a proposal regarding a certain action, you can screen it against the policy statements. Policies must be the basis for decisions about compensation matters. Policies must also be specific and comprehensive enough that they become important communication tools.

## Accountability to Employees

Part of being a health and fitness manager is providing accountability when necessary, including accountability to employees. Answering compensation-related questions by saying "I'm sorry, but that's our policy" might have worked 50 years ago, but it doesn't work now.

Because pay is such a personal matter, managers have the obligation to justify, report, or explain any issue related to compensation. Being accountable means having the authority to act if needed. For example, if an employee talks to other personnel about a policy that he or she believes to be unfair, management has the responsibility to investigate and act on the concern in a timely manner.

Being accountable to employees is not meant to restrict or dilute the manager's position. The final decision maker in any compensation issue is always the manager. However, being accountable reinforces that the organization wants to show fairness and a commitment to its employees.

## COMPENSATION PROGRAM BASICS

Every health and fitness setting is unique not only in terms of the type, size, location, and services offered but also in more subtle ways. For example, different settings have different management styles, tasks are performed differently, and decisions are made in various ways. As a result, managers in each setting should tailor compensation programs and practices to fit the specific situation.

Successful compensation plans are simple in design yet adaptive to the management philosophy. The procedures for providing employee pay should be easily understood and implemented by the payroll administrator and be flexible enough to facilitate the employees' needs. Employees enrolling into the compensation plan should be able to specify their pay rates for different job segments, if applicable. For example, managers

will often cross-train employees to work in two or more divisions of an organization. The pay associated with working in separate divisions may differ; consequently, the compensation program must be flexible enough to identify the areas worked and provide the appropriate pay. This is just one example of the importance of a payroll system that is adaptive to the needs of the organization.

## Grouping Employees

Before establishing a compensation plan, make a list of every employee position. This list will assist you in determining how to group employees into various classifications to establish compensation rates and packages. See the Employee Positions in Health, Fitness, and Wellness Facilities sidebar later in this chapter for an example.

The next step is grouping employees into an organizational structure that is easy to administer and classifies employees based on the goals of the organization. Various job categories may require different pay programs and practices.

For management purposes, group jobs so tasks and responsibilities are appropriate for each category and the training and recruiting methods required to fill the jobs are similar. Once you complete this, you can develop many personnel practices, such as recruiting, training, employee communication, and payroll, to meet the requirements of the job.

In a typical health and fitness club structure, there are at least four groups of employees to consider: full-time staff (salaried), full-time staff (hourly), part-time staff (hourly), and independent contractors. Within each category, there are subgroups that include employees from various divisions of the organization. For example, the full-time salaried staff category includes the general manager, sales and marketing director, group fitness director, personal training director, and tennis director. Employee subgroups vary depending on the type and size of the organization.

## Independent Contractors

A significant percentage of workers in the health and fitness field are neither full- nor part-time employees but are **independent contractors.** Some are contracted for specific tasks, such as group fitness or specialty program instruction,

# Employee Positions in Health, Fitness, and Wellness Facilities

## Management and Administrative Staff

- Owner or ownership group
- General manager or executive director
- Operations manager
- Manager on duty
- Administrative assistant
- Accounting or business office manager
- Accounts payable services
- Member accounts services
- Accounts receivable coordinator
- Data-entry clerk
- Human resources director

## Membership and Marketing Staff

- Membership sales director
- Membership representative
- Member relations staff
- Front-desk manager
- Front-desk attendant
- Marketing director
- Marketing assistant

## Program Staff

- Sports or athletic director
- Fitness director
- Fitness center instructor
- Personal training director
- Personal trainer
- Group fitness director
- Group fitness instructor
- Group fitness training coordinator
- Health coach
- Medical exercise specialist
- Program director
- Sports camp counselor
- Aquatics director
- Head lifeguard
- Lifeguard
- Aquatics instructor
- Aquatic fitness coordinator
- Aquatic fitness instructor
- Youth program director
- Martial arts instructor
- Gymnastics director
- Gymnastics instructor
- Court sports director
- Squash and racquetball pro

- Head tennis pro
- Tennis pro
- Tennis-desk attendant
- Basketball coordinator
- Basketball monitor

## Facility Services Staff

- Housekeeping supervisor
- Locker-room attendant
- Maintenance assistant
- Building engineer
- Assistant building engineer
- Pool maintenance staff
- Food and beverage manager
- Snack bar attendant
- Pro shop manager
- Pro shop sales staff
- Child-care supervisor
- Child-care attendant

## Spa Staff

- Spa director
- Spa estheticians and technicians
- Massage therapists
- Spa service-desk representatives

massage therapy, or personal training, and others are companies hired to provide specific services, such as major building repairs, landscaping, legal counsel, information technology, and marketing.

There are advantages and disadvantages to using independent contractors. An advantage is personnel placement becomes the responsibility of the contractor instead of the contracting organization. A disadvantage of using independent contractors is the lack of internal loyalty associated with being part of the staff. Contractors leave the premises once they have completed their class, client session, or task, so it is difficult to establish communication lines and develop a sense of camaraderie or cohesiveness among coworkers. If a full-time employee is passed over for a position that was assigned to an independent contractor, this could result in resentment.

It is critical that club owners understand the differences between employees and contractors so they know which they are employing. The following are the basic differences between employees and contractors:

- Contractors set their own schedules instead of working on schedules determined by the company.
- Contractors set their own rates for services instead of adhering to company pay policies.
- Contractors receive no employee benefits, such as health insurance, vacation time, or overtime or holiday pay.
- Contractors are not covered by company insurance and must provide their own liability insurance.
- Contractors are responsible for paying their own income taxes and Social Security and Medicare taxes. In the United States, contractors receive 1099-MISC federal tax forms from the company (depending on income earned) instead of W-2s.
- Contractors' actions are not controlled by the company beyond the extent of specific contractual obligations.

As you can see, there are considerable differences between employees and contractors. In the United States, health clubs that attempt to pay people as independent contractors but treat them as employees are at risk for substantial fines from the Internal Revenue Service (IRS). The IRS website provides documents and information regarding federal regulations on working with independent contractors.

# Approach for Developing a Compensation Program

A recommended approach for developing a compensation program follows. This traditional approach is used in many businesses.

## Identify Compensation Needs

Developing a compensation program begins with identifying needs. Organizations in the start-up phase need to create an initial pay program, whereas other organizations may need to change their compensation systems due to problems or new opportunities. Whatever the reason, identifying the needs is the most crucial aspect of compensation. Although there are many ways to identify needs, it is critical to have a reliable process that you can use to obtain the information you need.

Some methods for determining specific compensation needs include the following:

- Observe the compensation experiences and problem areas that employees encounter in their work.
- Use opinion or focus polls with managers and employees.
- Perform personnel audits in which you question all aspects of personnel management (not just compensation).
- Use statistical analysis and personnel data to determine needs. Obtain benchmark surveys from industry organizations IHRSA, IDEA, American Council on Exercise (ACE), ClubIntel). Consider using an information bank with job titles, responsibilities, and salary levels from similar settings to determine compensation rates.

## The Bottom Line

Identifying compensation needs involves regular monitoring and observation, feedback from reliable sources, and obtaining information on current trends in the industry.

## Develop Goals

Meeting the compensation needs of a health club starts with setting specific goals. Because much of personnel management is based on knowledge obtained from experiences, it is sometimes difficult to set specific goals. Goals that are difficult to measure, such as improving employee morale, providing greater internal consistency, or creating a better-quality work environment are often used to by inexperienced managers. Unfortunately, these nonspecific goals are meaningless and can confuse rather than clarify a specific intent.

Set specific, quantifiable goals, such as reducing the employee cost of health care by 10% or delegating pay decisions to department heads or supervisors. Once you have identified goals, set up appropriate systems to evaluate cost and value.

## Construct the Program

Based on the needs assessment and the stated goals, the next step is to construct the compensation program. Developing a formal compensation system in which everything is spelled out for every possible situation is highly unlikely. However, it is a good idea to establish standards in writing that can guide individual pay decisions. Such elements of a compensation program should contribute to better decision making, more consistency, and greater fairness. Neither the program nor its procedures can be the decision-making process.

These are five standards to follow when developing a compensation program:

1. *Align compensation programs to fit the way you manage the business.* As with any business, health and fitness organizations have their own unique practices, concerns, and issues. Management styles, operating systems, and personnel concerns vary from setting to setting. A properly tailored compensation program reflects each of these factors and is developed with these values in mind.

2. *Make the program flexible.* A compensation program should adapt to a rapidly changing world. Develop the program so you don't have to reinvent the wheel every time you make a change. Whether you incorporate wage scales, cost-of-living increases, performance-based pay, or commission-based pay, each of these is subject to change at any time.

3. *Keep the program simple.* Consider all the supervisors and other managers who must support and administer the plan. It should make their jobs easier rather than more difficult.

4. *Have a way to measure results.* There is no way of incorporating pay for performance if you can't measure performance. Use measures based on the goals of the organization. Possible measurements may include financial performance, department productivity, economic value, quality control, and customer service ranking.

5. *Don't let* compensation *be a bad word.* Help employees understand the compensation process. This doesn't mean sharing privileged pay information, but it does mean communicating and updating employees on the process. This will help motivate employees.

You should also use two cornerstones of compensation management—surveys and job pricing—to obtain specific pay comparisons and lists of current salary levels. Using these methods ensures that pay is sufficiently competitive and fair to employees.

Compensation information is the basis for determining competitive pay and is vital for establishing fair pay. In response to the need for more and better compensation information, the health and fitness industry has invested a great deal of time and effort in developing survey information to improve compensation management. As a result, a variety of information is available for managers in all settings to review and compare before establishing a compensation program.

When compared with more established businesses, the health and fitness industry is still relatively young with regard to salary data. Professional journals and industry organizations have primarily been responsible for salary surveys. The data obtained from these surveys can assist you in establishing comparative benchmarks when recruiting and conducting performance evaluations. Keep in mind that pay variations exist between similar positions depending on the region, type, and size of the facility and whether it is considered a low-revenue performer (25% less than average industry earnings) or a top performer (25% greater than average industry earnings). Table 6.1 illustrates the average compensation rates of several common full- and part-time positions in health fitness facilities according to IDEA (2015) survey data.

A word of caution when using published salary information: It is essential that the data obtained from any survey be closely scrutinized before adjusting or setting wages and salaries. You need to know the size of the survey and how, when, and by whom it was conducted. Determine the sample size of the organizations participating in the survey. The goal is to find reputable and reliable surveys used by most health and fitness managers.

Perhaps the most common method for establishing wages and salaries is **job pricing.** First, identify all compensated positions and write a brief description of each (usually one paragraph). Next, prepare an organizational flowchart that illustrates position hierarchy and establishes a career path for employees to follow. Once you have compiled this information, start pricing the jobs based on management's experience and salary information obtained from similar settings.

**Table 6.1** Average Compensation for Fitness Industry Professionals

| Position | Annual salary | Hourly rate |
|---|---|---|
| Fitness or program director | $43,317 | $25.00 |
| Personal training director | $43,051 | $32.00 |
| Group fitness director | $37,871 | $25.00 |
| Personal trainer | $31,250 | $30.50 |
| Fitness floor staff | $27,320 | $12.25 |
| Group fitness instructor | $18,000 | $27.50 |
| Pilates or yoga instructor | $27,817 | $31.25 |

Data from IDEA (2015).

Methods of obtaining compensation information include personal visits to other clubs, questionnaires, and telephone interviews with other managers.

## Test the Program

After designing a compensation program, you must test it. A major component of testing is reviewing and questioning its legal and tax implications. This process often requires working with an attorney and an accountant to make sure the organization complies with the U.S. Fair Labor Standards Act.

During this time, you need input from all levels of employees. Take a what-if approach and question each aspect of the plan, and then decide on any changes before implementing it.

## Implement the Program

Implementation means putting the program into operation and establishing the various procedures and necessary reviews. Ongoing application of the program shows whether it is achieving the original goals established by management and employees. Implementation is dynamic, so expect regular changes and modifications. In addition, the nature of administrative and operational work involved in implementation will change, and the staffing required to perform the work must similarly change to meet new requirements.

## Review and Revise the Program

Continual review of a compensation program will undoubtedly necessitate revisions or major changes. Causes for these revisions may be changes in operations, management, payroll regulations, or financial status. Stay abreast of economic conditions that affect inflation. Each quarter, monitor changes in factors such as cost of living and consumer price index fluctuations. Review the state of the industry annually. Are pay rates for all positions staying constant, or are they oscillating? Is the number of employees needed to operate various sizes of facilities staying the same, or is a downsizing trend occurring? Is there still a high demand for health and fitness professionals? Is the overall growth of the industry continuing to reflect a positive change, or has growth slowed? Consider all these factors when reviewing and revising compensation programs.

Making changes to an established compensation program is never easy, especially if the program has been successful and is understood by management and employees. However, waiting too long to make revisions may cause larger problems over time, so it is necessary to make regular revisions and act on them.

You can adapt this process for developing compensation programs to fit any health and fitness setting. Although you can use this process as a basic management tool, the real challenge is to make the program reflect the personality of the business. Because fitness centers are unique and dynamic, you must clearly understand the profile of the club, including short- and long-term goals and objectives.

## The Bottom Line

To remain innovative, you must update technology, stay in compliance with changing payroll laws, and adapt to the ever-changing needs of the organization.

## Process for Developing Compensation Programs

1. Perform a needs analysis. Identify questions, problems, or opportunities by doing the following:
   - Hold discussions with department heads or supervisors.
   - Hold discussions with employees.
   - Examine member- and staff-reported issues.
   - Perform personnel audits.
2. Develop goals.
   - Ensure goals are specific and measurable.
   - Consider the impact on all phases of the operation.
   - Consider the schedule format.
   - Determine whether enough staff members are available to meet these goals.
3. Construct the program.
   - Align the program to fit the way the business is managed.
   - Make the program flexible to change.
   - Keep the program simple.
   - Have a way of measuring results.
   - Don't let compensation be a bad word.
4. Test the program layout.
   - Consider the legal, tax, and accounting ramifications.
   - Consider what-if and worst-case possibilities.
   - Determine whether it will stand the test of time.
   - Compare the program against alternatives.
5. Implement the program.
6. Evaluate the program's effectiveness.
7. Review the program.

## PERFORMANCE-BASED PAY

**Performance-based pay** is a salary or wage paid to employees based on how well they perform the tasks required of their jobs. Whereas other pay strategies are designed to reward tenure and rank in the company, performance-based pay systems reward employees based on merit, which is typically measured by the attainment of specific goals or performance milestones. Many companies in all types of industries use performance-based pay systems for evaluating employees, setting salaries, and determining periodic pay increases. In a performance-based pay system, any pay increases or bonuses given to employees are based on evaluations of their performance, usually on a biannual or annual basis. The logic behind performance-based pay is that improved performance should result in greater employee productivity, which in turn should result in improved business results. As the fitness industry has grown and matured, owners and managers have realized that by rewarding individual performance, the company and the employees benefit. Over time, employees understand that their productivity is linked to their success and income and to those of the company as well.

Performance-based pay systems start at the beginning of each fiscal year with employee goal setting. Throughout the year, the system calls

# Developing a Performance-Based Pay Planning and Evaluation Form

The following is an example of the various sections and components of a form used to summarize an employee's annual performance and evaluation plan.

1. Opening section
   a. Employee name
   b. Job or position title
   c. Department
   d. Name of supervisor
   e. Date of midyear review
   f. Date of annual review

2. Instructions section
   a. This performance summary focuses on key aspects of job performance and should be completed at midyear and at year-end. It permits the supervisor to assess an employee's performance and comment on overall levels of achievement in fulfilling the position responsibilities. Recommendations given to improve performance and develop abilities should also be documented.
   b. To maximize the effectiveness of the performance summary, the supervisor should carefully and thoroughly prepare a review and discuss it with the employee twice a year.
   c. The employee is encouraged to make written comments on any aspect of the review and should sign the form after reading it and discussing it with the supervisor.
   d. A performance summary should be completed for all personnel. Supervisors should use this form as the basis for coaching discussions with employees.

3. Responsibilities and performance standards section
   a. List the individual performance objectives and primary responsibilities. Use the position description as a guide.
   b. Assign a priority to each responsibility using the following scale: H = high, M = medium, L = low.
   c. Describe specific results and achievements for each objective at midyear and year-end.
   d. Rate the performance for each objective using the following scale: EE = exceeds expectations, ME = meets expectations, BE = below expectations.

4. Closing section
   a. Taking into account the ratings for each objective, determine an overall evaluation rating using the same scale used to rate each objective: EE, ME, and BE.
   b. Write a short performance improvement plan and list any areas in which the employee could improve performance along with specific steps to be taken.
   c. Describe any special circumstances that prevent conducting a performance review at the appropriate time.
   d. Provide an opportunity for the employee to comment on the performance summary and ratings.
   e. Sign and date the form, and have the employee do the same. Include space for appropriate management or human resources personnel to review and sign as well.

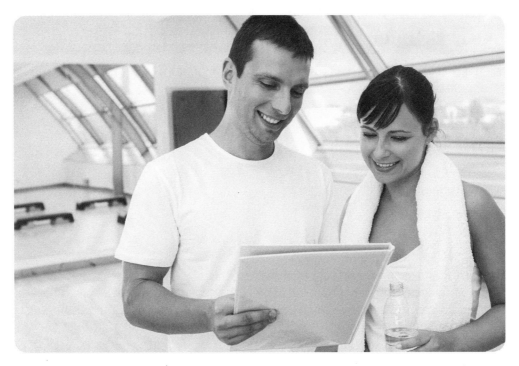

Some club employees, such as the program director, aquatics director, and general manager, will be paid salaries that might include bonuses and benefits. Other employees are compensated with an hourly wage, and still others are considered independent contractors.

iStockphoto/Lajos Répási

for regular discussions between supervisors and employees on performance issues. In this way, the system becomes integral to the daily management of the company. At the end of each year, the process concludes with a performance review in which ratings are given based on how well the employee has performed compared to the plan (see chapter 5). Because performance-based pay systems are directly linked to employee performance evaluations, annual or periodic pay adjustments are generally divided into three categories:

1. *Outstanding performance.* Employees who exceed job expectations receive the highest pay increases or other financial rewards to acknowledge their contributions to company success and to motivate continued high performance levels.

2. *Average performance.* Employees who meet but do not exceed job expectations receive moderate pay increases or rewards designed to encourage them to be more productive to receive higher pay increases in the future.

3. *Low performance.* Employees who fail to meet job expectations receive no pay increases or rewards and are typically warned that performance must be improve or they will have to leave the company.

While pay for performance can be an effective strategy for improving employee productivity, it is important to acknowledge that job motivation does not solely come from monetary rewards. Employees are also motivated by other factors, such as personal pride in working hard and accomplishing job goals, a desire to see the company succeed, achieving work satisfaction, or making significant contributions. Companies often find that focusing on individual performance goals and periodic job evaluations are just as valuable as pay increases. The discipline of working through a regular performance evaluation process helps a company not only focus on achieving important goals but also communicates to employees the specific expectations of each job and the company priorities. The rigorous assessment of job performance and individual accomplishments used as the basis for pay increases can be as motivating to high-level performance as the financial rewards themselves. Finally, employees appreciate working for companies in which performance is rewarded, accomplishments are acknowledged, and the pay system is viewed as fair and impartial.

## Key Terms

benefits

commission-based pay

independent contractors

job pricing

performance-based pay

salary

wages

# MEMBER RECRUITMENT, RETENTION, AND PROFITABILITY

As a manager or club owner, you need to be able to pay the bills. You would probably also like to get paid yourself. Part II presents an overview of the revenue-generating strategies you need to employ to be able to do both of these things. As competition has increased in the fitness industry, the best club managers realize they need to take a strategic approach when it comes to marketing and selling their services, while also developing sound programs that keep members coming back.

In chapter 7, you will learn how to effectively market your facility for maximum leads, branding, and traffic to your club. This chapter will help you navigate the ever-changing landscape of social media marketing and help you to maximize your efforts in promoting your organization and your programs.

Next, in chapter 8, you will learn how to build an effective sales system by incorporating the front desk, phone calls, and the face-to-face sales process. Consumers have a multitude of choices in most markets. An effective sales person will effectively align the prospect's needs to the benefits the club has to offer.

The essential topic of customer service is covered in chapter 9, where you will learn how to effectively communicate with members by truly understanding what they want and then delivering it. In chapter 10, you will learn how to design programs that improve retention and keep members coming back for more.

Generating revenue outside of regular membership dues is no longer optional—it is a necessity for a club to be successful. In chapter 11, you will learn various ways you can generate ancillary sources of revenue within your clubs.

# CHAPTER 7

# Marketing Your Program

## Learning Objectives

After studying this chapter, you will be able to

- develop marketing materials for the purpose of promoting fitness-related programs,
- analyze marketing research data and trends within the fitness industry,
- identify and apply the best practices for strategic marketing planning,
- understand the dynamics and impact of digital marketing (including social media), and
- demonstrate the ability to evaluate marketing effectiveness using data analytics.

Brenna is a fitness manager who has a strong background in exercise science, nutrition, and training clients. She also possesses a few national certifications in personal training and strength and conditioning. However, Brenna has little experience in marketing. She has just been told by senior management that she will be responsible for marketing a new program called the 60-Day Transformation Challenge, starting in January. This new transformation program is expected to generate a significant amount of new clients as well as increase income from existing clients who want to get back on track with their fitness journey. Brenna asks senior management whether she can bring on a fitness management or marketing intern who has taken courses in digital marketing. After being told yes by senior management, Brenna offers an internship to Chelsie, and they begin the process of developing a marketing plan and the materials for promoting this new transformation program.

erhaps one of the biggest challenges facing fitness managers today in marketing the facility and its programs is standing out in a sea of advertising clutter. In January 2017 the *New York Times* estimated that an individual residing in a city viewed up to 5,000 ad messages per day (Story 2017), a big jump from the 2,000 daily ads that an individual encountered just 30 years ago, according to the market research firm Yankelovich (Story 2017).

Traditionally, companies have relied upon the foundation of the four Ps of marketing—product, price, place, and promotion—to guide strategic planning. However, with the emergence of innovative marketing solutions (e.g., social media, data analytics) to engage and measure activity with the consumer, many in the marketing profession see modern marketing as going beyond the four Ps. One issue in modern marketing relates to who has true control of the messaging. With consumers publically expressing how they feel about products and services through social media, one has to wonder who is really responsible for today's marketing strategies—the company or the consumer.

These examples demonstrate just some of the challenges fitness managers face today with the recent shift from **traditional marketing** to **digital marketing**. The new digital marketing methods offer the ability to target specific audiences through digital channels such as search engines, websites, social media, email, and mobile apps. Therefore, gaining an understanding of the real-time dynamics and impact of these digital channels is paramount for success in marketing your fitness programs. Just as fitness managers can view and generate quantitative fitness data reports, fitness managers can use the **data analytics** provided by the digital channels to evaluate their marketing effectiveness. This chapter is designed to equip fitness managers with the foundation, tools, and best practices to drive business performance using digital marketing.

## DEVELOPING STRATEGIC MARKETING PLANS

*"Attraction is the first step in leveraging #DigitalMarketing. Without it, your brand does not exist in the mind of the consumer."* #SMKT523

*@Guy Danhoff (posted on Twitter 7/1/17)*

There are a few key components that maximize the marketing arsenal. The first step is a situational analysis regarding your organization's current situation in the marketplace. Your programs and service offerings must be defined from a competition frame of reference so everyone knows what key differences you offer the market. In other words, it must be crystal clear to you, your competitors, consumers, and prospects exactly what you offer that distinguishes the brand. As we previously discussed in the chapter, conducting an SWOTT analysis can provide the situational analysis data needed to communicate this information within the organization.

The second step is to describe your target markets in detail, as discussed, using the identification model of primary, secondary, and tertiary markets paired with the demographics and psychographics information. Having this detailed information is similar to a sniper having a target in their line of sight using a scope: Once the target is in clear view, it is time to act. The third step is to establish and refine the marketing goals and objectives. As mentioned earlier, the key here is to ensure every goal is measurable.

The fourth step is the most crucial element of developing the strategic marketing plan, because this is where the marketing communication strategies are identified, as are the tactics to execute the marketing plan. (Think of the *Mission Impossible* series in which Ethan Hunt carefully and strategically accounts for every step of the process in order to execute a flawless mission.) Today, fitness managers have a plethora of tools and platforms at their disposal to plan and execute an effective marketing launch. Furthermore, fitness managers and marketers can greatly enhance their ability to make effective changes to the plan based on real-time data from their website, social media channels, and other information technology systems. The notion of "data drives decisions" couldn't be more relevant than in this marketing application.

The fifth and final step is to create a budget for your marketing plan. Most companies allocate a percentage of their gross sales to account for the marketing budget. In a start-up company, the money for the marketing budget can come from a variety of sources such as borrowing, self-funding, or acquired funding. The key is to invest in the marketing activities and tools that generate revenue. Fortunately, most social media channels are free. The social media enterprise platform Hootsuite is not free, but it offers features businesses can use to build their brand, grow followers, and manage social media. Hootsuite offers five different plans to match the size of the organization and its budget.

Developing strategic marketing plans begins with positioning your programs or services competitively and understanding your niche market. Entrepreneurs and marketers have suggested that "the riches are in the niches"—if the organization develops a strong strategic marketing plan and executes the plan properly. Not only does the fitness manager need to be able to articulate and define the market for the organization's programs and services, but he or she must also have a clear grasp of what the competitors are offering and have the ability to demonstrate how the facility's programs and services offer a superior value proposition. Because data drives decisions, the starting point, as in any marketing endeavor, is the collection of data.

## MARKETING RESEARCH

Have you ever taken a trip to a vacation destination such as Daytona Beach, Florida, and not known basic information such as the cost and availability of the lodging and transportation? Or have you ever written a research paper for a class without reviewing the scholarly literature on the topic? The obvious answer should be no. However, you would be surprised at how many organizations have said yes to the question "Have you ever crafted a marketing plan or campaign for a program without collecting and analyzing data in the internal and external environments?" Just like planning a great vacation or writing a compelling paper, marketing a program requires time and energy spent doing research. The data collected can be internal data like information from within the organization, such as past performance reports on revenue and retention, and **customer relationship management (CRM)** databases. Or the information can be external data such as analytics data generated from specific digital marketing channels, which is data gathered by other people or organizations.

Today, marketing scholars agree that companies need to collect and analyze external data but also need to go further by using information from across the industry: "the long-term survival of their business depends not only on

individual genius, but on the collective insights of many geniuses" (Davila, Oyon, Parmigiani, and Schnegg 2015, 62). In other words, although the fitness manager may take charge of creating and marketing a new program, the decisions made should leverage the experience and insights of other people. Data-focused fitness managers use collective information on how others in the industry manage the adoption of emerging technologies or launching new programs; how consumers respond, behave, or engage across digital marketing channels; and shifts in industry trends. Fitness managers need to rely on collective insights when beginning the process of collecting and analyzing data in the internal and external environments. These data and insights should drive strategic marketing decisions.

## Needs Analysis

The needs analysis process is the foundation for creating and marketing your program. It is critical to first establish a need, want, or desire that exists in the target market. The needs analysis utilizes information previously gathered in the initial research; however, this is the stage where the specific need, want, or desire for the program gets identified. A fitness manager can also incorporate the use of surveys, focus groups, and interviews with potential consumers and staff as another method to collect quantitative or qualitative data. In other words, this data collected should be designed and crafted to target a hierarchy of needs for growth potential and future programming. After collecting this data, the data should be analyzed in context, examining the size of the target market, the planned brand position, sales forecasting, retention, future programming, and profitability goals over a period of 1 to 3 years. The needs analysis must consider each contextual aspect in order to predict the results of launching a new program.

Now, let's suppose the fitness manager has identified the need for a new program, the 60-Day Transformation Challenge. The next step of the needs analysis is to provide a rationale that addresses the why, what, and how of the marketing communication message. Savvy marketers understand *why* they are promoting what they are promoting, *what* they are offering, and *how* one can participate. Once they know the why, what, and how, the fitness manager and everyone in the organization are now able to communicate and market a story around the 60-Day Transformation Challenge.

As leadership thought leader Simon Sinek said during a TED Talk, "People don't buy what you do; they simply buy why you do it." Fitness managers marketing their programs should communicate to the public *why* they offer what they do. This approach resonates with the market.

## Trends Analysis

A trends analysis is a key component of crafting any **strategic marketing plan**. Fitness managers should undertake this analysis using surveys, focus groups, interviews, and observations of consumer behavior. This analysis will provide fitness managers an understanding of the trends and behavior observed in the marketplace. Furthermore, the trends analysis report should serve the organization in determining the direction and viability of future products, services, or programs based on the data, driving decisions to establish future market projections. Many entrepreneurs attribute success in business to getting ahead of the trend in order to gain a competitive advantage. In the fitness industry, for example, some fitness facilities analyzed the impact of the 2008 recession on the U.S. market on fitness programming and began to offer more group training sessions, a more affordable choice than personal training sessions for their clients who had less discretionary income. Although this was a bold move to make, those fitness organizations saw a trend based upon data and implemented a model for semi-personalized training that still exists today. Another example centers around the baby boomer generation: A few years ago, we started to see an increase in programming for this target demographic due to a need that was identified through the trend analysis process. Can you think of any other trends?

A great tool that fitness managers can use to organize a part of the trends analysis is a **SWOTT analysis**. The SWOTT acronym represents **s**trengths, **w**eaknesses, **o**pportunities, **t**hreats, and **t**rends. Formerly called *SWOT analysis*, the term evolved to include another *T*—trends for where the organization is heading. SWOTT analysis is a concept covered in many other textbooks, and many resources offer guidance on how to conduct an effective SWOTT analysis. The important thing for you to know now is that this important analysis tool now benefits from keeping a pulse on the trends of a given industry.

In addition to trends in the industry, there can also be trends in the way we communicate and market. For example, *Forbes* reported that 65% of the adult U.S. population are visual learners (McClue 2013). Thus, a savvy marketer might look at whether other organizations are using more visual tools or digital platforms to connect or engage with their intended target markets. A trends analysis could reveal an increase in fitness organizations' using more social media sites such as Facebook, Twitter, Pinterest, and Instagram and using blogs with pictures and videos to communicate marketing content. Although marketing practitioners understand the importance of innovation, an organization must read the environment and then enhance the pool of possibilities; it is this combination of responsiveness and innovation that leads the market in a new direction.

Live-streaming video tools such as Periscope, Facebook Live, Instagram Stories, and YouTube Live have emerged as a trend that marketers are using to promote their brands, products, services, or programs as well as engage with their followers on social media channels. Current market analysis reveals that internet users have an average of 5.54 social media accounts (Ahmad 2017). This data might prompt a club to analyze the need to pursue the use of live streaming video as well as determine which social media accounts they should be putting video on. The best way to make use of a trends analysis is to organize and carefully examine the information.

The following list is an easy and consistently practical way to track emerging trends:

- Go to www.IHRSA.com and www.clubindustry .com for specific fitness management information and reports

- Follow @IHRSA and @clubindustry on Twitter

- Go to the conferences of professional organizations such as the American College of Sports Medicine and the National Strength and Conditioning Association, and follow them on Twitter

- Go to U.S. government websites such as www.cdc.gov and www.Nutrition.gov

- Follow @MayoClinic or @HarvardHealth on Twitter for their daily blogging information
- Follow fitness equipment companies that specialize in areas of interest to you on Twitter
- Follow universities that specialize in areas of interest to you on Twitter
- Follow professors or experts in the field of interest to you on Twitter

Can you think of any others organizations, groups, or people to follow that can provide information for a trends analysis report?

## Competition Analysis

A highly strategic marketing plan must include a competitive analysis. It is amazing to learn how many organizations in the fitness industry market their programs without an understanding of their competitors' strengths and weaknesses and these companies' products, services, membership, and programs. The competitive analysis in marketing can be compared to the game preparation in a team sport such as football. If you asked a student-athlete "What kind of activities did you engage in to gain intelligence regarding your opponent this week?," the answer may be something like this: "First of all, my coaches provided me with a scouting report that detailed the strengths and weaknesses of the team as well as a two-deep depth chart by position. Our offensive line coach had us watch previous game films so we could understand the opponent's tendencies, formations, stunts, and blitz schemes. Finally, during the week of practices, we scrimmaged against our scout team, and they ran plays similar to those our opponent tends to use."

To extend this football team analogy, let's think about what is in a scouting report. The marketing equivalent of this report would include a plethora of information that provides the fitness manager with a competitive analysis in the areas of **points of parity (POPs)** and **points of difference (PODs)** in the mind of the consumer. Once the fitness manager has assessed where the company is equal to the competition (POPs) and the competitive differences (PODs) that exist in the marketplace, he or she can refine effective strategies to improve the company's competitive position. The POPs and PODs model is about the perception of the consumer, because most marketing is based

upon a competitive frame of reference. In other words, the fitness manager should examine the program based on the *perceived* POPs and PODs.

The "previous game films" in our football team analogy represents listening to vlogs and reading comments about your competitors. Consumers now have the ability to publically express how they feel about their fitness experiences (e.g., program offerings, customer service, pricing) through social media conduits. This public two-way communication stream is one of the main differences between traditional marketing and digital marketing. Although collecting and analyzing this type of information about your competitors might take considerable time, depending on the competitor, this current information provides fitness managers with a more thorough competitive analysis. Keep in mind, though, that the claims made in comments about your competitors are not always reliable—there is a lot of false information on the internet.

Just as the football team examines the opponent's tendencies and plays, fitness professionals can study their competitors' tendencies by making side-by-side comparisons of marketing messages in each marketing outlet. For example, how does your Facebook marketing compare to that of your competitors' Facebook marketing? Some fitness organizations have the staff meet regularly to strategically discuss the latest information regarding their key direct and indirect competitors. It is easy today for fitness managers to take a screenshot of advertising or promotions posted on a competitor's website, blog, or social media page. Similarly, it is easy to follow competitor-generated hashtags or key words used in search engines to determine ranking.

It is important for fitness managers to understand the differences between direct and indirect competitors, because these differences affect strategic marketing planning. For the purposes of this chapter, direct competitors are those competitors that compete directly and offer the same (or very similar) products, services, amenities, and programs in the same demographic and geographic areas. An example of direct competitors would be Bally's Total Fitness, Life Time Fitness, Planet Fitness, and Gold's Gym facilities within a 10-mile radius in a suburban area. While each of these competitors certainly has some distinct differences, the consumer sees that they all offer memberships, cardiovascular equipment, strength training equipment, personal training, and a plethora of fitness assessments. An indirect competitor is an organization that offers some similar products, services, amenities, and programs in the same geographic area but to a different clientele in terms of demographics or psychographics. Within the same 10-mile radius, the indirect competitors would be the YMCA, the city's recreation center, the city's athletic club, and a specialized sports facility. The key point to remember is that any organization that can generate revenue from your target market is considered to be the competition. Classifying a competitor as direct or indirect requires a level of discretion, but competition analysis is vital to the success of your strategic marketing planning and brand positioning.

# IDENTIFYING TARGET MARKETS

The marketing efforts of any business start with understanding who your typical customer is and shaping your marketing accordingly. Sounds simple, right? Think again. Imagine the challenge of having a training center that specializes in custom fitness and in sports performance. The target market made up of 35- to 55-year-old business professionals looks completely different from the target market of high school and college athletes in explosive plyometrics development programs. This doesn't mean that an organization cannot serve both target markets; this scenario is meant to demonstrate the challenge of shaping or crafting your marketing efforts to your separate target markets. A common mistake some fitness organizations make is putting too much marketing focus on one audience—for example, heavily promoting, on their website and social media, amazing photos and stories of athletes improving their performance as a result of participating in the explosive plyometrics development program. Now a 50-year-old woman who uses Google to search for custom fitness or weight loss is taken to this company's website; she is bombarded with photos and video testimonials of 20-year-old athletes. Then, only after further digging on the company's website, she sees one small tab to click on to get custom fitness information. One of the greatest challenges many fitness managers face is identifying their target markets and aligning the

appropriate amount of marketing activity toward those specific target markets. The marketing challenge escalates if the facility is multipurpose such as an athletic club, the YMCA, or a recreation center. So let's now break down a simple system for organizing target markets.

By identifying target markets, an organization can focus its marketing budget and brand message on a specific market that has a greater potential to purchase the programs and services. It is possible for a smaller facility to compete against larger facilities by specializing in a niche market. However, many fitness organizations use a target market approach that is considered a much more affordable, systematic, and powerful method to reach potential clients and generate revenue. A common way to identify your target markets is to organize them as primary, secondary, and tertiary. The target markets are classified according to the percentage of revenue, for example: primary 70%-80%, secondary 15%-20%, and tertiary 5%-10%. By using this classification, everyone involved in sales and marketing can understand who is being targeted as a consumer and which target market should get the greatest focus. To reach this point in the marketing process, you must have first conducted extensive marketing research to understand exactly who the consumer is.

The next step is to carefully consider the **demographics** of the specific target. These are factors such as age, location, gender, income level, education level, marital status, ethnicity, and occupation. Then consider the **psychographics** (psychological characteristics) to target specifically. These factors include personality, attitudes, values, lifestyle, and interests. Fitness managers must select those relevant factors from the demographics and psychographics list and pair them with the primary, secondary, and tertiary target markets. Here is a simple example:

## COMPANY: BEYOND FITNESS

### Program: SilverSneakers
Primary target market: baby boomers

- Demographics: men and women; ages 51-69; living within a 20-minute radius of Chesterfield, Missouri; $150,000 family income
- Psychographics: interest in group classes, positive outlook on life, priorities of health and family

Secondary target market: Generation X

- Demographics: men and women; ages 35-50; living within a 20-minute radius of Chesterfield, Missouri; $150,000 family income
- Psychographics: interest in group classes, positive outlook on life, priorities of health and family, interest in exercising with parents

Tertiary target market: beyond baby boomers

- Demographics: men and women; ages 70 and over; living within a 10-minute radius of Chesterfield, Missouri; $50,000 income level; retired from the workforce; single or widowed
- Psychographics: interest in group fitness, positive outlook on life, priorities of health and socializing

# DEFINING MARKETING GOALS AND OBJECTIVES

Experienced personal trainers or fitness managers know how to establish goals for their clients that are measurable and identify objectives that support those goals. However, students or aspiring fitness managers who have never established specific goals and objectives may not even know where to begin when trying to make goals for marketing. Therefore, this section will provide a roadmap to assist in this process for marketing a program. The first step is making sure that all goals established are *measurable*! Measurable goals set a benchmark or target for everyone involved with the marketing process. It is paramount that goals be **SMART goals**: **s**pecific, **m**easurable, **a**ttainable, **r**ealistic, and with **t**imelines established. Marketing goals should fit into and reinforce the organization's big-picture business goals such as revenue, retention, profitability, growth potential, and branding. Objectives are the activities that support the goals. See the following page for an example of a sales goal for a fitness center offering personal training.

## Customer Relationship Management (CRM) Marketing

A customer relationship management (CRM) system helps fitness managers identify and target the organization's best customers, manage marketing campaigns with clear goals and objectives, track and measure details about customer behavior, and guide data-driven decisions and more profitable relationships. The CRM software allows fitness facilities to execute a sales strategy and repeat a sustainable process using a data-mining technology built for sales, marketing, and support. The CRM software is designed to generate more sales and to retain more customers. The better CRM systems provide a competitive advantage for customer service teams by keeping customers satisfied and loyal. Other advantages to using CRM are to manage marketing campaigns more effectively, boost efficiency, and deploy content in a cloud. CRM systems integrate seamlessly with existing customer applications. When considering this type of management tool, the best way to evaluate and choose a CRM solution is to define the requirements, establish budgetary considerations, research several vendors, and gain consensus from your organization.

## Data-Driven Marketing

Because advertising budgets in the fitness industry are often limited, fitness managers and marketers today are expected to do more with less. One of the biggest mistakes in health club marketing is overreaching the target market by spreading the net too wide. Traditional methods of advertising such as direct mail are beginning to be phased out due to the high costs; however, many owners and operators have a mindset of quantity over quality and still believe in the notion of marketing to the masses to increase revenue. This mindset restricts the organization's ability to expand their marketing arsenal with modern options such as social media, digital advertising, and referrals. Taking a quality-over-quantity approach to marketing, health clubs can stretch their advertising dollars by using technology to reach out to the most likely prospects.

**Data-driven marketing** is the strategic leveraging of customer information for precisely focused media buying and creative messaging. Marketing scholars and practitioners agree that data-driven marketing is one of the greatest innovations that the marketing industry has ever experienced. Before this technology, marketers had a limited capacity and visibility when receiving information to questions such as *who, when, where,* and *what message*. Today, those questions are answered utilizing the data from decision-making information technology.

## Goal 1: The personal training program will generate $100,000 per month in sales revenue.

**Objectives**

- Each trainer will engage in a minimum of six paid training sessions on each day of a 5-day work week.
- Each trainer will engage in one or two new member orientations on each day of a 5-day work week.
- Each trainer will procure a closing ratio of 70%. The closing ratio is a calculation of how many new clients purchased personal training sessions in comparison to how many complimentary sessions were completed.
- Each trainer will procure a retention ratio of 50%. The retention ratio is a calculation of how many existing clients purchased additional training sessions once their sessions was completed in comparison to how many were up for renewal.
- Each trainer will allocate 30 minutes of unpaid training session time toward professional development; this includes role playing with colleagues, reading books and blogs, viewing videos, refining presentation skills, knowing the company's why, and others activities that foster improvement and training in the area of sales.

A practical guideline for fitness managers establishing marketing goals and objectives would be three to five goals with three to seven objectives.

The following is an example of short-terms goals and objectives for marketing a branded personal training program:

*Goal 1:* Establish a 10% increase in website traffic and inquiries on a monthly basis

**Objectives**

- Post a new blog daily on the benefits of health or personal training
- Post weekly a new 60-second testimonial video that targets the primary market
- Use hashtags daily to drive social media traffic to website

*Goal 2:* Establish a 20% monthly engagement rate on Twitter

**Objectives**

- Post content related to health and personal training programs three to five times each day
- Post one or two call-to-actions (CTAs) each day using a Bitly link to track URL link activity
- Use the Twitter social media daily calendar for special posts: #MotivationMonday, #TransformationTuesday, #WellnessWednesday, #TBT (Throwback Thursday), and #FunFriday
- Post a weekly contest for best fitness selfie (the winner earns a gift certificate)

*Goal 3:* Procure a 20% conversion rate for first-time buyers on the website each month

*Goal 4:* Procure two new followers per day on Facebook, Twitter, and Instagram

*Goal 5:* Procure a 20% conversion rate for CTA incentive posts on Facebook

## Targeting Demographics Through Technology

Due to budget constraints, a Midwestern sports club was only able to mail a direct mail piece to 10,000 houses over the past 20 years, with just 500 houses receiving the marketing message each year. As of 18 months ago, though, the club began taking a new approach by using technology and data-driven marketing. By tracking trends and targeting based on demographic data, this sports club has now been able to reach 6,000 houses using 10 to 12 customized messages. Technology provides business and marketing intelligence to the health club operators in real time and helps them target and better reach their customers in a more cost-effective manner.

There are three main benefits to using data-driven marketing: buying the most appropriate paid media options based on projected value, targeting the right consumers, and strategically messaging audiences with relevant messages. Data-driven marketing is a natural evolution from CRM; these software systems opened the doors to a new category known as *marketing automation software*. (More information on marketing automation tools can be found in the Evaluating Marketing Programs section later in this chapter.)

## PLANNING THE COMPANY BRAND AND PROGRAM BRAND

Knowing the history of the company and its story seems like an easy task to accomplish, so it is surprising to learn that many fitness managers or those involved in marketing truly do not know the evolution and mantra of the organization they market. As stated earlier in the chapter, a company's *why* should play a significant role in corporate communication, branding, advertising, and promotions. The first step in understanding the company is learning about those founding individuals involved with casting the mission of the organization, and why they decided to pursue the opportunity. Fitness managers need to know the vision of the organization's founders to align the company values with that mission and vision moving forward. It is also imperative for a fitness manager to know and understand the importance of the company's **corporate social responsibility (CSR)** initiatives, because these contribute to the well-being of the communities on which the company depends. Most organizations in the fitness industry use their website and select social media sites to provide information about their CSR activities and their involvement in serving the community. Identify the CSR initiatives of your organization. Do those CSR initiatives align with the company's vision, mission, and values?

It is critical that aspiring fitness managers understand the role and importance of **branding**. A simple mistake many fitness managers and marketers make in creating and marketing a new program is not effectively branding the program. In other words, a fitness manager might communicate that the organization offers boot camps, but it is marketed generically with only the company's corporate branding associated. Stronger market positioning results from creating a specific program brand that captures the essence of the program and ties to the company's vision, mission, and values. What is the purpose of a brand? Peter Drucker would argue the purpose of a brand is "to create a customer" (Morgan 2015). However, a more modern view of a brand's purpose might be to create a culture. This culture is associated with a way of life that is true to the organization's beliefs, values, and personality. According to a 2017 ranking of top brands in *Business Insider*, based on factors such as consumer familiarity and loyalty, Disney ranked sixth, Nike ranked third, Google ranked second, and Lego took the top honors (Rath 2017). Great brands are no accident, and they can significantly affect consumers' perceptions and behavior toward a product. Therefore, today's fitness managers must understand the concept of brand strength and brand value when creating a program brand that will resonate with the target market.

To illustrate this branding concept, the company Nike is a brand. The brand mantra of Nike is "Authentic athletic performance," their logo is

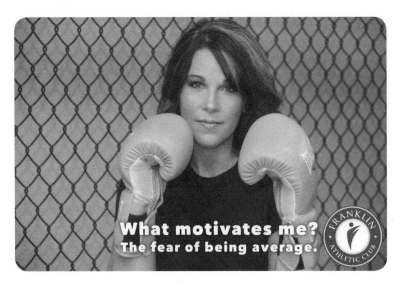

Example of a motivational fitness picture posted on social media for Franklin Athletic Club (Southfield, Michigan).

Photo courtesy of Franklin Athletic Club.

the Nike swoosh, and Air Jordan is a brand of footwear and athletic clothing produced by Nike that is endorsed by former Chicago Bulls basketball player Michael Jordan. Some popular program brands in the fitness industry are associated with personal training, boot camps, sport-specific training, Pilates, and yoga. SilverSneakers, a fitness class program that facilities across the United States offer to seniors, is an excellent example of a program brand.

## Company Name and Logo

The company name and logo plays a pivotal role in brand planning and marketing. This business name will be the company's first impression on the public and prospects. Therefore, strategically selecting a good name influences the ability to generate revenue. Choosing a good name that represents the brand makes it easier to spend more time on prospecting new clients, because you won't waste time explaining or justifying your company name. Business scholars agree that effective company names can be generated from a family name, such as Gold's Gym (founded by Joe Gold), or from the territory you work in, such as World Gym (also founded by Joe Gold). (As a side note, using your name as the company name has one major drawback: If you later sell the business to an outside group, your name will continue to be associated with a brand that someone else

controls.) A clever and appropriate name can wow your fan base; a dull name suggests a lack of creativity to the public. Some of the best company names are short and sweet, and some even invent their words. Nike, Under Armour, Aflac, Starbucks, Apple, Equinox, Planet Fitness, Life Time Fitness, Anytime Fitness, and Curves are all great names that meet these criteria.

The name of a company is paramount to gain a strong first impression when entering the market space. According to *MIT Sloan Management Review*, effective corporate company logos can demonstrate a significant favorable effect on consumer commitment to a brand (Whan Park, Eisingerich, and Pol 2014). Being able to differentiate your brand from your competition is pivotal to business survival. Furthermore, communicating the values and benefits of your brand is also a key for business growth. Crafting the right look and feel of a logo to convey a certain mantra is one area fitness managers cannot neglect if building a brand, a promise, to the intended target market, is a recipe for success. Therefore, as consumers continue to identify, differentiate, and draw favorable associations through an effective corporate logo, today, companies can leverage their logo as a *synthesizer* of the brand. An effective company logo makes it easier for the brand to stand out among all the media noise and clutter. One consideration when designing a logo is the connotation of the colors used: Each color reflects a specific image or message to the consumer. (The specifics of what associations' consumers have with various colors go beyond the scope of this chapter, but there are many resources available on this topic.)

## Program Name and Logo

As previously stated, the program name and logo play an important role in brand planning and marketing. Fitness managers must spend the research and creative time necessary to craft an effective program name and logo that will grab attention and resonate with the target market. An effective program name is appropriate to the business and unique enough to capture attention. Ideally, the program name should indicate the program's key points of difference to the consumer. As a side note, the program name should also be considered for use as a **hashtag** that the organization can use on all digital marketing platforms. (The use of hashtags will be discussed later in the chapter.) A great example of a program name is SilverSneakers; this program name associates a connection with their target market: baby boomers and beyond. The SilverSneakers name is matched with a highly identifiable logo that stands out from the crowd. Like the program name, the program logo should be attention getting. Also, the color of the logo needs to be considered; science indicates that emotions are associated with particular colors. (There are online resources available to view a color emotion guide.) The goal is to use the color associated with the desired emotion for the target market.

A best practice for a fitness manager or marketer is to conduct a focus group in which individuals view side-by-side comparisons of different program names and logos to see the initial perception of the brand logo and name. This type of comparison is quite conventional and is useful in most situations. However, in today's modern era of digital marketing and use of social media, another option to consider is to run a contest on Twitter, Facebook, or blogs, and let the followers weigh in regarding their reactions to the program name or logo. However, this strategy may be difficult in a start-up business because there will be few followers. Nevertheless, this is a strategy that can help drive engagement with the organization's followers on social media channels.

## Mantra

The mantra is an essential part of the brand planning. A brand mantra usually consists of three to five words that capture the essence of the brand. The brand mantra is considered internal to the organization, because it is not usually used as an advertising slogan. If you asked the average person what Nike's mantra is, most would answer "Just do it." But that's not their brand mantra! "Just do it" is merely an iconic tagline that works very well in print media, social media, and their world-class TV ads. Nike's actual brand mantra is "Authentic athletic performance." The purpose of the brand mantra is to assist Nike executives in the process of guiding future decisions regarding product introductions under the brand and what specific ad campaigns to launch. Another all-time classic brand mantra is that of Disney: "Fun family entertainment." A brand mantra is a crucial part of the brand planning and takes time to develop. It is imperative that fitness managers today take the necessary steps to develop a strong company and program mantra and then make sure everyone within the organization know them—the mantra provides guidance as to where the company should and should not go.

## SOCIAL MEDIA MARKETING

The explosion of social media use continues: Facebook alone is on the brink of reaching two billion monthly active users. And it is no surprise that most other social networking channels and apps are experiencing record-breaking numbers of users. Today, **social media marketing (SMM)** continues to evolve; there are seemingly endless possibilities to engage with followers across a plethora of channels, network, or apps. The concept of **social media engagement** has emerged as a hot trending topic among practitioners and marketing scholars alike as marketers leverage their social media marketing efforts to advance their brand, products and services, and business revenue performance. There appears to be a consensus among practitioners and marketing scholars that social media engagement is an important marketing objective and performance metric (Marketing Science Institute 2013; McKinsey and Company 2014; Mersey, Malthouse, and Calder 2010).

However, there currently is no consensus on exactly what constitutes this form of "engagement" (Syrdal and Briggs 2018). This creates an interesting situation for fitness owners, managers, and marketers in the fitness industry seeking to take advantage of and leverage the use of social media marketing.

Too many fitness organizations view and use social media as a traditional external marketing initiative; they lack the understanding that "to advance from social media advertising to social media engagement, your business needs to develop your tactical approach to harvesting social media content, how you will understand the message behind the content and isolate those conversations that are important to achieving your business goals, and how to respond to further develop that relationship so you achieve your objective" (Hiltbrand 2015, 10). A survey of top executives outside the fitness industry identi-fied digital customer engagement as the highest priority among a list of several possible digital initiatives (McKinsey and Company 2014). The key to success in using social media marketing is right there in the term itself: Just be social. As previously mentioned, the use of hashtags instantly allows organizations the opportunity to engage with their customers and prospects on social media channels by taking an active role in real-time conversations. Club owners, managers, and marketers have diligently worked for years on strategies to get people to interact and engage in their fitness facilities. Now it's time to make the shift from traditional thinking and strategy to social media marketing, which conveniently allows fitness facilities to interact and engage outside the four walls of the facility. Social media creates an opportunity for fitness managers and marketers the ability to reach and engage with your entire target market and beyond.

## Social Media Marketing

As a general rule, attraction is the first step for success in social media marketing (SMM). Therefore, here are five ways to craft engaging content that can be shared easily across social media channels:

1. *Vary your content.* Too many SMM content producers stick to their one favorite medium to communicate and connect with their audience. SMM experts suggest that diversifying your content through the use of videos, graphics, images, infographics, quotes, and streaming broadcasts is a simple way to produce highly creative and attention-grabbing content. In other words, you need to become the content equivalent of a Swiss Army knife.

2. *Keep it short.* This applies when using videos (other than live streaming broadcasts); YouTube states on their website that nearly 50% of all video viewers stop watching after the first minute. This also applies to text; after all, Twitter only allows 280 characters.

3. *Develop your social media voice.* Companies that have great brands write social media content that has a distinctive writing voice or style. Developing your social media voice and persona can add value to your SMM by offering new or creative perspectives to stale content.

4. *Create attention-grabbing titles.* Even if you have crafted amazing content to share, many people you're trying to reach will never read it, because social media users typically decide to read content based on the title. Here's a simple comparison of two different titles for the same content posted on Twitter: example 1: "The Four Latest Trends in Activity-Tracking Wearable Fitness Technology"; example 2: "Four Biggest Lies of Fitness Wearables Technology." There is certainly nothing wrong with the example 1 title; it communicates information a reader can understand. However, example 2 creates a stronger level of intrigue, especially to a reader looking for or interested in fitness wearable technology.

5. *Master the art of storytelling.* This is not as challenging as it seems if you have relevant personal stories or experiences and are willing to share interesting things that your readers do not know. Using the hashtag #TBT (the social media acronym for "throwback Thursday") is an appropriate way to share interesting content from the past that relates to the present.

It is a good idea to go to the website of each social media channel and learn about the features and benefits of the channel. It is also good to repeat this process on a regular basis, because it is common for these tools to be updated on a frequent basis as features, functions, and integrated applications may change. The changes and updates may affect your entire SMM strategy.

One of the most popular categories of photos in social media is the selfie. A **selfie** is easy: one person holds a smartphone away from him or herself and snaps a picture. There are inexpensive selfie sticks that can make it easier to take the photo. The following is a list of three ways to incorporate selfies into your social media marketing strategy.

1. Hold a contest for the best selfie of the week with your followers at your facility.

2. Hold a contest for the best selfie of the week using a branded frame at your facility that your followers can stand in front of to take the selfie.

3. Create an incentive program to encourage your followers to post a selfie on your social media channels such as Facebook, Twitter, or Instagram using your organization's or program's hashtag. The incentive might be a discount or a club gift card given to anyone who posts a selfie.

Live video has become a popular tool for social media marketers; as Facebook CEO Mark Zuckerberg revealed, "People watch live streams 300% longer and comment ten times more than regular videos" (Bullas 2017). From a marketer's perspective, incorporating live video into your SMM strategy would be game changing—as long as the video content is relevant to your brand and your followers want to consume the content. The most common apps on a smartphone to stream live broadcasts are Facebook Live, Periscope (owned by Twitter), Instagram Live, YouTube Live, and UStream. Keep in mind that each has differences, so a comparison may be needed to decide which app best meets the needs for a particular company and particular use. What types of content should be live streamed? Here are a few ideas to consider:

1. Stories
2. Events
3. Contests
4. Behind-the-scenes features
5. Demonstrations of new equipment
6. Launches of new programs

Fitness managers and marketers must understand that timing in social media marketing is paramount: When you post matters. What are the optimal times to make posts? There is no simple answer; it depends on the demographics of the audience and which social media channels are being used. However, a best practice to implement is to send messages or make posts when the audience is available to see and engage with them. Here is some helpful information and data to shed insight on the best times to post:

- A Facebook post reaches 75% of its projected engagement within 5 hours.

- A tweet on Twitter reaches 75% of its projected engagement within 3 hours.

- According to Hootsuite, the ideal time to tweet on Twitter is at 3 p.m. on a weekday (Monday through Friday). Live streaming via Twitter and Periscope can be very beneficial, especially when centered around events occurring on the weekends.

- According to Hootsuite, the ideal time to post on Facebook is between 12 p.m. and 3 p.m. on Monday, Wednesday, Thursday, or Friday and between 12 p.m. and 1 p.m. on Saturday or Sunday.

- A social media marketing management tool such as Hootsuite allows automatic scheduling to select the exact time to make a post appear.

The fitness manager or marketer should be aware of the pitfalls that often lead to less-than-desirable outcomes with using social media marketing. The following list reveals the top mistakes made by people involved with running their organization's social media channels.

## TOP 12 SOCIAL MEDIA MARKETING MISTAKES

1. Not establishing clear and measurable marketing goals and objectives

2. Blogging on topics beyond the scope of your business

3. Overusing the technique of newsjacking (aligning your brand with a current event)

4. Failing to respond to customer concerns

5. Not adding perceived value to your customer base

6. Making too many posts related to sales promotion

7. Not incorporating images and videos

8. Not creating a social media voice and lacking personality in posts

9. Not using a social media calendar

10. Regularly posting poor-quality content

11. Neglecting to monitor data analytics

12. Failing to build a marketing funnel

## Role of Social Media Hashtags

A hashtag is a word or phrase preceded by a hash or pound sign (#) and used to identify messages on a specific topic. Hashtags play a major role in social media marketing because they provide an easy method to search for specific content. Hashtags are analogous to key words used in an online search engine or key words entered into a database (the SPORTDiscus database, for example) in a university library. The hashtag provides fitness managers the ability to easily follow conversations about our brand and our programs and services. If used correctly, hashtags can also assist in keeping up with the latest developments happening in the fitness industry. Now, you're probably thinking to yourself, "I use hashtags all the time in my personal social media posts." That may be very true. However, you may not fully appreciate the scope and the enormous power of a hashtag, as thousands of messages are being sent all over the world every second of the day.

One of the main reasons to use a hashtag is to target a highly specific audience. If the fitness manager wanted to see the latest conversations about CrossFit training, then the hashtag #CrossFit can be easily searched on Twitter. But here's the key point: By using the #CrossFit hashtag as you create content and post a message, those following this specific hashtag now have the potential to find you or your organization. A second great reason to use a hashtag is to see what others are saying about your company's or program's reputation when you create the hashtag. Think of using the hashtag as a monitoring tool to hear real-time feedback. Using the hashtag as a monitoring tool helps the organization improve customer service by listening to the concerns of members or even prospects.

Another strong reason to use hashtags—and one of the more popular uses found within the fitness industry—is to promote your special events,

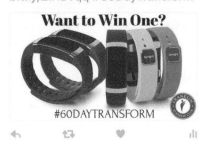

FranklinAthleticClub · 1/29/17

LAST DAY you can enter to WIN the world's first #wearable band that measures BF%. Click for info bit.ly/2iHBvqq #60DayTransform

**Want to Win One?**

#60DAYTRANSFORM

Social media call-to-action (CTA) content Twitter post using timeline-based incentive.

contests, or deals. Even those people who cannot attend the event can still follow the conversation and stay connected, giving you publicity that goes beyond the event itself. This is very true with the hashtag of a professional conference, such as #ACSM17 or #IHRSA17. The hashtag allows the fitness manager to stay connected and engage in the conversation while the event is happening live, even if not in attendance. Finally, hashtags allow the organization to keep current on the latest developments with their competition. Following the right hashtag can provide valuable information, especially when posting upcoming contests or deals on social media. In the modern era of social media marketing, the practical application of regularly using hashtags is paramount for the organization to maximize and leverage its reach using the social media channels.

## Creating a Social Media Marketing Calendar

One of the greatest challenges organizations face when using social media is keeping track of all content, messaging, images, videos, and URL links for each social media channel. Thankfully, fitness managers and marketers can use the free templates from the websites of HubSpot or Hootsuite or others for the purpose of creating a social media marketing calendar. These templates can greatly help with social media content planning for Facebook, Twitter, LinkedIn, Instagram, Pinterest, and Google+. Because every social media channel or network has its own nuances, a different worksheet should be used for every network, and the templates organize this for you. The templates are easy to use and relatively self-explanatory. However, you cannot just create one single social media update simultaneously. Although you do have the ability to promote the same piece of content across all six of those networks, you will need to figure out how to craft your update for each of them. Remember, one of the goals of using the templates is to leverage your social media strategy and connect the gap between where you are now and where you want to be in the pursuit of your social media goals. These templates will save you and your organization considerable time, energy, and effort.

Another reason creating a social media calendar is a good practice is that multiple people are involved in the process of providing input. For example, during the company's weekly social media calendar meeting someone may be put in charge of procuring photos, and once the photos are gathered another person is in charge of creating graphics with the photos, and then someone else is in charge of crafting the story and writing the attention-grabbing headline. The social media calendar can serve as the main hub for all personnel involved in crafting everything needed to make a tweet on Twitter or a post on Facebook, Instagram, or Pinterest. Because of the complexity of organizing several moving parts, it is imperative for the person responsible for the calendar to create a systematic process flow so everyone involved understands their roles and function, the rules of engagement, branding standards, and timelines. The social media calendar should include all planned social media messaging, organized by date and time.

The social media calendar's main function is to guide, organize, and plan all promotion using the social media channels or network. However, due to the real-time nature of interaction with live followers, social media engagement cannot always be planned ahead. Not all social media posts should rely solely on the content calendar. Let's say you have been promoting your upcoming 60-day Transformation Challenge for the past 60 days. Now, as people come into the facility to start the program, your staff is capturing photos or videos that you want to post in real time. Generally speaking, it is good to have a blend of automatically scheduled postings as well as real-time created content postings to further enhance engagement with your followers across the social media channels.

Social media platforms such as Hootsuite are valuable for managing multiple social networks, connecting with customers, and promoting the brand on social media. The Hootsuite "Social Media Management System" tool can be managed via desktop and with mobile devices, which will allow you to auto-schedule all your social network posts in one convenient dashboard. Using a social media management platform such as Hootsuite provides fitness managers or marketers the ability to easily schedule content, engage with customers, track social media campaigns using analytics, collaborate with team members to create messages, and listen to the things customers are saying about the facility, the brand, and even competitors.

## BEST PRACTICES IN MODERN MARKETING

The fundamental purpose of marketing is to grab the reader's attention. To do so, and to create a cohesive and forward-looking strategy that leverages social media and data analytics, fitness facilities should observe the following best practices.

### TOP 10 BEST PRACTICES

1. Identify and communicate what specifically makes your program different.
2. Start with your *why* in communicating your unique value proposition.
3. Master the art of storytelling in your marketing.
4. Create and use a functional social media calendar to organize your daily activity.
5. Always use Bitly.com to shorten URLs, measure traffic, and optimize links with real-time data activity reports.
6. Always use appropriate hashtags in your social media posts.
7. Craft attention-grabbing headlines for your posts.
8. Regularly monitor all social media analytics, website analytics, and CRM analytics data.
9. Use live streaming video broadcasts to connect and engage with your followers.
10. Use data to drive decisions in all marketing initiatives.

## Identifying What Makes Your Program Different

Differentiation plays a major role in consumer behavior and purchase decision making. Many organizations know their points of difference but do not properly communicate these differences to their intended audience. Consider this 2017 statistic by Statista: In 2016, there were 36,540 gyms (health clubs/fitness centers) in the U.S. market (Statista 2018). Now, imagine that a high percentage of those 36,540 gyms offer personal training, group fitness, and boot camps, and all those gyms are marketing those programs to compete for customers. Do you see where this is going from a marketing perspective? Consumers in some areas of the country are bombarded with personal training promotions. How can a facility differentiate themselves from 10 other local options, other than with price? Fitness managers looking to launch new programs must understand this marketing challenge of effectively communicating competitive differentiation to your target markets. How are you going to address it moving forward? What strategies are you going to implement and execute to cut through the clutter with your unique value proposition?

If you cannot distinguish your programs or services from those of the competitors, then how are they going to attract the specific market you're targeting? If the fitness manager or marketer has not identified what truly makes the programs or services different, then the public cannot possibly understand the differentiation.

Mastering the art and science of identifying and communicating what makes a fitness facility's programs and services different is paramount to effective marketing and is directly tied to revenue performance. Here are a few short strategies to consider when thinking about creative ways to communicate with your target market:

- Incorporate live streaming video broadcasts to show the public what makes your program different.
- Educate your followers using blogs.
- Use customer testimonials.
- Use social media to post examples of your differentiation.

## Reviewing Analytics

As noted earlier, an organization that engages only in social media advertising needs to transition to social media engagement to have the greatest impact on business performance. Club owners, managers, and marketers need to use the data generated in real time from social media analytics as a way to increase social media marketing power to increase profitability. Social media engagement has been associated with a plethora of positive outcomes, including increased sales (eMarketer 2015; Lake 2011) and increased brand loyalty (Powers et al. 2012).

There has been a remarkable shift in analytics technology over the past decade. The great news is that analytical technologies are now more powerful and more cost effective. The use of these technologies allows companies a greater capacity to store and analyze larger quantities and different type of data. As a result of recent technological advancements in analytics, analyses and recommendations are received nearly instantly due to the increased processing speeds. But due to the complexity of the data, expertise is required for optimizing these analytical tools, creating a need for organizations to develop specialists in data analytics and business intelligence. The advancements in analytics can greatly affect organizational success; however, to take advantage of the accessibility of the data, the organization's leaders must become more responsive and willing to change culture and strategy. Later in the chapter, we will examine analytics further in the context of evaluating marketing programs.

## WRITING AN EFFECTIVE MARKETING PLAN

Creating an effective marketing plan begins by answering the following two critical questions.

1. Who specifically is your target market?
2. How do they receive marketing information?

Once you have answered these two questions, you are then ready to move forward to the process of actually creating the marketing plan. Too many times marketing plans are created without a clear understanding of the answers to these two foundational questions.

Before we dive into the outline of the marketing plan, here are five essential factors to remember:

1. Identifying your target markets using demographics and psychographs data is a must.

2. Use of a social media calendar is a must for planning and executing SMM.

3. Establishing appropriate measurable goals and expectations for your SMM strategy is critical for success.

4. Using appropriate key performance indicators and analytics to monitor, measure, and analyze on a regular basis the effectiveness of your marketing plan will help you succeed.

5. Be willing to try new marketing strategies and tactics—each target market in a specific geographic area or market segment may interact and engage differently on various social media channels. (The age of a specific target market can affect social media engagement; research has shown millennials are not as active on Facebook as they were 5 years ago.) The key is to figure out how your audience receives their marketing information and use this to guide your communication.

The following outline for a marketing plan will help guide you through the process of creating your marketing plan.

# EVALUATING MARKETING PROGRAMS

When I teach undergraduate and graduate students about creating an effective marketing plan, I find it interesting that the topic of evaluation often challenges students. It is surprising, because exercise science majors in particular are usually exposed to a strong curriculum in the area of testing and measurement related to evaluating human performance biometrics ($\dot{V}O_2$max, body composition, etc.). This same concept of evaluation applies with marketing—the goal is to measure, using a plethora of tools, the effectiveness of the marketing plan. Measuring and analyzing the organization's marketing effectiveness are paramount to the success of the program. Let's take a look at some of the best ways to measure effectiveness using quantitative and qualitative methods.

1. *Marketing metrics.* These metrics include sales numbers, revenue, retention, return on investments (ROI), profit, and cost to acquire a new customer.

2. *Marketing goals.* To demonstrate whether the organization hit or exceeded your marketing goals, success could be measured in terms of whether there were any leads, sales, acquired users, converted customers, new followers on social media, or engagement rates.

3. *Marketing automation tools.* These tools measure website visits, page performance, blog hits, social media metrics, CRM reports, CTA clicks, and Bitly clicks.

4. *Surveys.* Surveys are still an effective way to capture invaluable information. The key is crafting a survey questionnaire in which the research objectives align with the questions posed. Research has shown that surveys that take only 5 to 10 minutes to complete yield the best results (Li, Pitts, and Quarterman 2008).

5. *Social media analytics.* Analytics data looks at impressions, profile visits, mentions, new followers, engagement, engagement rates, and social shares such as likes, shares, tweets, retweets, and commenting. Fitness managers and marketers can use the analytics data to understand the dynamic relationship between social media engagement and enhanced business performance.

6. *Google Analytics.* Google Analytics offers a variety of solutions to monitor website traffic, visitor engagement, and brand awareness.

7. *CRM analytics.* Using the analytics tools in CRM software helps you revisit your performance goals and the metrics you determined when implementing the CRM platform into your marketing plan.

## Electronic Surveys

Using online surveys is nothing new: For many years graduate students, faculty members, universities, and organizations have used online surveys to collect data, which they then analyze, make conclusions about, and sometimes publish in peer-reviewed journals. Although surveys are probably very familiar to you, you may not know some of the key elements that must be included in crafting a good online survey for marketing

## Marketing Plan Outline

1. *Executive summary.* Although this is the first content that is read, this section should be written *last*. The executive summary includes brief descriptions for the company and program; current status; products, services, and programs; market analysis; company objectives; financial ROI; top-level pricing; and funding plans.

2. *Introduction and rationale for the program.* This information includes the program name, logo, program description, rationale for program, competitive market overview (this includes communicating your program's point of differences), and benefits to the consumer.

3. *Goals and objectives.* This is the time to establish and articulate three to five goals and performance activities directly related to the goals.

4. *Scientific foundation of program.* This information includes a detailed description of the scientific foundations for the program through a brief literature review as well as any marketing research data or statistical information on trends.

5. *Target market identification.* This section lists the primary, secondary, and tertiary target markets, including demographics and psychographic information.

6. *Marketing strategy and tactics.* This information provides a strategic overview and details the tactics to be used in the marketing plan. This section includes the identification of marketing promotional items, a 6-month timeline and budget for marketing rollout, and direct and indirect competitor analysis and descriptions (including POPs and PODs).

7. *Social media marketing strategies.* This section establishes the goals and objectives for using SMM. It will identify which specific social media channels you plan to use to attract and engage each of your target markets. This section will explain how you plan to diversify your content through the use of videos, graphics, images, infographics, quotes, and streaming video broadcasts. Finally, this section will articulate how you envision using the social media analytics tools and social media content calendar.

8. *Social media content calendar.* In this section, you will provide an actual 30-day calendar that is completed based on the program you plan to market.

9. *Social media content.* Include examples of the content that you will share through social media, such as images that introduce the program, a video blog that introduces the program, a promotional image that offers an incentive or contest, tweets, and Facebook posts that use attention-grabbing titles.

10. *Sales projections.* This section should have a spreadsheet with a 1-year forecast for sales projections and 3-year projections of ROI. The key is to include the rationale behind the incremental increase or growth factor in years 2 and 3.

11. *Retention strategy.* This section should describe three or more retention strategies, with one example such as an actual survey.

12. *Educational materials.* The educational materials for the program could include a flyer, a 60-second education video, or a squeeze page that can be shared on social media.

13. *Marketing program evaluation.* This section would include the specific methods you plan to use to evaluate the effectiveness of your program.

14. *Call-to-action summary.* Other than the executive summary, this section is the most important section in the marketing plan because it provides the reader your call-to-action intentions. It tells what you are seeking. The purpose of creating a marketing plan is to get approval from someone in the organization so you can take action with your marketing strategies, so here is where you ask for that approval and the resources you will need.

15. *References.* This is a reference page that is formatted in APA style (*Publication Manual of the American Psychological Association, Sixth Edition*).

purposes, or the advanced ways a survey can be deployed. Therefore, let us begin this section by identifying a few key elements found in excellent survey questionnaires:

1. At least five research objectives of the questionnaire must identify and align with the questions posed. The importance of creating well-defined research objectives is the cornerstone for the survey questionnaire to specifically explore or examine what the data intended to collect. The researcher should consider asking as the following the: What is the purpose of this study? What do I need to know because of collecting this data? Why is this survey necessary in the first place? How will this data be disseminated and used? Is the data information accurate and timely? Finally, it is highly recommended the researcher refrain from asking a question that would be "interesting to know" if the question does not fall within the research objectives. In other words, as a best practice, the research should collect only information that is pertinent or relevant.

2. Avoid using a *yes* or *no* response when asking questions related to feelings, perceptions, or preferences. Using a five-point or seven-point Likert scale will produce better results and then can be used as quantitative data for future comparisons.

3. The optimal length of a survey should be between 5 and 10 minutes. (Avoid using too many open-ended general questions, which can create time issues for the respondent and the person reading the responses.)

Once you have created an excellent questionnaire, you need to decide on a method of deployment. The surveys can be given to the public via mobile, web, and social media.

## Google Analytics

Google Analytics is a free service that offers club operators the ability to track their website traffic and conversions. It uses a tracking code, which is created for the club upon sign-up. The Google Analytics tracking code provides club operators the ability to view the quantity of users visiting the site, the quality of users visiting the site based on variable parameters, and, most important, intelligence on how those users are attracted to and interacting with the site. Google Analytics provides a plethora of reports to meet your business goals and expectations. One report, the convenient audience overview, is a quick way to access and view the most information. There are many online tools to help you get the most out of the audience overview report. So take some time to familiarize yourself with this powerful tool, to review the capabilities of the various reports, and integrate them into your marketing goals and your strategic planning. In conclusion, using Google Analytics will greatly help you understand the activities that generate increases in traffic.

## Social Media Analytics

The best way to know and understand each social media channel's analytics is to go to the channel's website, where there is a wealth of information about the functional capability of each tool. Analytical data is easy to access and can be used even on the first day on the job. One of the best starting points in using social media analytics is to create a baseline for future comparisons. Facebook offers Facebook Insights, which provides a report on page likes, post reach, and engagement for the last 7 days of your page's performance. Twitter offers Twitter Analytics, which provides a snapshot of the past 28 days of your page's performance in the areas of tweet impressions, profile visits, mentions, and followers in addition to individual tweet impressions and engagement rates. This data is a simple way to get started using analytics to drive future marketing decisions by analyzing the data reports.

## Key Terms

branding

corporate social responsibility (CSR)

customer relationship management (CRM)

data analytics

data-driven marketing

demographics

digital marketing

hashtag

points of difference (PODs)

points of parity (POPs)

psychographics

SMART goals

selfie

social media engagement

social media marketing (SMM)

strategic marketing plan

SWOTT analysis

traditional marketing

# Increasing Membership Sales

## Learning Objectives

After studying this chapter, you will be able to

- recognize the importance of the relationship between membership representatives and reception-desk staff,
- be successful when using the phone to respond to membership information requests,
- understand how to create urgency during the tour,
- appreciate the importance of properly preparing yourself to sell, and
- understand the benefits of selling to corporate groups.

With his new club scheduled to open in 2 months, Roberto met with his sales staff to discuss membership presales. At the meeting, he reviewed all the information and club features that the staff would need to sell enough memberships to meet an aggressive presales goal.

After 2 weeks, Roberto was surprised to see that out of the 80 people who had come in for information, only 20 had purchased memberships. He asked the staff why this was, and their answers ranged from "They wanted to think about it" to "It's too expensive." He brought the staff back together to review the club's features and asked them to push prospects a little harder. A week later, sales had improved slightly but were nowhere near as high as he had forecasted.

Worried about starting out behind budget, Roberto discussed the situation with a colleague, who recommended a consultant who had helped him improve sales. After Roberto hired the consultant, the first thing she did was watch how the sales staff performed during the actual sales process. It quickly became apparent what the problems were, and she prepared a report with a corrective action plan. The consultant's analysis included these points:

- Sales personnel were not spending enough time developing rapport with clients. Customers are more likely to buy from someone they feel comfortable with.
- Sales personnel focused on the features of the club, like the equipment, swimming pool, and classes, rather than on the benefits to the customer. People won't buy something unless they understand exactly how it will benefit them.

The author acknowledges the significant contributions of Karen Woodard Chavez to this chapter.

- Sales personnel were not comfortable overcoming objections, and they let people walk away if they said they wanted to think about it or it was too expensive.

The consultant offered the following solutions:

- Train staff on how to build trust and rapport with clients.
- Train staff on how to better discuss the benefits that prospects will experience once they become members.
- Train staff on how to overcome objections by creating value and to view objections as another way of seeking more information without pressuring people into buying.

Training was initiated, and within 2 weeks Roberto saw a positive change in the closing percentage. Before the training, memberships were closed 25% to 35% of the time, but after the training, this increased to 50%. By the time the club opened, Roberto was slightly behind his initial membership projection but confident he would quickly reach the desired level. More important, he now understood the importance of a thorough sales training program in a competitive market with many consumer choices.

---

This chapter details several functions of the membership selling process. Before those functions are addressed, however, it is critical to clarify these elements:

- *Strong sales skills are critical to the success of any venture.* Club operators often fall into the trap of believing that a beautiful facility with lots of equipment will ensure their success. However, the fitness market is very competitive, and only the best will thrive. Although IHRSA reported that there were more than 60 million health club members in the United States in 2017 (20.3% of the U.S. population age 6 years and older) (International Health, Racquet, and Sportsclub Association 2018), it is important to remember that most Americans are not physically active and do not like to exercise. Convincing people to join a club is not as simple as giving a tour and wowing them with a nice facility and equipment. Successful selling is about understanding the reasons people say *yes* or *no* to a more active lifestyle that includes exercise in your club and then creating a compelling reason for them to say *yes.*

- *Strong sales skills are not about technique or manipulation.* Strong selling skills are about being the leader and being a good communicator. As you will read in this chapter, these skills include listening, asking the right questions, providing the right solutions for each potential member, and creating comfort in the decision.

This chapter covers the following essential elements of selling health club memberships:

- Fostering the partnership between the reception or service desk and the membership department
- Turning telephone calls and email inquiries into appointments
- Maximizing the face-to-face selling process

It does not address company-wide marketing campaigns, which were discussed in chapter 7. Note, however, that being able to generate your own leads rather than relying on the advertising campaigns of the club will be critical to your success.

## FOSTERING A PARTNERSHIP BETWEEN THE RECEPTION DESK AND THE MEMBERSHIP STAFF

This section focuses on the importance of a partnership between the reception-desk staff and the membership staff and how business can be lost if there isn't one. In a **partnership,** two or more parties contribute to a joint interest and share the risks and profits. You have a solid partnership between the reception desk and the membership department if the reception-desk staff do the following:

- Have a clear understanding of their roles as they relate to membership sales
- Give accurate information
- Understand how much information to give

- Give consistently positive and friendly greetings to prospective members
- Create a good first impression with prospects, setting up **membership representatives** for success

If you see the following, however, you must put energy into creating or strengthening the partnership:

- Incomplete tour cards
- Inconsistent greetings
- Inconsistent verbiage
- Inability to take control
- Lack of knowledge
- Poor attitude toward membership representatives

# Tools to Strengthen the Partnership

Fortunately, there are several tools you can implement to strengthen the sense of partnership among your staff. Here I discuss communication, incentives, and relationship support.

## Communication

Communication is vital to a strong partnership. Follow these guidelines to improve communication between the reception desk and the membership department:

- Choose a liaison from the reception desk to attend membership staff meetings and elect a liaison from membership to attend reception-desk meetings.
- Issue a weekly update for the two departments that includes updates on promotions (e.g., where advertisements are running), upcoming membership events, and upcoming projects the department may need help with. You should address anything the staff members need to know that will make them feel like part of the process.
- Keep an appointment sheet at the reception desk. Membership representatives can log their appointments on the sheet and include special notes the front-desk staff should know. When the reception-desk staff know who is coming in, they can give more familiar greetings, which is a professional and proactive way to create a positive first impression with the **prospective member**.

## Incentives

Incentives are one of the best ways to create a direct relationship between behavior and results; that's why so many clubs pay commissions as a large part of the compensation package for membership representatives. Some sort of incentive can help the reception-desk staff pay more attention to the membership sales process and what it takes to make it successful. The following are some possibilities:

- Give a small percentage of total membership commissions to the reception-desk staff. The reception desk bonus can be split based on the percentage of total hours worked by each staff member. For example, if the reception desk bonus for membership hitting or exceeding the goal is a pool of $500, a staff member who worked 20% of the hours gets 20% of this ($100).
- Dinners, movie tickets, and club or spa services are also valuable incentives.
- Consider giving some type of incentive even if a membership sale is not made. The process has to consistently work well to have long-term success, so a lower-level reward could be provided if crucial aspects of the process (greetings, phone verbiage, proper receipt of prospective members, completing guest and tour cards, being accurate, tracking expiring memberships) are regularly practiced at the reception desk.

Make sure all staff who are eligible for an incentive are aware of it and know how to get it. People often assume that staff members have all the information they need to do their jobs well, but this is not always the case.

## The Bottom Line

Because reception-desk staff members are partners in membership sales, they should get some kind of reward or perk when the club reaches its membership sales goals.

## Relationship Support

The most important thing you can do to support the partnership is ensure that reception-desk staff receive appropriate training from the beginning. They are often trained by the reception-desk manager, the operations manager, or the owner, and the emphasis is on answering phones, receiving members and guests, scheduling, and so on rather than on the importance of the membership process and how to affect it positively. Have the membership sales director incorporate membership-related training into the reception-desk training program, which will facilitate a better relationship between the reception-desk staff and the membership staff from the beginning.

When reception-desk employees do something well, let them know and thank them. Even if improvements are needed, let them know they did it 90% right and tell them how they can make it 100% right. Be sure to model the behavior for them.

## Tour Cards and the Reception Desk

Through effective marketing and promotion initiatives, prospective members will be driven to your health club to look around or for trial visits. One tool for improving the initial experience so a visitor is more likely to join is the tour card, which is used to capture prospect information and guide staff as they **interview** the member and begin developing a relationship. Effective use of this card by the membership staff and the reception desk will improve the guest experience and increase sales success.

The **tour card** is a strong sales tool for the membership representative. Although most clubs have tour cards, they don't maximize their benefits. If designed and used correctly, they can be one of the best tools for building rapport, gathering needs and motivation information, and setting the sales process up for success. Some

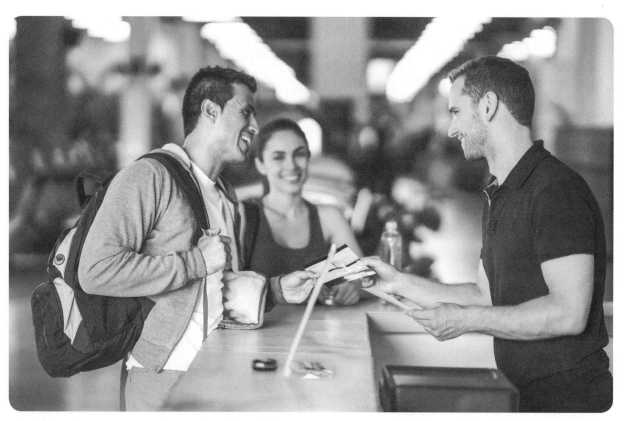

Reception-desk staff members are an integral component of the membership process. The relationship between the reception desk and the membership department should be considered a partnership.

Getty Images/andresr

prospective members will come into the club with a guest pass they received from a member or printed off your website. If the guest pass is already filled out with basic contact information, do not ask the person to repeat the information again on the tour card (a staff member can transfer that information).

## Characteristics of an Effective Tour Card

Effective and functional tour cards have the following characteristics:

- They should be big enough to capture relevant information about the prospective member but not so large that they are cumbersome or take too much time to complete. A good size for a print card is 8.25 by 5.5 inches (21 by 14 centimeters) or smaller. Some clubs have a digital tour card capture system. In that case, limit the content to one screen.

- They include space for the prospective member's name, occupation, and basic contact information—address, phone, email, and preferred method of communication.

- They include the following checklist that asks how the prospect heard about the club:
  - Friend, coworker, or family member
  - Digital marketing (e.g., Facebook, Google)
  - Radio advertisement
  - Newspaper advertisement
  - Television advertisement
  - Internet or social media advertisement or article
  - Local event
  - Billboard
  - Other _____

- They ask for the name of the person who made the referral. Mentioning the referring member allows the marketing representative to begin to develop a comfortable relationship with the guest. Early in the conversation, say, "I see that Tricia Smith referred you to the club; she's been a member here for years. How do you two know each other?"

- There are sample questions for staff to ask the prospective member printed on the back of the card, as well as space to record their responses. Questions can include the following:
  - What motivated you to come into this club today?
  - Are you currently a member of a health club? If so, what activities do you pursue?
  - If you are currently a health club member, why are you considering another club?
  - Do you currently exercise? If yes, what kind of exercise do you enjoy? If no, what factors would help you start an exercise program?
  - What are your health goals?
  - Are there activities that are of interest to you (e.g., yoga, running, strength training, swimming)?
  - How much time do you have today to learn about our club and the benefits it offers?

- There should be a **liability waiver** statement and a place for a signature on the card. This waiver is only for the visit; once the prospect joins, be sure a separate liability waiver form is completed. A full health history questionnaire is not needed as part of the tour visit, because most guests coming in to tour the club will not complete a full workout.

Too often, when a guest approaches the reception desk and requests membership information, the reception-desk staff member responds in a somewhat apologetic tone: "Sure. Would you mind filling out this card first?" This makes the task sound burdensome. Instead, when a guest inquires about membership, reception-desk staff should be trained to say "We are happy to tell you about membership! While you take a minute to complete this information, I'll get a membership representative to answer all your questions." When the staff member takes the position of directing the guest rather than asking the guest, the guest is less likely to be irritated by the process and more likely to provide complete information. Reception-desk staff also should be trained on the purpose of the tour card so they can explain it to a questioning guest. More details and tips on club tours and using the tour card are discussed in the Maximizing the Face-to-Face Selling Process section later in the chapter.

## *The Bottom Line*

An effective tour card can be a strong sales tool, because it provides information to help staff build rapport and better understand the potential customer's needs and motivation.

## TELEPHONE BEST PRACTICES

Mastering phone skills is critical to membership sales success. It is often the first step in transforming an interested party into a prospective member and ultimately into a full-fledged member. Certainly, face-to-face sales skills are also important but lack of good phone skills can push membership prospects away and possibly toward competitors.

There are many potential pitfalls when it comes to phone skills, including rudeness, indifference, inattention, poor information, and pushiness. Fortunately, there are some simple, proven ways to avoid these relationship-building killers.

When people call the club, you know they are at least interested in learning more about it. Perhaps they saw your ad, scanned your website, or were prompted by a friend. Many people who call a business to ask questions already intend to buy the product or service, but they don't know who they're going to buy it from. If you handle incoming calls properly, you can increase the chance that the caller will set up an appointment for a visit and tour. When you have an appointment with someone who is already seriously considering joining a health club, you are one step closer to having a new member. Therefore, it is critical to set yourself up for success from the beginning. The following are some telephone best practices you can implement immediately:

- During regular business hours, all phone calls should be answered by a person.
- Use the automated answering system only when the facility is closed or during nonbusiness hours. The outgoing message should be updated regularly with current information.
- Answer the phone in three rings or fewer.
- Answer with a proper greeting that includes the name of the club and your name (e.g., "Hello, West Side Health Club, this is Emilie.").

- Do not transfer a phone call unless the caller requests it or the caller gives permission.
- Do not place a caller on hold without permission (e.g., "Can I place you on hold, or would you like me to call you back?").
- If the caller would like to leave a message, offer to transfer the call to voicemail or take the message personally.
- Talk to the caller in a friendly and personable voice.
  - Speak in a pleasant tone of voice.
  - Speak clearly.
  - Speak at a reasonable and understandable rate.
- Speak to the caller with a professional and pleasant attitude.
  - Be courteous.
  - Be helpful and take initiative.
  - Show interest in the caller's needs.
- Use listening skills in phone conversations.
  - Listen before responding.
  - Respond to any questions asked.
  - Ask questions.
  - Offer options to engage the caller in conversation.
- Use appropriate sales skills when a caller asks about membership or a program.
  - Explain the benefits of membership.
  - Explain any current offers, if applicable.
  - Invite the prospective member to come in for a tour.
  - Explain program offerings if the caller expresses interest.
  - Record the name and basic contact information of the caller for follow up.
- Offer to return the call (or have someone else return the call) if further information or follow up is needed.
- End all phone calls with a pleasant closing (e.g., "Thank you for calling West Side Health Club and asking about our services. Please feel free to contact me if you have further questions, and we hope to see you here soon. Have a great day!").

How that prospect is served during the initial phone call will often determine whether the person visits the club. If the person answering the phone is friendly, professional, knowledgeable, and welcoming, the caller is more likely to come in. If the caller receives poor service or the call is ended before the caller receives the desired information, you may have lost a new customer.

With this in mind, club management must know how calls are being handled and train the staff to treat each caller as if he or she was standing at the front desk. Associates should never treat calls as annoyances. One effective tool for measuring telephone service is the secret shopper. A **secret shopper** is someone hired by a business to pose as a prospective customer to evaluate the quality of customer service provided (on the phone or in person). To obtain the most unbiased review of the shopping experience, the staff person being evaluated should not know the identity of the shopper and his or her purpose. Many professional organizations offer secret shopping services for as little as $15 to $25 per call, based on volume. These companies work with a business to determine the expectations for the staff answering the phone and handling membership inquiries, create a list of questions for the secret shoppers to ask, and look for opportunities to help the business improve those expectations by using an audit form to capture the responses to the questions during the call (see Sample Health Club Telephone Secret Shopper Questionnaire sidebar). After a number of calls are completed, the company provides a report to the client that details all the findings and gives a score based on the expectations stated by the business. This information will help the business gain a better understanding of the areas in which they are excelling and the areas of deficiency. By consistently monitoring customer service levels, you can coach staff members to improve low scores and reward them for the times they provide excellent service.

## The Bottom Line

Developing excellent phone skills is key in achieving sales success. Excellence in phone communication can be achieved through repetition of role-play phone calls and live phone conversations that turn callers into health club members.

## Sample Health Club Telephone Secret Shopper Questionnaire

1. Was the phone answered by a live person?
2. Was the phone answered in three or fewer rings?
3. Was the phone answered in a friendly manner?
4. Did the employee use his or her name and the name of the health club when answering the call?
5. Was the employee able to answer your questions?
6. If questions could not be answered, did the employee connect you with someone who could help?
7. Were you put on hold for more than 30 seconds?
8. Were you asked questions about your interests?
9. Were you encouraged to come into the club for a visit?
10. Were you told about special promotions or sales?
11. Did you experience any difficulties?
12. Did the employee seem happy that you called?
13. What was your general impression of the club after the call?
14. How would you describe your conversation with the employee?
15. What was the name of the employee who took your call?

## MAXIMIZING THE FACE-TO-FACE SELLING PROCESS

Meeting with a membership prospect for the first time and attempting to sell him or her on joining your health club can be a daunting task. However, understanding the sales process and why people buy from those they trust can create a more comfortable sales environment for both you and the prospect. When marketing your services in a face-to-face selling situation, you must develop a relationship with the prospective member and communicate why you offer what you do. The following are five simple steps to follow when engaging one-on-one during the sales process:

1. Build trust and a transparent rapport by sharing why you do what you do.

2. Ask probing questions to elicit why the prospect is there and what he or she is looking for.

3. Take the prospect on a tour of the facility and continue to ask probing questions.

4. Add value during the tour and hone in on what resonates with the prospect.

5. Offer the prospect at least three memberships types or options and include the price points. Be sure to ask how soon the prospect would like to get started.

The best membership sales representatives perform all these steps and use the tour to build desire by creating differentiation, showcasing the club's benefits, using trial closes, and handling objections so they can close the sale, all of which are effective sales techniques that will be discussed later in this chapter. Less-experienced sales staff start the tour before gaining an understanding of the prospect's needs, don't ask enough qualifying questions to build a rapport, fail to handle objections after the tour, and often do not close the sale.

How can you possibly build desire and show prospective members what they want if you don't know what that is? Strong membership representatives invest time before the tour so they know how to build desire for a prospective member. You should spend 3 to 5 minutes interviewing prospective member before the tour; this is just a friendly, informal conversation in which you use the questions printed on the tour card as prompts. During the interview, it will become clear how you should customize the tour to the needs of the prospective member.

This interview should take place in a relatively quiet part of the lobby away from the busy reception desk and out of the line of traffic. A sitting area or café in the lobby works well for this quiet conversation. Sitting is preferable to standing. Don't take prospective members into a sales office; many people have had experiences in which they felt trapped in a sales office, and they don't like it. During this time, use your tour card as a guide for asking qualifying questions and recording the information provided by the guest.

Taking a prospective member on a tour of your club is a unique opportunity to have a relaxed conversation, sell your club, gauge interest level, and begin to build a personal relationship. Think of the tour as an opportunity to continue your informal interview with the prospective member. Using the questions on the back of the tour card as prompts and conversation starters.

## Building Trust and Rapport

All successful sales philosophies have one element in common: building a good relationship with the prospective buyer. When buyers feel they have a relationship with you, there will be less tension, defense, and fear of exploitation. Instead, there will be trust, **rapport**, and more sales!

Building trust and rapport starts with the staff at the reception desk and continues with you and the other contacts made during the visit. This is why the membership sales department and the reception desk must have a solid and seamless working relationship. Once the reception desk has passed the prospect on to you, you will continue to work on relationship building.

## The Introduction

A strong introduction is simple and includes the following process:

1. Use the prospective member's name.

2. Extend your hand first for a handshake—be the leader.

3. Use your full name in your introduction.

4. If the person doesn't have an appointment and doesn't know who you are, state what your position is with the club and offer to answer any questions.

5. Avoid starting a conversation by asking "How are you today?" It is a nervous filler question that is irrelevant to the scenario, especially if it is the first time you are meeting this person.

6. End the introduction with a question that is relevant to the process, such as "What are you most interested in at our club?" Take the lead.

By starting the process with a strong, simple introduction, you set the stage for your professionalism and credibility. This is critical in the process of building rapport. Have you heard that people decide in the first 7 seconds whether they like you? This makes it challenging to get off on the right foot. Think about your own experience. People often make quick decisions based on appearance, initial action, tone of voice, or conversation. In sales, this can be deadly if done poorly. In addition to your introduction, the following factors can affect how the prospective member perceives you:

- Breath
- Oral hygiene
- Physical hygiene
- Physical appearance
- Choice of clothing
- Vocabulary
- Presentation skills
- Voice tone and volume
- Eye contact
- Nonverbal skills
- Facial expression
- Energy
- Attentiveness

All these factors affect your relationship with the prospective member, but your energy level is especially important. You should gauge the energy level of the prospective member and adjust your own energy to be at a similar, if slightly higher, level. Think of energy on a scale of 0 to 10 (0 = asleep, 10 = bouncing off the walls). If the prospective member comes in at level 4, you want to be at a 5. If you were at a 10, the prospective member would be overwhelmed. Take a few seconds to read the prospect's nonverbal communication (e.g., facial expression, posture, fidgeting,

curiosity) to gauge energy level even before you approach.

## *The Bottom Line*

Meet people where they are rather than expecting them to come to your energy level right away. As trust builds, they will move in your direction.

To initiate conversations with prospective members, use the questions on the tour card and the answers the prospect provided. Be sure you use vocabulary that is appropriate for the prospective member. If the person is wearing something of note—a shirt with a college or team logo, a fitness brand of clothing, something unique or recognizable—you might want to comment on it and develop a conversation if you perceive a level of comfort with the topic. Most important, be present and listen to the prospective member.

## Effective Listening and Communication

The process of selling a membership should not be mechanical or interrogational; it should be a relaxed conversation. This means you need to be an expert listener. As you ask questions, listen and then respond based on the customer's answers. Don't simply ask the questions on your list regardless of what the person says.

In a sales situation, getting customers to open up starts with asking good questions. You should ask open-ended questions (discussed in chapter 3) to elicit responses that will help you better understand the customer's needs and goals. Open-ended questions are important in building collaborative relationships because they initiate discussion and invite the speaker to express personal ideas, wishes, and plans. In addition, asking open-ended questions encourages you to become a better listener. A good learning exercise is taking common closed-ended questions and turning them into open-ended ones (e.g., change "Do you enjoy group exercise classes?" to "What do you enjoy about group exercise?").

Being a good listener is directly related to building the relationships that are necessary for sales and for being a professional in the fitness business. **Listening** is the receiving part of communication. We receive information through the ears and eyes and attach meaning to it, and then decide what we think or feel about that communication. Listening requires an attitude of honoring and seeking each person's perspective. It can be thought of as a genuine interest in getting to know people and hearing what they have to say. Truly listening for understanding means being open and giving full attention while another person is talking instead of being distracted or thinking about what you are going to say in response.

Renowned management consultant Peter Drucker offered this keen perspective: "The most important thing in communication is hearing what isn't said" (BrainyQuote.com 2018). A classic study done by Dr. Albert Mehrabian at UCLA found that 7% of communication comes from the spoken word; 38% comes from vocal qualities such as voice, pitch, tone, and emphasis; and 55% comes from visual qualities such as appearance, facial expression, and body language (Mehrabian 1972). Therefore, to be an effective communicator, you must consider these three dimensions of communication. Failing to listen costs a great deal in lost sales and causes misunderstandings between members and staff and among staff members. Inexperienced salespeople tend to spend too much time talking; they falsely think that if they tell prospective members all the features of the club, people will jump at the chance to join. But how do you know what information the customers are seeking if you are constantly talking and not asking questions and listening? To be effective, you should be listening more than you are speaking. As a learning experience, listen in on your coworkers as they give tours and have them listen to you, and then give each other feedback on the ratio of listening to talking during the tour.

Listening is a powerful but underused communication skill. To become a better listener, practice focusing only on listening; don't think about talking. This can help increase your awareness of your listening behaviors. This is also a good training tool to use with staff members.

Becoming a good listener is challenging because listening is multifaceted; in a matter of seconds, you must hear information from the speaker, interpret what he or she is saying and its true meaning, determine how you feel about it, and respond appropriately.

1. *Hear.* When conversing, let the other person speak with no interruptions from you. Fully focus on the speaker and keep an open and focused mind. Give the person plenty of time to talk; even if the speaker pauses momentarily to think, resist the urge to jump in. This may be difficult for those of us who are not so comfortable with momentary silence.

2. *Interpret.* After you hear what has been said, you internally interpret the message. Interpretation comes from not only the words that were said but also the tone, nonverbal cues, and your own filters. Filters include your perceptions, memories, biases, expectations, attention span, feelings, needs, and so on.

3. *Reflect.* Once the speaker is done and you have interpreted as well as possible, start your part of the conversation by reflecting back what you think you heard to be sure you've got it right. Reflections are rarely used in most conversations. They often start with words such as *so* or *it sounds like* or *you said*. They are not questions. In a reflection, your tone of voice must go down at the end; if your voice goes up, the words become a question. Reflections are subtle and powerful; they express care, show that you are listening, communicate understanding, and demand less of the speaker.

4. *Check for meaning.* Before responding, ask any clarifying questions you have based on the speaker's response to your reflection. This ensures you don't jump to conclusions. Remember, the way you interpret the speaker's words may be very different from the speaker's intended meaning.

5. *Respond.* After you hear, interpret, reflect, and check for meaning, you can confidently make thoughtful responses that reassure the speaker that you heard, understood, and properly evaluated the message.

Be sure to have an open posture, make eye contact, and avoid distractions while a prospect is speaking; these are powerful nonverbal messages that convey interest and an intent to listen. Embrace a desire to listen, remember the benefits of good listening habits, and practice listening whenever you can. If you have only been listening 30% of the time and you improve to listening 70% of the time, that is a 130% increase in effectiveness. A 130% increase in effectiveness can have a significant effect on your membership sales production.

## Emotional Connection in the Sales Process

When prospective members don't join the club on the first visit, you might think it is for one of the following reasons:

- They lack motivation.
- They need to discuss it with a spouse or partner at home.
- They don't see how an exercise program could work in their schedule.
- They aren't financially qualified.
- They have to get in shape before joining the club.

These are external reasons, meaning they appear to have nothing to do with the membership representative. The following are some internal reasons prospects don't join on the first visit:

- You didn't prepare properly.
- You didn't ask the right questions.
- You didn't create and sustain trust.
- You didn't create value.
- You presented the buying question too soon.

This section will focus on complementing your professional sales skills with emotional connections that inspire prospects to join on the first visit. The goals in creating an emotional connection are to facilitate the buying process, build trust, keep the new member as a long-term member, and create a referral stream. As you read

on, keep this thought in mind: You can earn a commission using a sales technique, but you can earn a fortune building relationships.

**Trust Busters**   There are many reasons prospective members might not trust you. The following are several trust busters:

- Preconceived notions the prospective member has about the fitness industry or salespeople in general
- Preconceived notions you have about the prospective member
- Inappropriate appearance (e.g., you are dressed unprofessionally)
- Inappropriate demeanor (e.g., you use vocabulary that is too technical, abrasive, or negative; you keep prospects waiting; you don't follow through on what you say you're going to do; you fake answers you don't know)
- Pushing to make a sale rather than focusing on getting the prospect involved in the best program

Selling styles can also be trust busters. Table 8.1 compares trust-busting styles with trust-building styles. Review them and see where your sales style falls.

**Trust Musts**   Trust musts, which build emotional connections, include the following:

- Listening to understand rather than to reply
- Analyzing needs rather than forcing a fit with the club
- Maintaining warm, focused eye contact
- Showing respect for prospects
- Talking to them on their level

**Table 8.1**   Comparison of Sales Techniques

| Trust busters | Trust builders |
| --- | --- |
| *Focus on closing:* disregards any rapport building, needs assessment, qualifying, or customization and puts a lot of energy into the tail end with the close; feels like a hard sell | *Focus on the front end:* focuses on building rapport, needs assessment, qualifying, and customization; addresses needs and solutions; feels genuine to the buyer |
| *Pitch products:* becomes canned and focuses primarily on features; offers a fast answer for everything; often irrelevant to the buyer | *Listen and learn:* zeroes in on the details the buyer wants most; customized to the buyer |
| *Overcome objections:* doesn't give the prospect a chance to express emotions or real concerns; can become adversarial; often involves outdated closing techniques | *Resolve concerns:* invites the buyer to open up; focuses on investigating or consulting rather than providing quick answers; reaches a natural conclusion and mutual commitment that joining is the right fit for the buyer |

- Repeating points that are important to them by restating them in your words
- Having a visible passion for what you do
- Maintaining composure at all times, especially when they express objections
- Offering guarantees you can support (e.g., satisfaction, programs, pricing)

**Building Connections**   Once you have used trust to create an emotional connection, the following tips will help you further build a connection throughout the selling process:

- Know prospective members' true motivations (not just their interests and needs), and use this knowledge throughout the tour to build desire. For example, when someone tells you what their goals are, your next question could be "It sounds as though you're very clear about your goals. What's your motivation for getting there?"
- Use feeling questions throughout your introduction and club presentation. An example would be "Tell me what it's like for you when you feel your absolute best. When was the last time you felt that way?"
- Help people visualize their results and being a part of the club.
- Genuinely agree with them when appropriate.
- Build urgency based on motivation, programs, and promotions throughout the tour.
- To create a stronger bond and a more immediate feeling of belonging, introduce staff and members who are relevant to the prospective member's needs as you tour the facility.
- Have a genuine interest in prospective members' success in achieving their health and fitness goals. When you are only looking for your own immediate gratification (i.e., commission), that success is short lived. When you have a hand in someone else's success, that connection can last a lifetime.

Certainly, there are many ways to sell memberships. To get the least resistance and the highest return, examine your selling style for the following qualities and professional sales skills: preparing, asking professional questions, creating value, building rapport, building trust, creating emotional connection, and asking for the sale.

# Performing a Personal Interview and Asking Qualifying Questions

Assessing needs and asking qualifying questions are two critical elements in the sales process that often end up being rushed or skipped altogether. They allow you to investigate what will and will not allow a prospective member to join the club today. In addition, the information elicited will allow you to do the following:

- Build desire on the tour
- Create urgency
- Understand the prospective member's concerns before they become objections
- Handle objections while on the tour

## Interview Questions

Interview questions should help you find out why the prospective member is interested in joining. They cover interests, needs, and motivation and should be asked before and during the tour. And interview might go something like this:

*Membership representative: Luis what would you like to do at the club?*

*Luis: Well, I'd like to run on the treadmill, maybe swim a bit, and lift weights.*

At this point, the membership representative has discovered what Luis is interested in but has not yet uncovered Luis's needs. To do that, the conversation should progress as follows:

*Membership representative: Well, Luis, we certainly can provide excellent programs and equipment for you in those areas. Tell me, what is it that you want to accomplish with running, swimming, and weights?*

*Luis: I'd like to lose some weight, strengthen my heart, and improve my strength.*

The membership representative has now discovered Luis's true needs. Read on as the representative uncovers the motivation:

*Membership representative: It sounds like you have some pretty clear goals in mind. That's good news, because most people aren't quite so clear about their goals. Do you mind if I ask what is motivating you to have those goals?*

# Preparing Yourself to Make the Sale

The time you spend mentally preparing for success in the **sales process** is critical and has an exponential effect not only on that day but also on each day thereafter (and therefore on your career). We are all constantly bombarded by other people's actions, thoughts, and words, most of which may not be positive. In addition, your own self-talk creates your reality. If your self-talk is not constructive, supportive, and forward moving, then you will end up degrading your own image. Therefore, you must continuously prepare yourself to be the best. The following are some tips that will help you stay focused in the sales process:

- *Love selling.* Selling is a choice; don't accept a sales position because you don't *mind* selling. Truly excellent membership representatives love the sales process.

- *Know your big picture.* Think about what you want for yourself in the next year, 5 years, and 10 years and break your goals down into five categories: personal, physical, financial, spiritual, and relationships. Write out your goals in these areas to stay on track.

- *Keep visual reminders of your life goals.* Magazines, websites, social media sites, and photos are good resources for visual images that reinforce what you want. When you find an image that fits what you are working toward, save it for reference later.

- *Know your sales goals and stay on track.* Know what your monthly goals break down to on a daily basis, and never let yourself get more than 2 days behind before you catch up. It is a lot easier to make small corrections than it is to make a big one.

- *Read industry publications and stay connected through social media.* Stay abreast of what others in the industry are doing to confirm what you're doing right and to get new ideas.

- *Read sales books and watch sales videos.* There is an abundance of industry-specific and nonindustry sales material that will rocket your performance ahead.

- *Listen to motivational speakers.* Motivational talks can help break you out of a rut and see things in an entirely new light.

- *Role-play with your coworkers.* Many membership representatives don't like to spend time role-playing, but it can shorten the learning curve and improve sales results. Try using a role-playing exercise as a warm-up at staff meetings, or take 20 minutes once per week and role-play whatever aspect of the sales process you want to improve.

- *Have weekly sales meetings.* When done correctly, these meetings can provide significant individual and group motivation. When you attend, be prepared to participate, share, ask, and be open to learning new skills and techniques.

- *Proactively seek help with your sales performance.* Don't wait for the sales director to tell you that you are not performing to the expected level. "I need your help" will be music to your sales director's ears and hasten your success.

- *Use the club.* Working out at your club might seem obvious, but using the club's entire range of services can build empathy for a potential new member and give you experiences and information to share while giving a guest tour. Don't do the same activity and use the same equipment all the time. Try everything in your club. Use all the equipment, take a variety of classes, swim in the pool, have a massage—the variety will help you to talk about and ultimately sell those areas even better.

- *Brainstorm on urgency.* Think about all the reasons a prospective member should join today versus coming back. By creating urgency in the sales process, you build momentum.

- *Eat well and get rest.* In selling, you have to be on all the time. Be sure to take breaks throughout the day, and don't skip meals or eat poorly. It's hard to stay motivated when you are starving and exhausted.

- *Commit to your own success.* Promise yourself that you will do whatever is ethically and legally possible to be successful in your position. Commitment doesn't guarantee success, but lack of commitment guarantees you'll fall far short of your potential.

- *Practice keeping yourself motivated daily.* If you don't, your sales could suffer.

You usually get what you expect in life, so expect the best for yourself.

*Luis: Well, I used to play basketball in high school, and we have our 20th reunion coming up. People remember me as an athlete, but I've put on a few pounds and am not very active these days.*

Too often, membership representatives mistake the prospect's interests or desired activities for needs. You need to continue to probe for the needs and motivation. The motivation is imperative, because it is what causes people to act on something. Knowing the motivation allows you to build urgency without seeming pushy, because you are using their motivation rather than your own.

Read on to see how the prospective member's motivation can help create urgency:

*Membership representative: Okay, your 20th reunion, that sounds like fun. So, you want to feel good about yourself as well as look good. How much time do we have to accomplish your goals?*

*Luis: The reunion is in 3 months.*

*Membership representative: Your timing is great, Luis. If we start now, we can make it happen.*

## The Bottom Line

Using a prospective member's motivation to join makes the process much more genuine and more powerful. If you use your motivation (making a sale), it comes across as pushy.

## Qualifying Questions

At this point, the membership representative has enough information to know what will make Luis say *yes* but not enough information to understand what will make Luis say *no*. This is where **qualifying questions** come in to uncover any concerns before they become objections after the tour. You never want to give an energetic tour and build rapport and then lose your momentum because a bunch of objections are thrown at you later. By asking qualifying questions before the tour, you can uncover problems and have more time to work through them while you are on the tour.

## Pretour Power Questions

Review the following questions that will help you to uncover needs, motivations, and qualifications. Incorporate these into your interview to maximize your success.

- How did you hear about us?
- How much time do we have today?
- Most people join the club for one of four reasons: medical or rehab, sport performance, appearance or fitness, or social interaction. Which of these would you say is your main motivation? Tell me more about that.
- When was the last time you felt really good about your fitness level? What's changed?
- Would you like to go back to that same level or somewhere in between?
- Will this membership be just for you, or will someone else be involved?
- What is your time frame for making a decision?
- Picture yourself as a member 6 months down the road. Ideally, what would be different with your health and fitness?
- Where are you in your decision-making process?
- Tell me about your past club experiences. What did you like most at your last club? What did you like least?
- What recreational activities are you planning on incorporating into your fitness program?
- How often will you be using the club?
- What most interests you about our club?
- What could you see today that would tell you this is the club for you?

Qualifying questions uncover the five major areas of concern before they are expressed as objections.

1. Eagerness and motivation to join
   - Questions: When are you planning on making your decision to start a fitness program? When do you want to start your membership?"
   - Concerns expressed: I want to think about it; I'm shopping around; I'm not sure I can commit.

2. Decision-making ability
   - Question: Is there anyone else you need to consult in making this decision?
   - Concern expressed: I need to talk with my spouse (doctor, insurance company, employer).

3. Time availability
   - Questions: How many days per week are you planning on using the club? What time of day works best in your schedule?
   - Concerns expressed: I don't think I can make time in my schedule; I'm too busy.

4. Financial ability
   - Question: Our membership rates range from _____ to _____. Does that fit with what you have in mind?
   - Concerns expressed: I can't afford it; it costs too much.

5. Other limitations
   - Question: Assuming you feel the club works for you, is there anything that would keep you from joining today?
   - Concerns expressed: I just moved here and am still getting settled; I am recovering from an injury; I have to get in shape before I join.

These qualifying questions will help you to uncover any concerns that may exist. When you uncover the concerns, you should not always handle them at that moment. This is information may come out before the tour, but other details may be revealed as you walk around. Remember, it is fairly early in the sales relationship, and you don't want it to feel adversarial. Concerns or objections are best handled as you strengthen the relationship during the tour.

# Building Desire on the Tour

The purpose of the club tour is twofold: to create differentiation between your club and the other facilities in town and to build desire for the prospective member to purchase membership. This section will cover some of the most effective ways to build desire. Too often, people become rote tour guides and give tours that are informative but are not very exciting for prospective members. When you build desire, you are taking the information prospects have already provided and using it to build anticipation for them to become members.

Once you have built rapport, conducted a strong interview, and asked qualifying questions, you have the platform to build desire. The following are some of the tools you can use to accomplish this goal:

- Show genuine excitement and enthusiasm for how the club will work for prospective members. Vary the tone in your voice, and use other nonverbal skills, such as facial expressions, smiling, raising the eyebrows, and so on.

- Customize the tour by first taking prospective members to areas that are of particular interest to them. Show them what they want to see, not what you want to show them. Avoid doing the same canned tour every time.

- Know their motivation and verbalize it frequently on the tour. Using their motivation to join is much more powerful than using your motivation.

- Introduce prospective members to other staff throughout the tour. The purpose of this is to bonds early in the process, so prospective members feel they are already a part of the club. Your staff should be warm and welcoming. Be careful, however, when introducing prospective members to current members; this can backfire if you are faced with an unhappy or grumpy member. Be sure you know the member well before making introductions.

## Create Urgency

One of the most important ways to build desire is to create urgency. When you create urgency, you are reminding prospective members why they should join today. This element is missing or is done incorrectly on most tours. When it is done incorrectly, it feels like pressure; when it is not done at all, it delays the sales process and you can lose the sale to another facility. There are three ways to create urgency: promotions and price, programs, and personal motivation.

The health and fitness industry has historically used promotions and price to create urgency. It sounds like this: "If you decide to join today, we can waive your enrollment fee [or add an extra month of membership or enter you into our drawing]". This is not the most effective method, because it is based on the club's motivation rather than the buyer's.

Program urgency can be effective in some situations. It is based on the start time of a program, league, class, or other offering. Although many clubs have ongoing classes that do not have a specific start dates, some specialty programs may run on a cycle. If the prospect misses the opportunity to sign up now, it would delay involvement for another 6 to 8 weeks (or however long the program lasts). Program urgency is only effective if it speaks to the needs or motivation of the buyer. It sounds like this: "Tyrone, you mentioned that you wanted to start playing tennis again and need some help. Well, your timing is perfect—our beginning player clinic starts this Tuesday, and we have a space available. Let's get you in there!"

Personal motivation is also very effective. It is based on the reason the prospect gave for needing the club. It is a gentle and encouraging reminder not to delay results any longer. When you discover the buyer's needs, always find out if there is a time frame for accomplishing the goal. This can be a great tool to create urgency based on the buyer's terms. Here is what it sounds like: "Alicia, I am so glad you're here. I was thinking about what you said earlier about wanting to lose some body fat, tone muscles, and improve endurance before the summer biking season. This is the perfect time for you to start. If you start now, you'll be seeing results within a few weeks. After all, tomorrow's results start today!"

The most effective way to create urgency is to use a combination of these methods (when appropriate) and use them throughout the tour rather than just at the end. If you create urgency throughout the tour, it feels more encouraging and builds excitement for the buyer.

## Create Differentiation From Your Competitors

Most clubs have competition within their community, and most clubs don't close 100% of their sales on the first visit. Therefore, most clubs need to be able to create differentiation in the market and in the minds of buyers.

Clubs attempt to create differentiation in their marketing messages but often forget to do so in their tours. They sell their club, but they don't sell how their club is different from the competitor. In creating differentiation, you should establish in the potential members' minds that this is the club for them. The best tools to accomplish this are establishing and using your unique selling position, knowing your club's exclusive features, and knowing your competition.

**Establishing and Using Your Unique Selling Position**    Your **unique selling position** refers to the characteristics that favorably differentiate you from your competitors. It is an honest benefit statement that caters to the specific needs of the prospective member. It is based on six elements: programs, services, staff, equipment, facilities, and philosophy. Within these six categories, you need to determine what your club does or has that is unique. Most facilities base their unique selling position on features rather than on philosophy, which can be dangerous. Your competitors can duplicate your features, but it is more challenging to duplicate your philosophy and its delivery. Your philosophy typically focuses on who and how you serve. Take some time to develop and articulate the philosophy that makes your club different. Once it has been articulated, the entire staff should understand it and be able to deliver it verbally and through their actions.

You can integrate this unique selling position into your tours and conversations like this:

*Ahmed, you mentioned earlier that you're concerned about not coming to the club regularly and getting the value from your membership. What you will find makes us different from the other clubs in town is that we print a monthly report of all members who have not been in the club during the previous month. We then contact those members to help them figure out how they can best use their memberships. What that means to you is we don't forget about you, and we help you get the most out of your membership. Does that sound like it would benefit you?*

**Knowing Your Exclusive Features**  Exclusive features are similar to the unique selling position, because they can only be found at your facility. Focus on features that address the specific needs of the buyer; otherwise, they are irrelevant. Features can be mentioned in the following way:

*Alison, you mentioned you spend most of your time performing functional strength training. You'll be interested to know that we are the only club in the city with a room dedicated to functional training, complete with a full line of individual-use equipment and machines designed for that purpose.*

**Knowing Your Competition**  The only way you can develop and use a unique selling position or exclusive feature is if you know your competition. Visit your competitors once or twice a year and research their programs, services, staff, equipment, facilities, and philosophies. Also check out their websites and social media pages. It is critical to stay abreast of your position in the market. The best way to approach this is honestly rather than sneakily. Before going to another club, phone the manager or owner and say the following:

*Hi, [name], this is [your name] with [your club]. I'm calling because we would like to come over and see your club. I'd like to have you show me around, and I'd like to schedule a time for you to come over and see our club as well. When would be a good time for both?*

By being honest and upfront, you minimize the defensiveness of the competitor and maximize the results of your visit and the relationship. Before you appointment, see figure 8.1 so you know what to look for. Do not take the form into the club with you.

Using these tools, you will be able to not only sell your club but also sell how your club is different from the competition and ensure buyers that they need not look further. When you create differentiation, you expedite the sales process in a gentle and educated way.

## Ask Trial Close Questions

Trial close questions are terrific tools you can use to test the waters and monitor the interest level of the prospective member during the tour. The purpose of the trial close is to

- affirm the buyer's enthusiasm,
- uncover any remaining concerns,
- handle those concerns, and
- give you the perfect opportunity to ask the prospective member to join.

All these points are critical in the sales process. However, most membership representatives don't ask any trial close questions at all. Therefore, when they finally ask prospective members to join, they have no idea about their enthusiasm levels or concerns. By asking trial close questions, you expedite the sales process because you know exactly what the prospective member is thinking and feeling at the time and you deal with it immediately.

Depending on the size of your club, you can ask five to nine questions as you tour the facility. Be sure you vary the questions so you don't sound redundant. In addition, when you ask trial close questions, you want the delivery to be conversational rather than confrontational. Thus, you need to practice asking the questions so you are comfortable enough to deliver them conversationally.

The best times to ask trial close questions so they come across naturally include the following:

- As you show a part of the club: Marcela, this is our yoga studio. How does it feel to you?
- As you leave a part of the club: Thomas, does it look like our free-weight area has what it takes for you to get the workout you want?
- Hallways or transition areas: Sofia, from what you've seen in the club so far, does it feel like the club will work for you?

As you can see, trial close questions can be open ended or closed ended. Notice how the three sample questions would reveal the prospective member's level of enthusiasm or concern and give you an opportunity to address any concerns. In addition, trial close questions give you an opportunity to ask the prospective member to join if the time is right. The following are more examples of trial close questions:

# CLUB COMPETITOR DATA

Evaluator: _____ Date: _____ Time: _____

Club name: _____ Phone: _____

Address: _____

| Price structure | Enrollment | Monthly dues | Annual dues |
|---|---|---|---|

Individual: _____

Couple: _____

Family: _____

Facilities

Group exercise rooms #: _____ Approximate ft² (m²): _____

Floor type: _____ Classes/wk: _____

(Attach schedule)

Free weights (selection rating 1 2 3 4 5 6 7 8 9 10)   Size S M L XL

Resistance training machines: Type: _____ #: _____

Specialty training area: _____   Size: S  M  L  XL   Type of equipment: _____

Circuit training area: _____ # of stations: _____ Type of equipment: _____

Classes/wk: _____

Cardio area equipment type and # of each: _____

_____

Group cycling studio size: _____ # of bikes: _____ Classes/wk: _____

Aquatic facilities: Indoor lanes #: _____ Outdoor lanes #: _____

Racquetball: _____  # of courts: _____  Charges: _____

Tennis: _____  # of courts: _____  Charges: _____

Basketball: _____  # of courts: _____  Charges: _____

Track: _____ Laps for 1 mile (1.5 km): _____

Child watch: _____ Hours available: _____ Charge/child: _____

Massage: _____ # of rooms: _____ Charge: _____

Fitness testing services : _____ Charge: _____

Personal training : _____ Charge: _____

Pro shop : _____ Types of products : _____

Food service/beverage bar : _____ Beer, wine, juice, smoothies : _____

**Figure 8.1**   Sample form for club competitor data.

*(continued)*

**154**

Spa services: _____

Sauna: _____ Men's: _____ Women's: _____ Coed: _____

Steam: _____ Men's: _____ Women's: _____ Coed: _____

Whirlpool: _____ Men's:_____ Women's: _____ Coed: _____

Locker-room size: _____ Amenities: _____ Condition: _____

Other facilities not listed: _____

| Rating | Very poor | | | | Average | | | | Excellent | |
|---|---|---|---|---|---|---|---|---|---|---|
| Outside appearance | 1 | 2 | 3 | 4 | 5 | 6 | 7 | 8 | 9 | 10 |
| Cleanliness | 1 | 2 | 3 | 4 | 5 | 6 | 7 | 8 | 9 | 10 |
| Atmosphere | 1 | 2 | 3 | 4 | 5 | 6 | 7 | 8 | 9 | 10 |
| Attitude of staff | 1 | 2 | 3 | 4 | 5 | 6 | 7 | 8 | 9 | 10 |
| Attitude of members | 1 | 2 | 3 | 4 | 5 | 6 | 7 | 8 | 9 | 10 |
| Energy of club | 1 | 2 | 3 | 4 | 5 | 6 | 7 | 8 | 9 | 10 |
| Equipment condition | 1 | 2 | 3 | 4 | 5 | 6 | 7 | 8 | 9 | 10 |
| Location | 1 | 2 | 3 | 4 | 5 | 6 | 7 | 8 | 9 | 10 |
| Visibility | 1 | 2 | 3 | 4 | 5 | 6 | 7 | 8 | 9 | 10 |
| Parking | 1 | 2 | 3 | 4 | 5 | 6 | 7 | 8 | 9 | 10 |

**Figure 8.1**    *(continued)*

From M. Bates, M.J. Spezzano, and G. Danhoff, *Health Fitness Management*, 3rd ed. (Champaign, IL: Human Kinetics, 2020).

- Is the club what you expected?
- Where do you think you'll be spending most of your time in the club?
- How does the club feel to you?
- On a scale of 1 to 10, where is the club for you?
- Does it look like we'll be able to meet your needs?
- Do we have what you're looking for?
- Is this the kind of class that would work for you?
- So, do you think you'll join?

Of equal importance to asking the trial close questions is how you respond to the answers.

When you ask a trial close question, listen for one of three types of answers: very enthusiastic, lukewarm, or negative. If you hear an enthusiastic answer, terrific! This is a green light for you and the prospective member. If you hear a lukewarm or apathetic answer, probe it rather than letting it go. For example, when you ask Marcela how the yoga studio feels and she responds unenthusiastically with "Uh, it's nice," don't just let it go; you could say, "I thought you would be more excited about our yoga studio. Tell me what you're thinking." Trial closes help you move forward, so don't allow yourself to stumble by not probing when you get an answer that is less than enthusiastic or even negative.

When you ask the appropriate number of trial close questions throughout your tour and probe the answers to understand how the prospective member feels, you will know when it is time to invite that person to join. Trial closes allow you to get to this step smoothly, professionally, and confidently.

## Handle Concerns or Objections on the Tour

Most membership representatives handle concerns and objections at the end of the tour or not at all. Often they have not asked questions to determine what the concerns are, or they simple don't want to hear *no*. Handling objections at the end is predictable and tends to build pressure for the buyer and the seller.

You can enhance your sales skills by handling objections during the tour. The benefits of this approach include increased comfort, less pressure, a more conversational style, and a lighter energy, which all add up to a more conducive buying scenario. Picture this: You are walking through the club with a prospective member who has a concern about whether she can fit club use into her schedule. At that point, a conversation such as the following may be appropriate:

*Membership representative: Maria, I was thinking about what you said earlier about being able to get into the club as much as you want. It strikes me that with how much you like this area, it will motivate you to come into the club. What are your thoughts on that?*

*Maria: You're right; I do love it. But I'm still a bit concerned that I'll join and not come in enough to get my money's worth.*

*Membership representative: Hmm. I can see what you're saying. It sounds as though it is a value concern for you. Is there anything else that might hold you back from feeling that the club would work for you?*

*Maria: No, that's it.*

*Membership representative: Okay. Would it be all right if we took a few minutes to see how this could work for you?*

*Maria: Yeah, I would really appreciate that.*

*Membership representative: Great—I'm glad you're willing. Let's start with small steps. We want you to be successful and feel good about your*

*decision with the club. Let's figure out where we can find an hour twice a week in your schedule. When do you typically have the least amount of activity or demand on your time?*

*Maria: That's a hard one. I'm always on the go. I have meetings in the evenings and my lunches are usually scheduled as well. I'm all over the place.*

*Membership representative: It does sound like you're busy. Maria, let's go for two mornings a week before work. If you can come in by 6 a.m., we can make sure you get your spin class in and have a strength workout before we get you to your office by 8 a.m. How does that work for you?*

*Maria: Six a.m.? I can't commit to that twice a week!*

*Membership representative: Okay. Let's do one day during the week at 6 a.m. and then a weekend day of your choice for a more leisurely pace. How does that sound for starters?*

*Maria: Oh, I like that. I can do that.*

*Membership representative: Excellent. I know that you'll be happy with that decision.*

In this conversation, the membership representative quickly handled the concern while touring an area of the club that was particularly appealing to Maria. This type of conversation could occur while you are standing in an area of interest or while walking and talking. This allows you to skip the pressure of sitting down after the tour to go over concerns or handle objections. In addition, the membership representative proactively brought up the concern rather than waiting for Maria to bring it up at the end. This eliminates pressure because the element of surprise is removed; you are simply discussing a point that was brought up earlier.

To successfully handle objections on the tour, you should do the following:

- Ask qualifying questions before the tour. Qualifying questions tell you what might prevent the prospective member from joining today. The sooner you have this information, the more time you will have to work through the concerns on the tour.
- Ask five to nine trial close questions on the tour. These questions assist you in accomplishing four things: affirming enthusiasm, uncovering remaining concerns, handling

objections on the tour, and assessing the buyer's position.

- Follow these seven steps for handling a concern:

  1. Listen to the concern without interrupting.

  2. Reflect or paraphrase the concern so you know you understand what was said and the prospective member knows you understand.

  3. Determine whether this is the only concern or there may be others.

  4. Ask whether it is appropriate to find a solution to this concern.

  5. Continue to probe and ultimately come to a solution that works for the prospective member and the club. The solution may be right on the tip of your tongue, or you may need to be a little more creative. Take your time here; it is not a race to see who can speak first or fastest.

  6. Confirm that the solution you offered works for the prospective member.

  7. Make the offer to join once the solution has been confirmed.

By handling the prospective member's concerns on the tour, you change the entire dynamic of the sales process, which results in a more comfortable buying scenario and typically in more buying. When buyers trust the seller, they are more likely to purchase. Handling objections on the tour makes you more trustworthy and professional, and it differentiates you from your competitors and produces more first-time closes than handling objections at the end of the tour. To incorporate this style into your sales presentation, practice the simple steps described in this section. Give yourself 30 days to become proficient with this style and you will experience a noticeable difference in your sales results.

## Presenting the Price

You've just done a fabulous job with a prospective member. You built rapport to a point where you both felt comfortable, the trust was high, you qualified him, and he's a hot prospect. You masterfully did the pretour interview to determine his needs, and you know the club can meet them. On the tour, you escalated his desire even higher.

You tested the waters with trial closes, and he's ready to sign up. When you sit down to do the price presentation with him, however, the energy changes. He decides he needs to think about it for a while, and he leaves without joining.

What happened here? Aside from not handling the objection, it could have something to do with how the prices were presented. This section will focus on how you can present prices to improve your first-time closing rate.

A smooth and confident price presentation can make or break the close. Presenting the prices is not the close; the close should take place long before you go over the price details. If you wait until the price presentation, you make price the focus of the close and put yourself at a disadvantage. When presenting prices, follow these seven steps:

1. *Get out of your head.* Oftentimes, people apologize for the club prices. You might not think the club is worth the price, or you might not be able to afford a membership yourself. This attitude comes across and poisons the way you sell.

2. *Financially qualify the prospective member within the first 3 to 5 minutes.* You should ask your qualifying questions before the tour to uncover concerns before they become objections. A good question to uncover any financial concerns would be "Malcolm, what price range are you considering for membership?" The prospect will either say he's not sure and will ask how much membership costs, or he will tell you what he has in mind.

If he is unsure what he can spend, say, "Our memberships start at $45 per month and go to $75 per month. Does that fit with what you have in mind?" If it does, he's qualified and you can continue with your other qualifying and needs analysis questions. If at any point before you go on tour he starts to ask detailed questions about the different memberships in the range you just gave, simply say, "Since it looks like our range fits with your range, let's wait to go over those details until after you've seen the club; it'll make a lot more sense then."

If he responds with a number that works with the pricing structure, then your response should be something like "Excellent! We have several options that will work for you." If he responds with a number that does not work with your pricing structure, you should say. "Our memberships start at $45 per month and go to $75 per month. Are you firm at $35, or can you stretch a bit?" If he can stretch, you'll know he has just qualified himself financially and price will not be an issue.

If the pricing does not fit with what he had in mind and if he cannot stretch, then you may want to say, "Malcolm, I can understand that the membership price may not work for you, so we have two options at this point. If you don't want to take the time to see the club, I understand; however, know that I would love to show you the club." By doing this, you are gracefully giving him an option to leave without feeling embarrassed, and you are letting him know you want him to see the club. If he leaves, that's okay; he wasn't financially qualified.

3. *Relax; the prospect already said yes.* You've already verified that pricing isn't an issue, so if you aren't confident in presenting the pricing, the prospective member will get a mixed message. Continue to support the decision to join with positive language and genuine enthusiasm. The more comfortable you are with the numbers and membership options, the easier this becomes. In addition, slow down when you speak. Being able to relax during the price presentation simply takes practice, so you should role-play this frequently.

4. *Have a professionally printed price sheet with options.* List no more than four options on a price sheet. If there are too many options, it's too much to think about to make an immediate decision. Simplify your pricing structure and printed presentation to encourage an easier decision-making process. Clubs that offer only one option, however, end up shooting themselves in the foot; without options, the only choice is whether the membership works.

5. *Always start with your most expensive membership, and if it is your most popular membership, say so.* Often this will be the most popular package because of all that it includes without extra fees. If that membership doesn't work, you can go down to the next option. If you start in the low or middle range, however, you've limited your options. In addition, it may appear that you are tacking on extra fees for additional services. When you start high and from the perspective that this is the best membership package, you will sell more of them, and if you need to go down it will be received more positively.

6. *Break the information down into smaller pieces and test the waters as you go along.* Sometimes the numbers can get confusing, so be sure to break it down and not get too far ahead. Presenting all the options all at once and speaking too quickly can leave the prospective member confused.

7. *Close each option before you move to the next one.* How many times have you presented one price only to have the prospective member ask about another price on the sheet? The problem with this is you don't get any feedback on the first price, so you don't know whether it will work for the prospect. The best way to address this issue is to say, "I'd be happy to tell you more about that membership. Before I do, though, tell me what your thoughts are on the price I just went over."

Take a look at all seven steps in action:

*Malcolm, I'm excited you've decided to join the club today. I know you'll get what you want and more from your membership, so let's see which one works best for you. We have a few options, and the one I'm going to recommend first is our full-service membership. It's our most popular membership because it's our best value, and here's why: It includes everything you've seen in the club today plus towel service, and you get privilege pricing on tanning, massage, and pro-shop items. Can you see why this is our best value?*

*Now, there are two ways you can take care of your membership: You can choose the annual program or the monthly dues program. Which would you like to hear about first?*

*All right, the way the monthly dues program works is we start your membership today with your enrollment fee of $125 and the monthly dues of $55. How does that work for you? Great, then let's go ahead and finish up the details.*

That's all the price presentation needs to be. If Malcolm wants to know more about the annual plan, you would find out exactly what his thoughts are on the monthly dues, handle anything that needed to be handled, and then proceed to close him on the annual plan. By creating this flow, you will make price a detail and not the point of the conversation, and you will notice a significant increase in your first-time closing skills.

## Closing the Sale on the Tour

Most membership representatives wait until the end of the tour to close the sale, and some never even ask prospective members for their business. Remember, the answer is always no until you specifically ask for the sale. There is an abundance of business for membership representatives who are willing to ask for it. The following are some reasons representatives wait to ask for the sale or don't ask at all:

- *Rigid training.* Some clubs are locked into a traditional, inflexible style of sales by training that does not allow for any spontaneity or adjustments based on the prospective member. (Membership representatives who do too much talking and not enough listening are often the product of this rigid training.)

- *Fear of offending.* Some membership representatives feel that asking prospective members for their business will somehow offend them. However, prospective members expecting you to ask for their business; if you don't, you are sending a mixed message that their business is not that important to you.

- *Philosophy or style.* Some clubs have a philosophy of not directly asking for the sale. Clubs

are something that people want to feel a part of. Prospective members want to be invited to join and feel that they are important.

The benefits to closing during the tour include the following:

- It relieves pressure on the buyer and the seller.
- The presentation is more conversational and thus spontaneous and natural.
- It creates more differentiation between your club and your competitors.
- It expedites the sales process.

When you ask prospective members to join and they say yes, be prepared to sign them up without finishing the tour. For example, you could say, "That's excellent! Would you like to see the rest of the club, or would you prefer to get your membership taken care of and see the club later?" That may seem shocking, but most prospective members come into the club ready to buy.

## After-Sales Service and Follow-Up

When you sell a membership, you start a new long-term relationship that will be pleasurable and profitable. Often, clubs believe that all they need to do is get the members. Believe it or not, that's the easy part. The hard part is keeping the members or **retention**. The opposite of retention is **attrition**, which refers to losing members.

Attrition is one of the biggest problems most clubs face. The cost of getting a new member is much higher than the cost of keeping current members. New members are assets that needs to be taken care of by the club staff. The following is a list of things you can do to ensure new members are happy with their decision and remain with the club for years to come:

- When a new members joins, schedule a complimentary training session or fitness assessment within 24 hours, if possible. For new members who are not already practicing fitness enthusiasts, you want to get them in the habit right away.

- Get members involved with other things, such as classes, lessons, or social functions.

- Introduce them to as many staff members as possible so they immediately feel like part of the club.

- Send a personal, handwritten thank-you note the day the member joins.

- Call a week later to check in to be sure the new member is comfortable and enjoying the club. The reception you get from this call will likely be positive. However, if there is a problem, be prepared to deal with it immediately rather than passing the buck to someone else. How expediently and gracefully you handle potential problems here will determine the propensity for longevity.

- Call or email members on the first day of the month to review the club's referral program for their friends and colleagues.

- Email them every 2 months from the date they joined. It is crucial to maintain this relationship with your members. That way, if they have any problems, they know who to come to for resolution. In addition, they will bring their friends to you as referrals.

These are low-cost ways for you to have a positive effect on member retention and increase your referral base.

You will close more sales if you ask prospective members to join during the tour. Closing on the tour reflects confidence, professionalism, and comfort in your delivery that is a refreshing departure from the canned sales styles of the past.

## The Bottom Line

A club tour with a prospective member is usually the best opportunity to create differentiation between your club and others, build desire to purchase membership, develop a relationship with the client, provide all requested information (including price), and close the sale.

# CORPORATE AND GROUP MEMBERSHIP SALES

One way to sell several memberships at one time is to negotiate deals with local businesses and organizations for employees to become club members. Many health clubs make arrangements with companies to provide **corporate and group memberships** so employees can join the club at reduced rates and with customized services. The club usually requires a minimum number of employees who commit to joining in order to qualify for a group rate. This section will focus on corporate and group membership sales and membership structures for these groups.

## Benefits to Corporations

Since the mid-1970s, corporations and businesses have demonstrated that taking steps to keep their employees healthy through exercise is a good return on investment. According to the Centers for Disease Control and Prevention (CDC), maintaining a healthy workforce can lower direct costs, such as insurance premiums and worker's compensation claims, and positively affect many indirect costs, such as absenteeism and worker productivity (CDC 2015). Rather than making the significant financial investment required to develop their own exercise facilities on-site, many businesses opt to work with local health club facilities to negotiate group membership rates for employees. The benefits of a corporate or group membership include the following:

- The health club benefits by increasing its membership, gaining more publicity, and working with corporations. Having a working relationship with corporations often creates good public relations and establishes the quality of the club's programs and its emphasis on caring for members. In very competitive markets, that foot in the door can be very useful for future business relationship expansion.

- The corporation gains healthier employees, who tend to be more productive, have lower health care costs, take fewer sick days, and deal with stress better. Physically active employees tend to cost less per year than sedentary employees. Also, offering the fitness program makes an employer more desirable to potential employees.

- The employee reaps the social and health benefits of a club membership. In addition, employees who exercise frequently have higher job satisfaction scores (CDC 2015).

## Setting Up a Corporate Membership

There are several ways to set up corporate or group membership sales packages. The specific sales promotions can vary slightly depending on the needs of each corporation, but a club should be consistent in the basic group policies, membership structures, and incentives offered. Consider the following elements:

- *Joiner or enrollment fees.* Offering a discount on the joining or enrollment fees is a common incentive that health clubs offer to groups. This provides a financial incentive that is not available to the general public but still ensures consistent income through monthly dues.

- *Membership dues.* Many clubs are reluctant to offer monthly membership discounts to groups. One option to consider is suggesting that the company subsidize a portion of each employee's membership dues. This way, the employees receive discounted memberships, but the club receives the same monthly rate. A club can also create a program in which the company pays for a set number of employees to join the club for one year, and the club offers a discounted rate for that group of people. The company pays the fee upfront and therefore has an incentive to recruit employees to join. The club benefits from gaining a new, predetermined revenue source. If the number of employees who join exceeds the established number for the negotiated period, additional payment is made to the club. The deal can be modified for subsequent years.

- *Number of employees.* Clubs may choose to offer discounts on dues or joining fees on a sliding scale based on the number of employees who commit to joining (e.g., 10% discount on dues for groups of fewer than 50 and a 20% discount for groups of 50 or more). To gain a significant yield on corporate membership sales efforts, clubs may want to focus on corporate sites with large numbers of employees, 500 or more, for example. That way, if a relatively small percentage of employees join, the effort will still be worthwhile.

- *Additional services.* Corporations may look for group membership packages that offer additional programs and services such as stress management, weight loss, fitness assessment, personal training sessions, back exercise, health-risk screening, and health fairs.

- *Reporting.* Corporations may ask for reports on general employee usage patterns and attendance in specific programs. Reports on employee usage provide the corporation with insight into the value of the relationship and how much employees are using the benefit. Companies may also be able to use this data when discussing insurance rates and benefits with their health insurance providers.

- *Payment options.* Corporations typically prefer that health clubs offer more than one option for fees and billing. Negotiations for group membership packages often include options for dues sharing with employees, payroll deductions, and corporate rates.

## Developing Corporate Membership Sales Tools

Having professional sales materials is an important component of selling health club memberships to local businesses and organizations. Companies expect top-quality printed materials and slide presentations that reflect well on your club and highlight the value of corporate memberships. An in-person presentation to company leaders should be professionally prepared, tell the story of your club, and integrate information on the benefits of good employee health for the corporation. Be sure to take the time to customize each presentation for the corporate audience, and have leave-behind materials, such as brochures, which should contain a website address for more information. Be sure your presentation and sales materials focus on the benefits and the value to the company, not on the price or on discounted rates.

### The Bottom Line

Health clubs have many options for developing corporate membership proposals and plans for group sales. Work with company leaders to tailor an employee membership plan to best meet the company's needs to improve the health and morale of their workers.

## Key Terms

| | | |
|---|---|---|
| attrition | membership representatives | retention |
| corporate and group memberships | partnership | sales process |
| interview | prospective member | secret shopper |
| liability waiver | qualifying questions | tour card |
| listening | rapport | unique selling position |

# CHAPTER 9

# Focusing on Customer Service

## Learning Objectives

After studying this chapter, you will be able to

- recognize the importance of customer service and building loyalty,
- understand avenues of training to enhance customer service,
- explain essential communication skills for exceptional service, and
- monitor the success of customer service.

Owning and operating a fitness center may sound exciting, being your own boss and helping people become healthy. But the hard work of providing great customer service has to happen every day by every staff member. How you treat each member is the key to determining whether or not you stay in business, making customer service your highest priority. The people you employ must also share the philosophy that the customer is always first. Hiring people who are friendly and genuinely like people is a good start, but some situations will test even the friendliest staff. Let's see what happens when a top service staff is confronted with a difficult situation you might recognize.

Lauren is a front-desk manager who seems to teach her associates new things about customer service every day. In addition to providing tips, strategies, and techniques to provide exceptional service, she regularly demonstrates good service in her actions. The staff marvels at her ability to have even the most difficult situations result in positive outcome. Her secret? She listens. She always hears the client out to better understand the situation from his or her perspective and then works to find an acceptable solution. One of the many things she has learned along the way is that an unhappy customer is often angry and frustrated about many things and dumps that emotional baggage on the first person in a position to listen.

One day a member was angry because the lap swim times had been changed due to a scheduling conflict. Lauren listened as the woman berated her for the schedule change and said, "I've had it with this place and am never coming back, and I'm telling everyone on Twitter how awful it is here!" When the member seemed to have said all she was going to say, Lauren calmly said, "I am so sorry that we have inconvenienced you today. Your time is valuable and I know that being able to exercise is important to you. What can we do to make this right?" Still too angry to respond, the woman stormed out the door. Several

The author acknowledges the significant contributions of Terry Eckmann to this chapter.

minutes later she came back to the desk and said, "I'm really sorry. I behaved badly and I appreciate you taking the time to listen to me vent." She went on to tell Lauren that she had been upset with some work-related issues and realized that she got carried away. She thanked Lauren again for listening, more calmly discussed the situation, and continued to be a loyal customer for many years to come.

---

Have you ever received the wrong order in a restaurant? Maybe it was something as simple as asking for a glass of water with a slice of lime and receiving water with lemon instead. How did it make you feel? For some people, it's not a big deal; others, however, see it as their request being ignored. If customers continue to order lime but receive lemon, over time this becomes a significant service issue. In the fitness industry, managers and front-line employees are constantly being bombarded with seemingly small requests from members, and they sometimes don't properly fulfill these requests. These small things can be important to members, and over time the neglect of these requests can come across as poor customer service. It's not enough to think or say that customer is always first.

People who run businesses of all types realize the importance of good customer service and how it can build long-term customer loyalty. Research has shown that when you solve a customer's problem, you create a loyal consumer who will tell 10 to 16 other people about your company. If you fail to make a customer happy, however, that person will each tell an average of 28 people about the terrible experience (Freeman 2013). Like all service businesses, health fitness organizations must provide great customer service. Fitness professionals with stellar customer service skills will excel, and the fitness organization will be successful if its foundation is exceptional customer service. This is because the fitness industry sells services. A product is tangible; it takes up shelf space, has a shelf life, and can be inventoried, depreciated, and taxed. A service, on the other hand, doesn't exist until a person requests or requires it. A **service** is an action that helps another person achieves a goal or objective. A **customer** is any person who requests or requires these services. **Customer satisfaction** and loyalty occur when a service meets or exceeds a customer's expectations and when problems are resolved quickly and easily.

This chapter provides an overview of customer service. Topics include the importance of customer service and how it can build customer loyalty, the two categories of customers, what the customer wants, training staff to provide exceptional service, communicating with customers, dealing with difficult customers, and monitoring the effects of customer service.

## RECOGNIZING THE IMPORTANCE OF CUSTOMER SERVICE AND LOYALTY

We live in a rapidly changing world that continually bombards us with information. Fitness clubs continue to be challenged by economic uncertainty, more competition, changing demographics, technology, new research, and whatever the latest exercise fad seems to be. Club members are continually trying to balance the demands of work and their personal lives. These challenges make exceptional customer service in the fitness industry an important practice for all staff members all the time. The goal of customer service is to create a friendly, comfortable, clean, and well-maintained environment that meets members' needs and solves their problems, retains members, and brings in new members. **Exceptional customer service** is exceeding the customer's expectations by going the extra mile and adding that special touch. Serving members well must be the number one priority in health fitness organizations.

Customer loyalty is often linked to customer service. When it comes to service, businesses create loyal customers not only by providing the level of service they expect but also by helping solve their problems quickly and easily. When confronted with a customer service issue, staff members should ask themselves how they can make it easy for the customer. This simply means removing obstacles. Customers resent having to waste a lot of time complaining about something, having to repeat information, and being shuffled to different people for a resolution. Telling frontline staff to exceed customers' expectations sounds like a good strategy, but it can be confusing if staff don't take the time to understand what those expectations are. Customers expect problems to be solved; empowering staff to focus on solving problems quickly and easily is often more straightforward and satisfying to both parties. Great customer service people are quick to express empathy, let customers know they've been heard, and find resolutions to problems.

## The Bottom Line

Successful organizations anticipate, meet, and exceed customer needs and build customer loyalty by providing great service and solving problems.

Ameyo is a call center and customer experience management company that examines the current research on customer service trends from companies such as American Express, Accenture, Deloitte, McKinsey, and Salesforce and creates lists of important statistics. According to their 2017 summary of customer experience data, 70% of buying experiences are based on how customers feel they are being treated (Gautam 2017). The following are other key statistics Ameyo has compiled (Gautam 2017) on customer loyalty and service:

- Customer experience will overtake price and product as the key brand differentiator by the year 2020.
- Fifty-five percent of consumers would pay more for a better customer experience.
- A customer is four times more likely to buy from a competitor if the problem is service related versus price or product related.
- Eighty-nine percent of consumers have stopped doing business with a company after experiencing poor customer service.
- Eighty-two percent of customers say that getting their issue resolved quickly is the number one factor in a great customer experience.

- Forty percent of customers begin purchasing from a competitor because of their reputation for great customer service.

Reprinted in part from N. Gautam, *50 Important Customer Experience Statistics You Need to Know* (Sunnyvale, CA: Ameyo Blog, 2017).

Companies that focus on meeting customer expectations and solving problems quickly will experience the most success in gaining new customers and in keeping current ones. As mentioned in chapter 8, it is cheaper to retain customers than acquire new ones. Many marketing studies in various industries have shown that it can cost between 5 and 25 times more to acquire new customers than it does to retain existing ones (Gallo 2014). This demonstrates why customer service and satisfaction are important. Fitness businesses typically spend thousands of dollars on marketing and promotion in the hopes of acquiring new members. Keeping someone who is already sold on your company makes solid business sense.

## The Bottom Line

Customers reward companies that deliver on their promises to deliver quality products, provide great service, and solve problems, and they punish those that don't by leaving and telling others about their unsatisfactory experiences. Managers need to work hard to keep customers satisfied to retain them as well as appreciate and learn from customer complaints.

## IDENTIFYING YOUR CUSTOMER

Organizations have internal and external customers. **Internal customers** are all the people who work in an organization. The front-desk staff, personal trainers, group fitness instructors, program directors, building engineers, cleaning staff, managers or team leaders, and any other people who work every day to make your operation a success are internal customers. Internal customers usually rely on information and assistance from each other to fulfill their job duties; for example, a sales representative would need help from a fitness staff member to learn how equipment works.

By serving each other, employees of an organization create a positive atmosphere. Strained internal relationships, however, can adversely affect company morale and member satisfaction.

In a fitness center, the front-desk staff welcome members and set the tone for the member experience. The front-desk staff may also be responsible for member sales and service, customer concerns, problems or questions, and keeping members updated on happenings in the club. These staff members also provide a service to all other employees by creating a positive feeling at the first point of contact and through new-member sales and service.

Group fitness instructors provide a service to other employees by reducing overcrowding on the equipment during peak hours, for example. The workout options available through group fitness classes give customers variety to keep them interested in getting and staying fit, so the group instructors are providing a service to the membership staff.

These are a couple examples of how the network within a fitness center can provide internal customer service that will affect the service provided to external customers. Providing strong internal customer service creates a positive atmosphere of teamwork and collaboration.

**External customers** are the people who purchase an organization's services. External customers are essential to the success of any business because they provide the revenue stream. Satisfied external customers often make repeat purchases and refer their family, friends, and colleagues. A customer who has a negative experience with a business, such as being treated rudely by an employee, can also dissuade others from patronizing the business. Customer service is, therefore, a wise investment in short- and long-term marketing. Customer satisfaction is like an election that is held every day. Customers vote with their feet, and if they are dissatisfied, they will walk out your door to a competitor. If they are satisfied, however, they will continue to walk into your facility.

The manager must lead by example and provide exceptional customer service. Employees often mirror the behavior of their leaders. A good leader is out there meeting, greeting, observing, and listening to customers. A good leader provides training for employees so they are prepared to deal with difficult situations and people, and good

leaders empower employees to make decisions in response to customer needs. A leader focused on customer service will consistently review policies and procedures to keep the organization focused on the changing needs of the customers and changes in the fitness industry.

Common reasons for poor service include uncaring employees, inadequate employee training, poor handling and resolution of complaints, employees who are not empowered to meet customer needs, and differences in what the organization thinks customers want and what customers actually want. Managers must stay focused on these issues to help to prevent difficult situations and angry customers.

Many business owners have a natural tendency to focus on relationships with external customers because they purchase the products and services. Savvy managers, however, will take steps to improve internal relations by training employees to think of their coworkers the same way they do external customers and to provide the same high level of service. Managers can set an example by showing appreciation for their employees' efforts and encouraging their feedback.

## *The Bottom Line*

A customer is any person who requires or requests your services. An internal customer works for the organization, whereas an external customer purchases the organization's products and services. Providing great service to both types of customers is vital to the health and success of the organization.

## UNDERSTANDING WHAT THE CUSTOMER WANTS

In the fitness industry, a customer might be called a *client*, *guest*, *patron*, or *member*. Whatever term is used, it is essential to understand and respond to the wants and needs of the customer. The fitness industry is competitive, and there are many options available. If your organization does not meet or exceed customer expectations, the customer may do business with a competitor, purchase home exercise equipment and virtual training tools, or not exercise at all.

Differences between what a business thinks customers want and what customers actually want can result in failure to meet expectations and poor service. It is necessary to keep in touch with customer advisory boards, focus groups, and personal conversations to see what they are thinking about the services provided by your business. Surveys are also useful tools for finding out how customers are feeling. The survey responses can provide valuable information on what is going well and what might need improvement. See figure 9.1 for a sample customer service survey card.

What customers want and what they need are sometimes two different things. The task of a sales representative is to first listen to what customers say. Customers will tell you whether they are looking to fulfill a want or a need by the way they approach the purchase. If they immediately state what they want, that is what they intend to buy. If they appear indecisive, that is when you ask about the intended use, which will help you determine what they really need. This short encounter will help build trust and a relationship with customers. Most customers share general wants and needs such as the following:

Dear Member,

It is important for us to know how satisfied you are with your visit to our club today. Below is a short questionnaire that we would like you to complete. Answering the questions will take you less than a minute. As always, we welcome your comments and suggestions.

Your responses will serve as valuable feedback as we continually strive to provide great service to our members. We want to know how we're doing so we can recognize areas we are doing well and improve poor service as quickly as possible.

Please deposit your completed card in the designated box at our service desk.

Thanks for your help!

Club Manager: _____

Date of visit: _____  Time of visit: _____

**Scoring scale**

1 = Excellent
2 = Good
3 = Fair and needs improvement
4 = Poor and needs immediate attention

1. Staff courtesy _____
2. Staff responsiveness _____
3. Cleanliness of facility _____
4. Quality of programs _____
5. Met your expectations _____
6. Did any staff member call you by name? Yes   No
7. Did any staff member ask you about your progress (e.g., reaching fitness goals)? Yes   No

If you were the club manager, what would you improve?

Name (optional): _____  Email (optional): _____

**Figure 9.1**  Customer service survey card sample.

From M. Bates, M.J. Spezzano, and G. Danhoff, *Health Fitness Management*, 3rd ed. (Champaign, IL: Human Kinetics, 2020).

- *Customers want to feel welcome.* A warm greeting gives the customer an immediate sense of appreciation. Greeting customers with a friendly hello and a smile while making eye contact is the foundation of a greeting; addressing the customer by name is something extra that can make a big difference. Customers need to be the first priority. If staff members are spending too much time chatting with coworkers or using the computer, customers will feel overlooked and unimportant.

- *Customers expect a clean environment.* Staff must clean equipment regularly, and members need to be educated about doing their part to keep equipment clean. Treadmills, elliptical machines, rowers, exercise bikes, resistance training machines, free-weight equipment, and individual mats and exercise props all accumulate dust and dirt. Vacuuming and wiping down the equipment keep the environment clean and welcoming for customers and increase the life of the equipment. Cleaning staff must also perform an hourly bathroom check; keep a cleaning checklist on the inside of the bathroom door to show customers you are committed to a clean environment.

- *Customers want efficient service.* People have busy schedules and do not like to wait for service. A quick and easy check-in system allows customers to access the facility with minimal wait. The facility should open on time, and group fitness classes or personal training sessions should start and end on time. During peak hours, use a sign-in system for cardio equipment to help more members have access to the equipment for at least 20 to 30 minutes; it should be simple and monitored by staff so a customer doesn't have to ask another person to get off a machine. Enact guidelines to prevent customers from monopolizing resistance training equipment during peak times. Having an adequate selection of equipment during peak times is an expected component of fitness center customer service. In addition, the club should minimize out-of-service equipment through preventative maintenance and quick repairs.

- *Customers appreciate solutions to problems.* Customers need to be heard and understood when they come to you with problems. For example, if a customer has a bad experience with a personal trainer and is not happy with the service provided, you must listen, gather all relevant information, empathize, and determine an equitable solution for the customer. You may need to work with management to resolve the issue, but don't pass the customer off without helping him connect with the appropriate staff member. Customers want to be heard when they have problems, concerns, or questions and want their problems resolved quickly.

- *Customers expect a variety of programs and services that will help them reach their goals.* To meet a customer's needs, you must consider why that customer is a member. A customer may want to lose weight, increase lean muscle mass, decrease body fat, reduce blood pressure, lower cholesterol, improve strength, increase flexibility, improve overall health, feel better, meet people, or any combination of these. Information gathered from a new member at the time of registration can identify goals, wants, and needs so you can help that member succeed. For the facility to succeed, it must be a customer service–driven environment with programs and services that will attract a wide variety of people. A customer-focused, friendly, unintimidating environment will be more attractive to clients who are new to exercise and initially uncomfortable in a fitness setting.

- *Customers expect knowledgeable, friendly, and helpful staff.* It is important to make members feel welcome and comfortable when they walk in the door, and it is essential that they feel at ease as they enter a personal training session, fitness class, resistance training area, or any other place in the facility. When an employee observes signs of confusion or frustration from a member, the employee should approach that member and offer assistance. Not many people are comfortable asking for help; taking initiative can help them feel comfortable.

## The Bottom Line

Understanding the specific wants, needs, expectations, and goals of clients provides opportunities to meet and exceed them and is a template for organizational success.

A staff that is well trained to meet the needs of a variety of customers is essential to the success of the organization. Every member interaction is a moment of truth in the fitness industry. When staff meet the needs and wants of members, they are satisfied and loyal.

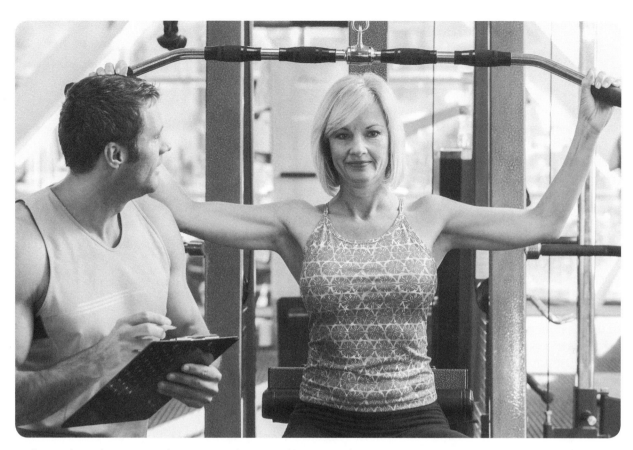

Understanding what your members want and expect is key to providing exceptional customer service. Members of your club will certainly expect the staff to be knowledgeable, friendly, and willing to help them get the most from their membership.

Monkey Business/fotolia.com

## TRAINING STAFF FOR EXCEPTIONAL CUSTOMER SERVICE

One of the common reasons for poor service is inadequate employee training. Providing excellent customer service does not cost the company much more than providing poor service. The company is already paying staff to work, and it is also spending money to train staff. After hiring friendly and engaging employees, providing training specific to a customer-focused mission is the next step toward ensuring members receive the level of service they expect. To deliver exceptional customer service, you first need to train employees to understand what exceptional customer service looks like, sounds like, and feels like. Staff members who are well trained and deliver exceptional customer service are more likely to feel helpful and fulfilled and will stay with the company, which benefits the employee and the company.

Every company should have a clear customer service philosophy that staff and members understand. Orientation of new staff should include comprehensive customer service training exercises (e.g., role-play) to reinforce the expectations of staff from the outset. Ongoing training is also necessary; this can include in-service sessions conducted by a staff member or other professional, required reading materials regarding customer service (in print or online), attendance at training seminars, and other methods. However, the most effective technique for teaching good service is staff modeling of exceptional customer service every day. (For an overview of training techniques, see chapter 4.)

# What to Teach

The reputation of a fitness business is only as good as how members feel about the services they receive and their interactions with the staff. Customers will come away from every encounter with an employee feeling neutral, happy, or unhappy. A careless word or an indifferent attitude from an uncaring staff member can ruin a customer relationship forever. If an employee is helpful, friendly, and concerned, however, the customer will likely have a positive impression of the entire organization. All staff members have the power to make the organization successful based on how they treat people; thus, it is important for every staff member to be concerned with excellence in customer service and to receive proper training in how to provide this service.

It is also necessary to train all employees on certain aspects of fitness center operation. For example, training for personal trainers should include information on front-desk operation and facility cleaning, because clients may come to them with service-related issues—and the client doesn't want to wait for 10 minutes while the personal trainer tries to find someone who knows how to refill the soap dispenser. Likewise, fitness instructors should understand membership options, hours of service, services provided, club guidelines for safety and efficiency, emergency procedures, and how to correctly use equipment.

A customer service training checklist is a helpful way to break down all job-related tasks and ensure that new employees understand what they need to do. Below is a sample checklist of customer service performance criteria with specific tasks for both relationship and service skills.

## RELATIONSHIP SKILLS

- Immediately greets all members and guests
- Greets all members personally using their names
- Has an on-stage mentality and gives full attention and energy to members
- Shows an interest in members by being warm, friendly, and willing to help at all times
- Initiates interaction with and between members
- Asks members if they need help or assistance

- Gets to know members personally by asking about family, job, hobbies, and so on
- Introduces members to other staff and members
- Invites members to participate in other programs

## SERVICE SKILLS

- Is clean and well-groomed and wears the proper staff shirt and name tag
- Asks satisfaction questions about programs and services
- Listens to suggestions and responds immediately
- Addresses complaints and concerns immediately
- Has thorough understanding of membership policies and rates
- Knows how to access information in the member database
- Is readily available and prepared for facility tours
- Has attended customer service staff training

One technique that a fitness center can use to reinforce how important customer service is to members and staff is to have a staff pledge regarding service criteria. A pledge serves as a visible reminder to staff of the expected behaviors, and it also notifies members of the level of service they can expect. For example:

*As a staff member I will:*

- *Smile and say hello. I will provide a friendly welcome to everyone I see.*
- *Help build friendships. I will make a personal connection with our members, introduce members to each other, and meet someone new each day.*
- *See it and own it. I will take responsibility for correcting any problem I see.*
- *Give thanks. I will make each day special for members and staff by having a positive attitude and by appreciating others.*

*Then, I will do it again tomorrow!*

Having employees involved in establishing customer service criteria and goals is a good management technique, and this involvement will increase commitment to achieving the goals. Seeking ways to improve customer relations can lead to a healthier work environment.

## Accountability

Checklists for training and performance assessment ensure accountability. Accountability for customer service and other job-related tasks is essential to maximize employee performance and professional growth. Employees need specific and immediate feedback and should be rewarded when goals are met. Be consistent in catching employees doing things right, and praise them immediately.

### *The Bottom Line*

A well-trained staff that meets customer's needs is essential to the success of the organization so customers are satisfied and loyal members. Regular customer service training ensures that all employees understand service expectations. A training checklist with specific expectations will help focus service delivery.

Staff rewards can be simple and inexpensive. Although tangible rewards are always appreciated, managers should remember that the best rewards are often immediate recognition and positive reinforcement for a job well done; all employees like to hear that they are doing a good job. Other rewards can include personal thank-you notes; a photo posted in the facility, newsletter, or local paper; a paid day off; movie coupons; a massage; lunch with the boss at a favorite restaurant; attendance at a local, regional, or national workshop; a free car wash; or a gift certificate to a local business. Brainstorming with staff regarding desired rewards gives employees ownership in the plan. See chapter 5 for further discussion of incentives and rewards.

If an employee continually provides inadequate customer service, you must document specific situations and provide opportunities for change. Giving feedback through conferencing can help get the employee on the right track to providing exceptional customer service. Generally, there are three types of **instructional conferences**:

1. *Instructional conference used to accelerate growth and accentuate the positive.* The purpose of this conference is to identify and discuss the employee's customer service skills. This conference increases the probability of those behaviors continuing and improving and works best when the customer service skills are effective, the customer service representative is relatively new, and immediate feedback is possible.

2. *Instructional conference used to address deficiencies and develop alternatives.* The purpose of this conference is to identify ineffective customer service skills and develop alternatives that will increase effectiveness and performance. Employees are often unaware of their ineffective customer service skills and do not know how to correct the problem. The employee and manager brainstorm more effective ways to deal with weaknesses, or the manager gives specific direction on how to improve. This conference is best used when the employee is relatively new or there have been observations of or complaints about poor service.

3. *Instructional conference used to ask why that employee is in the position.* This conference is used when the employee is consistently providing unacceptable customer service, the situation is or will soon be out of control, and the employee has made no attempt to correct the ineffective behaviors or skills.

### *The Bottom Line*

Providing rewards and feedback to staff regarding customer service delivery is essential to building a service culture. The best reward is often recognition and positive reinforcement for a job well done. The most effective feedback is specific, immediate, growth oriented, and preserves the dignity of the employee.

## Communicating With Customers

**Communication** is a two-way sharing of information that results in an understanding between the receiver and the sender. Because people process everything they hear and see through a filter system of values, experiences, beliefs, and culture, perceptions of what a speaker says may be different from what the listener hears. It has been long recognized that person-to-person communication is both verbal and nonverbal. While the relative amount of each component is debated, it is fair to say that nonverbal communication is significant and needs to be understood to maximize customer service delivery.

## Be Conscious of Nonverbal Communication

**Nonverbal communication** can send a clear message to its recipient; for example, a simple sigh can suggest annoyance, frustration, or impatience. It is possible to communicate messages through body language and vocal inflection without intending to. A person's facial expressions, eye contact, body posture, and gestures all send out messages.

A calm, concerned, and sincere facial expression sends the message that you care about what the customer is saying. A smile sends a welcoming and friendly message, but smiling when a customer is expressing anger may communicate a mocking attitude or indicate that you don't take the customer's message seriously. Facial expressions often affect inflection, even when you are talking on the phone. Placing a mirror by the phone with a reminder to smile can actually improve phone communication. The eyes also communicate a great deal in conversation. Making eye contact indicates an interest in the customer and shows that you are paying attention. Rolling eyes can indicate disgust and should be avoided.

Exhibit good posture, such as standing and sitting straight and tall, in a work setting. Slouching or putting your feet up on an object or desk indicates an inattentive, disinterested, and overly relaxed attitude. It sends a message that you don't want to be bothered. Maintain a nonthreatening, open body posture and be sure not to invade a customer's personal space. Body movement can also affect perception of interest. Moving slowly, especially when working with a customer who is upset or waiting for service, can send a message of disinterest. Gestures can also send messages; for example, crossing the arms in front of the body is a defensive stance that may suggest an unwillingness to listen. Resting the head in the hands indicates you are tired and unconcerned.

Avoid chewing gum or eating while you are on the phone or in the fitness center, because these behaviors can be distracting and irritating to a customer who is trying to communicate with you. In addition, eating in front of customers gives the impression that you don't want to be disturbed because you are busy with a personal matter, which discourages customer interaction. Chewing food can also be noisy and unappealing.

Personal habits of dress, grooming, and cleanliness also send out messages regarding professionalism. Hair, hands, fingernails, and teeth need to be clean. Clothing should be appropriate for the setting. Inappropriately showing skin and undergarments is unprofessional and should be avoided. Although tattoos and body piercings are popular, their appearance in work settings may be controversial. Fitness organizations should develop policies regarding acceptable dress and grooming practices in the workplace so there is clear understanding among employees.

## The Bottom Line

It is not what you say but what is heard. It is not what you mean but what is understood. There is no one reality, only perception of what is said and heard.

## Focus on Listening

Chapter 8 discussed how good listening skills can help build relationships with prospective members. Listening is also critical in providing great customer service. Efficient listening can mean the difference between your members feeling satisfied or dissatisfied with some aspect of your business. To deliver high quality, consistent customer service, all staff members should receive training on how to improve their listening skills.

By focusing on listening, customer service representatives can better understand members' immediate needs or issues. Listening also helps staff respond appropriately to those needs, which results in a higher level of customer satisfaction. In addition to the tips discussed earlier, the following are three key ones to focus to improve service to members:

1. *Avoid distractions.* Tune out all forms of distraction that could cause you to shift your focus from the member you are assisting. At this moment, helping the member is the most important work you have to do.

2. *Paraphrase what the customer said.* One way to practice active listening is to paraphrase what the customer said after listening to the concern. This helps make the customer feel heard and shows that you are genuinely concerned and willing to assist. It is also a way to be sure you understand exactly what the customer said and verify the customer's primary concern or problem. This simple yet effective step often allows you to provide the needed assistance and solve the problem quickly.

3. *Ask questions.* Asking the right questions ensures that you understand the customer's needs and overall concern. This will help you find the best solution.

## Portray a Positive Attitude: The Power of One

In the eyes of a customer, each employee in an organization *is* the organization. Everything an employee does is a reflection of the organization as well as the person. One person can make a positive impact on the organization, and one person can make a negative impact. Unfortunately, it is the negative experience that will be most talked about and remembered. A positive attitude in customer service is essential for organizational success.

**Attitude** is a reflection of how you think about something or someone, and how you think about the customer is how you will treat the customer. If your attitude is positive, you will handle difficult situations more effectively. To develop a positive attitude, you must realize you have control over your attitude. Attitude is a state of mind influenced by feelings, thoughts, and action tendencies; thus, it influences three things that you can control: what you think, what you say, and how you behave. We all choose our attitudes about ourselves, other people, and work. The quality of your work is a reflection of your attitude.

The hiring process is the critical first step in employing people with positive attitudes. Fitness professionals and support staff need to genuinely believe in the positive benefits of fitness and have a desire to connect with people.

## Power Talking

No one likes to hear the word *no*. People don't want to hear what you cannot do for them. *Yes*, on the other hand is a powerful word that can turn a negative customer into a positive customer. A response that begins with a *yes* creates a positive perception and sends a message that you are working to accommodate the needs of the customer. For example, responding to a request for help with "No, I'm busy with another client" sends a very different message from "Yes, I'll be happy to help you in a couple of minutes." Power talking is a way to use positive words to tell the customer what you can do. It involves avoiding blame and striving to understand the listener, as you can see in the following sample phrases.

| Instead of this | Say this |
| --- | --- |
| Your problem | This situation |
| You have to | I'd appreciate it if you'd |
| Don't forget | Please remember |
| I'll have to | I'll be glad to |
| I can't | I can |
| But | And |
| Spend | Invest |
| I disagree | I understand |
| You'll have to ask | I can help you by |

## DEALING WITH DIFFICULT CUSTOMERS

Despite best efforts, customer service will fail from time to time. It is best if the employee responds to the dissatisfied customer on the spot or as quickly as possible. Empowered employees can better serve the customer and resolve conflicts. Employees with an understanding of the importance of customer service and knowledge of how to effectively and efficiently resolve customer concerns will create an environment of customer satisfaction.

Everyone has heard that the customer is always right. Of course, the customer is not always right, but the customer is always the customer. Every customer complaint is an opportunity to create a positive relationship. The goal is to reduce the number and frequency of complaints, but complaints are opportunities to improve service and build positive relationships by turning unhappy customers into happy and loyal customers.

One of the most important strategies for dealing with an angry or difficult customer is to listen. Listening for understanding will often diffuse a difficult situation. Some people simply want to be heard and understood. You can't fix the problem until you know what it is, and if you are waiting for your turn to talk instead of seeking to understand the customer, you may miss the real problem. To effectively listen, you must keep in mind that it is not a personal attack, although it may seem personal. Effective listening requires you to let go of preconceived notions about the person and the situation and seek to understand the angry customer. People speak approximately 125 to 175 words per minute (Slowik 2000) and listen at a rate that is about four times faster, so a listener can easily think ahead and lose the underlying message being sent by the speaker.

When you are working with an angry or concerned customer, make sure that you do what you say you are going to do. If you are going to check on a policy or the possibility of another membership option, check it out and get back to the customer as soon as possible. Prompt service is key to customer satisfaction. It is also important to be flexible. Policies are necessary, but they can become outdated and may not apply to every situation. Be sure to question policies that often create customer dissatisfaction and anger.

A policy that once had a purpose may no longer be necessary. If there is question about a policy among staff or with members, ask why it exists, whether it still serves a purpose, and whether it needs to be modified or eliminated to better serve members today. Don't lose members over a bad or outdated policy.

There will be times when angry customers are right about their situations. This is an appropriate time to go the extra mile with a complimentary service or an extension of membership. It is also important to follow up with a phone call or note to thank the customer for taking the time and energy to provide you with the opportunity to fix what went wrong.

There will be times when an unhappy customer is in the wrong and will not be satisfied by anything you do, but they will be few and far between. An angry, irrational customer can create a negative environment that makes employees and other customers uncomfortable. If this happens, a manager will likely need to step in to defuse the situation and address the conflict. When all else has failed, you may have to suggest that the customer might be happier elsewhere. It is best to cut ties with that customer than to risk losing other customers.

## CUSTOMER SERVICE BEST PRACTICES

Developing a culture of excellent customer service in an organization is a challenging, ongoing process. This section addresses several categories of customer service best practices for fitness centers that will drive staff behavior and support your company's stated customer service philosophy.

### STAFF

- The reception desk has enough staff to give prompt attention to prospective members.
- Reception-desk staff smile and greet all visitors and members personally (i.e., using names).
- Staff members are clean, well groomed, and dressed according to the uniform standards.
- Staff members wear name badges while on duty.
- Management staff are visible and regularly circulate throughout the facility greeting members and guests.

## RECEPTION DESK

- All point-of-contact areas are clean and free of clutter, such as food, beverages, newspapers, and staff belongings.
- The reception desk is used only by authorized staff.
- There is a back-up system staff member when the reception desk gets busy.
- The organization's commitment to service is prominently displayed.

## TELEPHONE

- Incoming telephone calls are handled by a person dedicated to that task; other people are assigned to greeting and serving members and guests.
- Experienced staff are assigned to answer the phone. All incoming calls are answered by a person rather than an automated service.
- The phone is answered promptly by the third ring.
- A standard caller greeting has been developed and is used by staff.
- Staff check back with callers on hold every 15 seconds.

## INFORMATION FOR RECEPTION DESK

- There is a system for keeping up-to-date information near the phone and easily accessible by reception-desk staff.
- The reception-desk information includes all current club brochures or program flyers.
- The reception-desk information includes recent news releases and other information that callers may refer to.
- The reception-desk information includes a current roster of all management staff, program instructors, and facility staff.
- The phone receptionist and reception-desk staff should have list of management staff whom they can contact easily.
- Staff members have easy access to all emergency phone numbers.
- The reception-desk staff has information on meetings and events held in and out of the building, including contact phone numbers.
- There is a system for referring and tracking all membership inquiries so membership staff members can contact prospects to schedule interviews and tours.
- There is a system for recording all membership inquiries and tracking those that have interviews and those who ultimately become members.

## FACILITY APPEARANCE AND CLEANLINESS

- All facility signs are visible, contain up-to-date information, and are well maintained.
- The atmosphere of the entire building is warm, friendly, neat, and clean.
- The club has sufficient numbers of custodial and maintenance staff to thoroughly clean the facility.
- The club shows members and guests that it is committed to cleanliness by posting the cleaning schedule so it is visible.
- The responsibility for cleanliness is part of every staff member's job description and daily duties.
- The building property manager and executive director regularly inspect the facility during times of peak use to see what needs improvement and assign staff accordingly.
- Cleaning solutions and towels or sanitary wipes are present in all exercise areas so members can clean off equipment after use.

## EQUIPMENT

- All equipment is inspected thoroughly on a daily basis.
- When malfunctioning or broken equipment is discovered, staff immediately determine whether a service call is required for repair.
- All staff members report broken equipment to appropriate staff using a repair form that is copied to appropriate management staff.
- The club has a staff member who is trained and certified in equipment maintenance to monitor all equipment and immediately make routine repairs.
- A supply of spare equipment parts that can be replaced by staff without a service call is kept on hand.
- All malfunctioning or broken equipment that cannot be quickly repaired is taken out of service or removed from the fitness center

until it is restored to working order. A sign is posted on broken equipment indicating that a repair service has been scheduled and when the equipment is expected to be back in operation.

- The club assigns staff members to make and document regular inspections of the facility.

## PROPERTY

- The outside of the facility is clean and well maintained.
- Interior and exterior signage is uniform and in good condition.
- If the facility has a parking lot, it should be well lit, safe, and secure; well maintained; clearly marked; and free of potholes, debris, and cracks. It must have the required number of handicapped parking spaces.
- All trash receptacles are secured out of sight to the extent possible.
- All facility landscaping is groomed, well maintained, and free of weeds and trash.

## INTERIOR APPEARANCE

- Club facilities are clean and well lit.
- Corridors and stairwells are clean and not used for storage.
- Carpeting is clean and fresh and is not worn with traffic patterns, spills, or frayed areas.
- Tile and wooden floors are kept clean, including corners.
- Lockers are in working order and free of scratches, dents, or graffiti.
- Locker rooms are well ventilated, odor free, clean, and well lit.
- The lobby furniture is clean and fresh and is not worn, torn, broken, or stained. The lobby should be furnished as a social place for members and guests.
- All doors and windows are clean and free of signs and other markings.

## MONITORING THE EFFECTS OF CUSTOMER SERVICE

Everyone in an organization is responsible for delivering and measuring customer satisfaction.

There are multiple ways a club can know whether its customer service efforts are working. When customer service is working, members are more likely to be satisfied and tell their friends and colleagues about your club; therefore, membership sales staff will notice an increase in member referrals. Word of mouth is a powerful marketing tool, especially when members use social media. (To take full advantage of members' social media use, managers can use incentive programs, as discussed in chapter 7, to promote the club through the members.) In addition to attracting new members, current club members will use the club more often and for longer periods of time if they feel welcome and comfortable in the environment. Former members are more likely to return if they have established relationships with club staff through positive customer service experiences. Club members and staff will be smiling and satisfied if the environment is conducive to having a good time and people are happy. Members will take pride in their club. You will see members wearing club T-shirts and hats or carrying water bottles with the club logo.

When customer service is working well, there will be more positive comments and fewer complaints. Focus groups will come up with creative new ideas rather than dwelling on what is wrong at the club. Customer service surveys will focus on the positive experiences more than the negative ones.

Staff members are more involved and engaged in a customer service–driven organization. They take pride in the club and create a team atmosphere when customer service is working, and there are fewer problems with absenteeism and staff turnover. Focus groups, customer satisfaction surveys and inventories, advisory boards, management by observation, suggestion boxes, social media engagement, and secret shoppers are some ways to measure the effectiveness of customer service.

## Focus Groups

Conducting focus groups of about 10 people who provide the club with general performance feedback or share feedback related to specific issues is a great way to improve customer service and increase retention. Focus groups held on a regular basis can offer valuable ideas for your facility and build strong relationships with club members as you include them in the improvement process. Listening to club members in a focus group sends the message that customer opinions are important. Make the focus group experience valuable by following these tips:

- Write clear goals and objectives for the meeting. Know what you want to accomplish and what open-ended questions you need to ask.
- Select 8 to 10 people to participate in the group. Initially, work with staff to identify 10 to 20 people so you end up with 10. The group should include clients who are regulars and those who come less regularly, people of different ages, men and women, and people with different cultural backgrounds. A diverse group will provide a wider perspective.
- It is wise to offer simple incentives to those who participate. For example, members of the focus group may receive healthy food and beverages during the group meeting and a voucher for a moderate membership discount on renewal or gift certificate for club merchandise.
- Focus groups are more likely to be honest and share thoughts and ideas if a facilitator who is not a staff member conducts the group. The facilitator will keep the conversation focused and flowing in an unintimidating manner.
- Thank the focus group at the end of the meeting and with a follow-up note informing them of the action taken in response to the meeting. Meeting notes can be posted on the club bulletin board or in the newsletter.

# Customer Satisfaction Surveys and Inventories

These can provide an opportunity to know what customers are thinking. They can be specific or general, depending on what you want to know from the customers. It is important to follow up with those who complete the surveys and inventories to show that the input they took the time to give you was considered. An action plan to implement legitimate suggestions and address common concerns can help build trusting relationships with customers.

## Advisory Boards

Advisory boards made up of club members can offer effective feedback on a regular basis to allow club owners, team leaders, and staff members to see the club from members' perspectives. An advisory board should consist of 10 to 20 people from diverse backgrounds and who range in age. The advisory board term can be from 1 to 5 years, and meetings can be held quarterly or monthly. Board members should receive an agenda before the meeting so they can provide input on the listed topics and consider other topics of concern or ideas for improvement. Board members should receive recognition in the club, verbal and written thanks, and a small gift for their efforts.

## Management by Observation

This leadership practice, commonly referred to as *management by wandering around*, is often used by successful business leaders. Managers and owners must do more than talk about customer service; they must demonstrate exceptional customer service and be visible throughout the facility. Managers, owners, and team leaders should walk around the club to provide performance feedback to staff and build relationships with members. Management by observation is one of the best ways to train staff, provide immediate feedback on staff performance, and consistently monitor customer service. A leader's mood and modeling can send a powerful message to employees.

## Suggestion Box

A traditional suggestion box at the club's front desk can be a good way to measure customer service efforts and find ways to improve service. The contents should be collected each day by the staff member in charge of addressing suggestions. Another effective option is a suggestion form on the club's website. An online suggestion box allows club personnel to communicate directly with members and work with them toward solutions instead of reading anonymous written notes that are sometimes scribbled in anger. Whether written or submitted online, suggestions need to be addressed in a timely manner.

## Secret Shoppers

Chapter 8 addressed how secret shoppers can be effective for monitoring staff telephone skills. They can also be used to gain perspective into a company's ongoing customer service practices. Secret shoppers can be used to perform specific tasks, such as using the club on a trial basis, participating in group exercise classes, asking questions, registering complaints, or behaving in certain ways, and then providing detailed reports or feedback about their experiences.

## The Bottom Line

Measuring customer service quality and customer satisfaction helps improve these areas. Everyone working in an organization is responsible for delivering and measuring customer satisfaction. Anything and everything that affects the customer should be measured. Performance standards and criteria that are quantifiable and can evaluate performance through hard data are essential to effectively measure and apply the process of continual improvement.

## Key Terms

| | | |
|---|---|---|
| communication attitude | exceptional customer service | internal customers |
| customer | external customers | nonverbal communication |
| customer satisfaction | instructional conferences | service |

# CHAPTER 10

# Retaining Members Through Program Management

## Learning Objectives

After studying this chapter, you will be able to

- understand how programs are crucial components of a member retention strategy,
- understand membership retention principles,
- know how to turn new members into long-term members,
- develop a retention plan using the logical progression of programming,
- use one program to promote another,
- understand the five steps to successful programs, and
- follow a complete programming agenda.

A large health club was experiencing a decline in member sales and an increased attrition rate. In an effort to turn things around, the club underwent a costly renovation of its equipment and facilities, which was accompanied by a substantial increase in dues. The hope was that the renovation would attract new members and improve the retention rate of existing ones.

As expected, the initial response to the renovation was positive. But club management noticed that once the initial influx of new members slowed and the excitement subsided, membership growth lagged again. Realizing that the addition of new equipment wasn't enough, they decided they needed to improve customer service and develop a more productive new-member initiation and engagement program. Less than half of new members took advantage of the existing program.

The club hired a fitness management consultant, who proposed training staff on how to professionally greet new and prospective members, promote registration for programs and services, track the results, and transition new members into personal training sessions. This strategy required the club to be more selective in hiring staff with good personal communication skills and to provide staff with quality customer service training.

Next, the club put up a registration board for new-member orientation. Members signed up for orientations in the areas of most interest to them (cardiorespiratory equipment,

The author acknowledges the significant contributions of Sandy Coffman to this chapter.

resistance training, or both) and had the option to meet with a group exercise instructor to discuss current classes. The new orientation program had the following significant improvements:

- Groups of up to 12 members could sign up for each time slot, which encouraged interactions among new members.
- Orientations were available in a variety of formats, each with a different focus, such as classes, general equipment usage, sports, cardio, and strength.
- Staff received customer service training on how to effectively conduct group activities.
- Membership sales staff promoted the orientation as a new-member service.
- Staff conducting the orientations had goals to meet, including providing a fun, social, educational experience, and increasing registrations for personal training or group exercise programs.

Within 2 years, these efforts to improve member engagement resulted in a 12.5% reduction in the attrition rate. In addition, the number of new members who participated in personal training sessions increased from 280 to 400.

---

Although most people understand that being physically active and exercising regularly can lead to better health, they will not maintain an exercise routine if they aren't enjoying the experience. If left alone to exercise without guidance, encouragement, or recognition, many people will give up because they don't meet an expectation, find excuses not to exercise, or experience an injury. When these things happen to club members, particularly new ones, chances are pretty good that they will quit exercising and quit the club. The reasons members give for leaving are pretty familiar to club managers: I'm not using the club enough, I don't have time, or it's not convenient to get to the club. The reality is that they are not using the club to exercise because the experience they've had at the club is not of enough value to them. Members who are left to work out alone with little or no direction and no connection to a group do not fully realize all that a club experience has to offer. The value of a club membership is in sociability, camaraderie, friendships, relationships, leadership, and group experiences. These are all things a club's menu of programs and services is designed to provide.

Membership retention is a result of having a variety of programs and services that offer different experiences and challenges to keep members active and engaged month after month and year after year. Members often become bored with the same routines, and their interest in exercise can wane. Exercise is a club's product, and club operators have to offer a variety of programs to help members achieve their health goals, including aquatics, group exercise, personal training, sports, competitive challenges, family programs, and social events. Having members engaged in different programs over the course of a year keeps them interested and returning to the club regularly. It may take involvement in up to six or eight different programs in a year to get a member committed to a club and a lifestyle that includes regular exercise.

The goals of **programming** are retention and helping members meet their goals. Therefore, the objective of every program is to get members to use the club, enjoy it, and feel at home there. Programming and retention go hand in hand, but they are often overlooked; if clubs put as much time, effort, and energy into programming plans for member engagement and retention as they put into sales and marketing, their bottom lines would significantly increase. Studies show that it can cost six to seven times more to get a new customer than to keep an existing one, and if clubs can decrease their attrition rates by 5%, they might be able to double their profits (Reichheld and Sasser 1990).

When you pay attention to members and provide them with programming options, they will use the club more and feel that it is an indispensable part of their lives. When members connect with other members and staff, they have a more enjoyable club experience and look forward to seeing these people regularly. Programming that facilitates engagement with other members and staff in a fun, social environment increases referrals and retention and decreases attrition. Programs and services must be designed to provide these experiences.

## MEMBERSHIP RETENTION

Membership is the financial and programmatic lifeblood of any club; without members, the club wouldn't exist. Although the sales function of a club is designed to bring in new members, it is the club's programs and services that retain long-term, loyal members. Membership retention is the process of engaging members in the club experience so they will use the club regularly and remain satisfied customers. Many club operators see membership retention as their biggest challenge. Club operators need to create an environment that keeps members happy and makes them feel confident that their gym memberships are worthwhile investments. Keeping members happy and satisfied will reduce the need to continually market to attract new members.

Retention is often calculated one year from the joining date (although checking retention rates at 3 and 6 months is also useful). In 2017, the retention rate of independent clubs that were not part of national chains was 79%, and the retention rate at national chain multipurpose facilities was 69% (International Health, Racquet, and Sportsclub Association 2017b). The following is a simple and popular method for calculating retention rate:

$$[(EM - NM) / SM] \times 100$$

where

EM = Ending members (the number of members at the end of the period)

NM = New members (the number of new members acquired during the period)

SM = Starting members (the number of members at the start of the period)

For example, if you have 111 members at the beginning of the month and 15 members cancel their contracts and 20 new members join, then you end the month with 116 members. Using the previous equation, the retention rate can be calculated as follows:

$$[(116 - 20) / 111] \times 100 = 86.5\%$$

Knowing which members are most likely to leave, and for what reasons, is a complex and critical issue for club managers. Members often leave a club without stating their reasons; they simply stop using the club and stop paying membership dues. Some members leave due to dissatisfaction with some aspect of the club, and others leave for reasons unrelated to the club experience (e.g., moving away). Efforts to determine why members leave can greatly improve retention. Strategies such as sending brief email surveys to members who quit or having regular discussions with members can provide insight into issues that might cause members to leave. Obtaining this information can help managers understand the club experience and develop plans to encourage members to stay engaged and committed to the club.

As mentioned in the chapter-opening scenario, new-member orientation programs can be vital opportunities to connect new members with staff and existing club members. According to a survey by IHRSA (2017a), 76% of people who left a club did so due to lack of relationships and connections (e.g., a favorite staff person left, the member did not fit in, the member did not find exercise partners, the member did not get involved a program). Personal connections between members and staff are a powerful tool, and creative, challenging, and enjoyable programs are a great way to create those connections. Here are a few other retention tips from the IHRSA *Member Retention Report* (International Health, Racquet, and Sportsclub Association 2017a):

- Nearly 90% of club members say they value communication from staff members.
- Social interaction affects renewals. The risk of cancellation was 56% higher among members who only use gym equipment versus those who exercise in groups.
- Your best salespeople are your fitness staff; they can generate 600% more income per

member than salespeople alone. Frequent interaction between fitness staff and members results in more member visits, and members who visit more often have higher renewal rates.

- Social interaction also affects overall member satisfaction; 70% of club members who made new friends through their memberships self-identified as club promoters rather than club detractors.

- Reaching out to a member—whether by phone, email, text, or social media—more than doubles the likelihood that the member will be a promoter rather than a detractor. In fact, the report states that "any type of interaction with a member at risk of cancelling can reduce the likelihood of dropping out by nearly 10%."

# Retaining New Members

As discussed previously, programs can provide numerous benefits to club members. Staff must be skilled in designing, conducting, and evaluating programs so they meet members' needs. The following sections address key factors in implementing programs that retain new members.

## Communication With Members

Staff should personally contact every new member who joins the club within the first week of membership. It has been proven that most new members quit a club before they start using it on a regular basis. It is difficult for new members, especially inexperienced ones, to enter the club alone and feel comfortable walking into a group exercise class or getting on a piece of equipment. A personal invitation to meet with a staff member at a convenient time is very effective. You can send a reminder postcard or an email, but a personal phone call is best. Members who are intimidated or inexperienced will probably not come in without reassurances from staff.

## Follow Up

Your work is not done when you call and invite a member to a program or meeting. Professional communication includes following up on your invitation or promise. You should follow up with an email or another phone call, especially if it seems the member is not sure about participating. A reminder 12 to 24 hours before the meeting or program helps ensure participation and reinforces the sincerity of your invitation.

## Recognition of Participants

It's imperative to acknowledge the work and achievements of new members who participate in programs or activities. Giving a compliment, taking a picture, or extending a sincere handshake can be meaningful to the member. You can also present an award or certificate to the member. Because programs are tools for keeping members engaged in the club, keep track of member attendance and recognize participation.

## Sociability

It is a common saying among club operators that most members join clubs for exercise and fitness, but they stay for the fun and social aspects. Sociability, camaraderie, and friendships are all key ingredients to a club experience. When people are in a group program, they are more likely to enjoy themselves, meet others like themselves, and form friendships. Group programs provide sociability, which is a major factor in retention.

## Commitment to a Schedule

New members must be committed to the program, to exercise, and to a new lifestyle, and some members are committed to a leader or the other members of a group. These are all good commitments that will help new members feel the sense of belonging that will keep them coming back. The one that is key to retention, however, is the commitment to a specific schedule or time frame, because it helps form an exercise habit. Retention occurs when members put the club into their lifestyles and come to the club on the same days and at the same times every week.

# ESTABLISHING THE PURPOSE OF PROGRAMMING

Health club programs, such as group exercise, sports, aquatics, and others, must provide one or more benefits to members. Program benefits

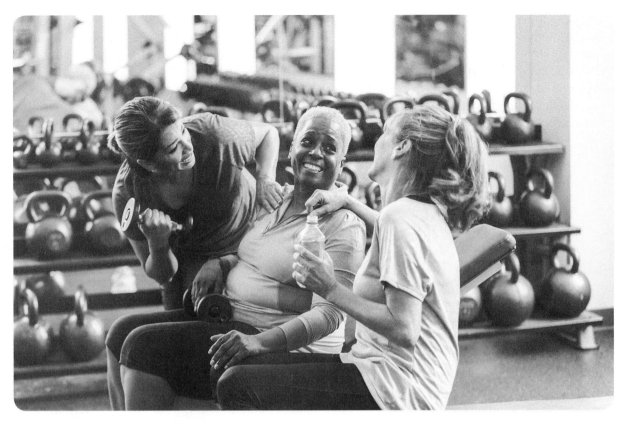

An important key to retaining memberships is implementing group programs that foster the formation of friendships.

kali9/E+/Getty Images

include meeting other members, learning new skills, or just having fun. To make sure members are reaping these benefits, program staff should track participation, give recognition for performance, and promote the other club programs. These good retention practices will keep members from becoming inactive and eventually quitting club because they aren't using it. Your responsibility in running quality health and fitness programs is to help members meet other members who have common interests, schedules, and abilities so that they develop a sense of belonging and commitment while experiencing a sense of achievement and purpose.

The success of programs as member retention tools is dependent on hiring qualified program staff, training them with the proper procedures, teaching them to use proven protocols to accomplish goals for every program, and holding them accountable for reaching those goals. Different programs need to be offered throughout the year to keep the member engaged, interested, and

coming back. Following are some best practices for programs that will retain members:

- Members who use the club regularly are more likely to remain members; ideally, members should be using the facility at least one or two times per week. On-going participation in programs ensures regular usage of the club, helping to keep members engaged and active.

- Members should have regular interactions with one or more staff members to create a sense of loyalty to the club and staff. Programs provide such interactions with an instructor or trainer, which creates loyalty, trust, and comfortable familiarity, all of which contribute to retention.

- Staff should aim to engage members in more than one program within the year. Once engaged in programs on an on-going basis, exercising in your club will become part of their lifestyles, and they will become loyal members.

Transitioning a new member into a loyal, retained member in part depends on the types of programs offered and their target population. Member populations can be categorized by gender, age, interests, skill levels, schedules, personalities, and lifestyles. All members can be placed in four general groups for programming purposes:

1. New members
2. Active members
3. Inactive members
4. Potential members

The overarching goal of every program is to integrate new members, diversify active members, offer new beginnings to inactive members, and create initial interest in potential members.

## DIVERSIFICATION OF ACTIVITIES

A major factor in retention is providing diverse activities for members throughout the year. Many people get bored doing the same routine or activity over and over, so new challenges, goals, and experiences will keep them interested or renew their interest in exercising. In addition, new members might be searching for that one activity that will really inspire them, so offering many options can aid in this quest. Cross-training is another reason **diversified programming** is so important. Cross-training typically results in better overall fitness results and helps prevent boredom, so diversified programming is both emotionally and physically beneficial. Diversified programming keeps members engaged and coming back, which is the goal of programming.

## PROGRESSION OF PROGRAMS

Progressing through a series of programs is the objective of the wheel of logical progression (explained later in this chapter). It ensures retention through an extended period of diversified programming. New members can begin their memberships with an introductory program and progress to more advanced instructional opportunities, which can prepare them for regular involvement in programs such as sport leagues, fitness challenges, personal training sessions, or group exercise classes. Participation in progressive programming is a significant factor in keeping

members active, interested, goal driven, and successful in their efforts. If you use one program to promote another, the progression will continue. The objective is for all members to become integrated in the club through introductory programs and services, become familiar and comfortable with them, and commit to activities that make the club part of their weekly routine.

## PROMOTION OF PROGRAMS

Professional promotion starts with a calendar of club events and services that offers a variety of activities and programs throughout the year. Programs can be promoted through posters, bulletin boards, website notices, and flyers no less than 3 weeks before the start of the program. Email campaigns, through which you invite members to a specific event, are productive if they are sent at least 3 weeks in advance and are followed up with a confirmation email sent 12 to 24 hours before the program begins. Programs should also be promoted verbally within the club. For example, the front-desk staff can promote a program to every person who comes in, group exercise instructors can promote programs in their classes, and personal trainers can promote programs to their clients. All promotions must be timely with the start of the program.

## RELIABILITY OF THE SCHEDULE

**Reliability** is a crucial issue that is often misunderstood or ignored altogether. Reliability means that you set a programming schedule that can be maintained. For example, a programming schedule that offers a beginner-level program on a Tuesday and an intermediate-level program on a Thursday should maintain that schedule for at least 6 months and preferably for a year or more. Members need to plan ahead, so your club should have consistent core program offerings to allow people to adjust their schedules to accommodate their programs of choice. When you change the same program to a different time and day, you eliminate the members who spent weeks preparing their schedules to make room for a class at 9 a.m. on Tuesdays only to find that it has been changed to Wednesdays. Keep several core programs on a consistent schedule to set a reliable precedent for members.

## ACCOUNTABILITY FOR GROWTH AND RETENTION

Every program must have a leader who is held accountable for these key elements of retention. The accountability structure of programming, if managed efficiently, is worthy of a program director's position. If a full-time program director is not feasible, there must be a leader assigned to each program who is capable, responsible, and held accountable for taking the program through the development keys. At the end of the day, the success or failure of a program is linked to how well these key factors were implemented. A program cannot run successfully without accountability for its presentation, growth, and effect on member retention. Programs that are professionally developed, implemented, monitored, and evaluated are the heart of membership growth and retention.

## *The Bottom Line*

Retention is not simply a goal; it is a vision for a vibrant, successful health club. Engaging members in the club experience results in them using the club regularly and remaining satisfied customers. Keeping members satisfied reduces the need for continual marketing to attract new members. Retaining members requires providing great service, having qualified staff who focus on meeting member needs, and having a variety of high-quality programs that are fun and challenging.

## PROGRAMMING BY LOGICAL PROGRESSION

Simply put, a membership retention strategy is a step-by-step plan to take every member in your club from orientation to involvement to commitment. You must provide opportunity, innovation, education, and leadership in a positive atmosphere that ensures ongoing program activity that results in fitness, exercise, and health. The operative word is *ongoing*. Unfortunately, working out for 3 months and then stopping will not provide the lifetime health and fitness benefits members need, but this is not uncommon among people who join a club with the idea of a lifetime commitment to exercise. Here I discuss a system of developing programs to achieve the goal of retention.

The **wheel of logical progression** is based on the theory of applied creativity used in the business world. It means following a logical progression of activities or programs to ensure that people will keep coming back. The theory is best illustrated by a wheel with six spokes (see figure 10.1). All the spokes must be in place for the wheel to work.

The logical progression of programming includes the three stages people go through when they join a club or begin any exercise program. Each stage is further broken down into two programming opportunity phases that lead to retention.

1. *Integration stage.* This includes the introduction and instruction phases.
2. *Acceptance stage.* This includes the involvement and achievement phases.
3. *Commitment stage.* This includes the improvement and fun phases.

This system is adaptable to any health fitness facility, recreational activity, or fitness program and to any participant ability level. People who are new to exercise or sport can begin their participation on the wheel of logical progression and continue on. In addition, a person who is experienced, active, and fit will find that the wheel offers the exact experience necessary for beginning a new activity or sport and will allow progression to occur at a higher degree of ability, experience, or skill. The steps to retention remain the same.

The following sections outline the three-stage, six-phase progression for engaging members during the first year of participation. You are most likely already doing some of these programming activities. The key is to identify any gaps in your programming system that can cause members to drop out. You will see where you can fill those gaps with the appropriate programs.

One of the major mistakes made in the health fitness industry is skipping programming phases. Skipping phases results in lack of achievement, lost interest, poor performance, or frustration. Work in order (starting at step 1), and don't skip any steps. Every program should be designed to promote and inspire participation in a follow-up program. This is more likely to occur, of course,

1. **Introduction**
   - Develop a new interest
   - Have fun
   - Experience success
2. **Instruction**
   - Learn more
   - Get better
3. **Involvement**
   - Leagues
   - Sessions

4. **Achievement**
   - Recognition
   - Award presentations
5. **Improvement**
   - Competition
   - Education
   - Diversification
   - Advancement in skills
6. **Fun**
   - Social events
   - Special events

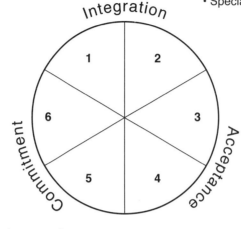

**Figure 10.1**    The wheel of logical progression.

© Sandy Coffman

if the programs are enjoyable, achievable, and successful.

You are undoubtedly beginning to see how the program sale begins after the membership sale. Each programming phase must be promoted and sold to members after they have bought the membership. The program director, instructor, trainer, or leader must be held accountable for selling the idea of progressing from one level to the next and for keeping the members involved in a program or series of programs throughout the year.

## First Stage: Integration

The **integration stage** is often called *orientation*. It gives members a beginning experience but must also be designed to encourage further participation and thus improve retention. New members typically receive an initial orientation or introduction to a program, have a goal-setting session, and then are left to fend for themselves. Most members who are handled this way don't use the facilities frequently and eventually drop their memberships. To prevent this, you need to give members a variety of reasons to keep coming to the club.

The integration stage begins that process. The two phases in the integration stage are introduction and instruction.

## Introduction Phase

The **introduction phase** of the integration stage is the most important, and it is usually the most poorly implemented phase. The biggest mistake made in the introduction program is giving too much information that members don't understand and that will be quickly forgotten. Don't confuse members, overwhelm them, or push them too hard too soon.

In the introduction phase, new members should develop new interests and learn new things, have fun and be encouraged and complimented by the staff, and experience some degree of success. The introduction phase might consist of a one-on-one orientation, an introductory class, a new-member social event, a beginners' exercise clinic, or some combination thereof. The best advice is to keep it simple. This is not the time to show off, try to impress members with an enormous amount of knowledge, or rattle on with unfamiliar terminology. The goal of the introduction phase is to connect with new members and create an environment that makes them eager to come back and learn more. An introduction program must leave the participants feeling confident, educated, and accomplished.

## Instruction Phase

The **instruction phase** introduces members to goal setting and gets them to start using the club on a regular basis. During this phase, you help members establish specific workout schedules and begin their education, which includes terminology, safety, correct form, and general dos and don'ts. In this phase, the objectives are for members to learn more and get better at their programs.

The instructor's teaching expertise is important to the success of this phase. Instructors must establish rapport and connection with beginning exercisers. They must also have empathy for beginners and a sincere understanding of their perceptions, past experiences, frustrations, and fears. The biggest fear is failure, and this is not the time to let members fail or even have the perception of failure.

Consider an introductory resistance training clinic as an example. If the trainer is a very accomplished lifter with a model physique, that might be fine, but it doesn't mean that person is the best teacher for new exercisers. A highly fit person might not have the requisite empathy or the desire to teach basic skills to new exercisers and may not be able to motivate the average person to exercise regularly.

The instruction phase should be a series of sessions over 4 to 8 weeks. You want new members to commit to a series so they will keep coming back to learn more. A series of less than 4 weeks doesn't have time to build momentum, and a series of more than 8 weeks can become redundant and boring. You will find that the dropout rate increases dramatically after 8 weeks.

Another great reason for the series is that participants feel a sense of belonging that encourages commitment. For example, if the program is in a group setting, some of the participants will connect and develop friendships, and this is a key to retention.

## Second Stage: Acceptance

The **acceptance stage** is when members become involved in an ongoing program and can be part of recognition events or participate in advanced program options.

## Involvement Phase

In the **involvement phase**, members start using the club on a regular basis. At this point, engagement and retention are really starting to occur. Involvement programs can include a series of classes or training sessions or participation in a league.

An involvement program is characterized as follows:

- New members are engaged in regular sessions, activities, or programs.
- The programs are scheduled on the same day and time every week.
- The programs have the same instructors or supervisors for each session.
- Most participants will be the same week to week, so they have opportunities to create friendships.
- Participants are encouraged to continue attending the programs or sessions.

One form of involvement programming is training sessions or a series of group exercise classes. The program consists of a variety of classes and exercises. Each class will have its own time slot every week with the same instructor. Most participants come to the same class every week, and they make it a priority.

Clubs must not lose sight of the fact that maintaining the quality of the program and the quality of the instructor will largely determine whether participants continue with any program. Regularly scheduled programs and activities of high quality are significant vehicles to keep members involved in the club, the important first phase in the acceptance stage of the wheel of logical progression.

Once members learn something new and start getting better at it, they will want to continue with the activity. One way to do this is through a league. For example, introductory classes in racquetball, tennis, or volleyball could encourage players to join leagues in which they play against other teams every week. Leagues are fun, social, and competitive. The players look forward to seeing familiar faces, competing with them, and enjoying some social time after the game. Members will make this experience a priority. This type of involvement program is critical to retention because it offers a sense of belonging.

## Achievement Phase

In the **achievement phase**, members are recognized for their participation or competition, and awards are presented by the leader in front of peers. The achievement program is pivotal in the wheel of logical progression. At this point, participants feel good about themselves and their new experiences, and encouragement and recognition from the program directors or instructors will top off the experience. The objective of this phase is to raise the self-esteem and comfort level of members and encourage them to participate in further activities.

The best achievement programs have award ceremonies or informal but visible and memorable presentations. Recognition for achievement can be as simple as giving out the awards, posting names on a recognition board, featuring members' names or pictures in the newsletter, or giving enthusiastic handshakes and asking for applause from the other participants.

This important phase is often eliminated because clubs tend to forget how powerful it can be or because clubs feel they can't afford the time or money. You can't afford *not* to give out awards. The awards need not be expensive; T-shirts, water bottles, or inexpensive gift cards are appreciated by participants. Nothing makes a person feel more important than recognition for personal achievement, and this recognition encourages retention.

Don't give recognition awards to only the best, fastest, or fittest members; this leaves out the members who want and need the experience most. For example, presenting an award based on attendance rather than performance will provide a wonderful experience to someone who wouldn't receive an award based on performance alone. Be creative, and find ways to recognize everyone for something. This is the goal of the achievement phase.

## Third Stage: Commitment

You know now that retention occurs only when members are committed to a program or service, a healthy and active lifestyle, and the health club. You've also learned that it takes a series of programs and activities to achieve that commitment. The objective of the **commitment stage** is to enhance members' commitment to the club by creating deeper levels of socialization and bonding between members and staff. During this stage, members get involved in club-wide events in addition to their regular programs, such parties or other social functions, competitions, tournaments, seminars, or health education sessions.

## Improvement Phase

It's important to assist and support members in their quests for higher levels of accomplishment and achievement in their exercise routines or sport activities. As members improve and attain goals, you'll want to help them establish new goals and diversify their activities. The beauty of getting to the **improvement phase** is that it provides you with another opportunity to recognize achievements and continues to build a sense of belonging that will lead to retention. Improvement programs include competitions; education, seminars, and clinics; diversification through new programs or activities; and more advanced exercise or sport programs.

When people are comfortable and confident in their ability levels, they are ready to learn more and accept new challenges. Improvement programs add new dimensions to previous programs. As participants gain confidence, they also get a heightened competitive edge. Even those who declared themselves to be noncompetitive will enter the improvement phase of programming comparing themselves with others in the program or simply competing with themselves to do better. The quest for improvement is exciting and will further solidify members' activities.

You must be aware of the psychology behind the improvement phase. The members have experienced a good deal of success by this time. If they had not gone through the first four phases, their club experiences may have left them unfit, lacking in knowledge, and uninspired. It's exciting to see a member willing to take on a new challenge with confidence and a positive attitude. At this point you know you've done your job. You've traveled yet another mile down the road to retention.

## Fun Phase

The last phase is the **fun phase,** which consists of social events. At the end of the day, it's all about enjoying what you are doing and having fun. Making fitness fun has been a mantra for the health and fitness industry for many years, and it is one of the most difficult parts of the business to accomplish.

If you host an all-club event, such as a holiday gathering or a member appreciation party, the scenario is almost always the same: About 90% of the attendees are active members who have been using the club regularly for more than a year and who have already made friends with other members or some of the staff. These members will come without too much cajoling, but new

members may need to be personally invited and encouraged. Therefore, focus your efforts on getting new members to attend events so they will feel wanted, accepted, and comfortable before they become inactive or quit. Feeling connected to other members through fun, social events within the club is a powerful retention tool.

Even though a club event is social, friendly, and fun, the newest members will not attend if they don't yet feel like they are part of the group, if they don't know anyone else there, or if they are not encouraged by other members or staff. You can't expect new people to participate without having had a friendly, fun experience in the club; this is why the previous phases of the program are so important. If the members who joined the club within the last 3 to 6 months attended an introductory clinic with other new members and have been participating in a regularly scheduled programs every week, they will likely feel comfortable

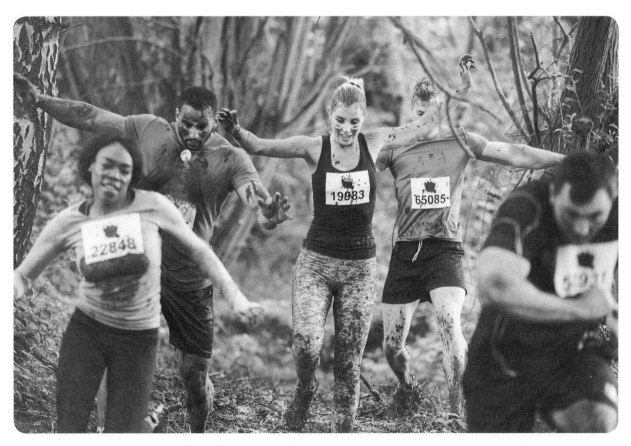

Social events that focus on making fitness fun are a part of the commitment stage, during which members become committed to the program, the lifestyle, and the club.

monkeybusinessimages/Getty Images/iStockphoto

attending an all-club event. If they do, you know that your programming efforts are working. You have nurtured their experiences using the wheel of progression, which has led to retention and a sense of belonging. These members will be committed to your club and their new lifestyles.

## *The Bottom Line*

When planning and implementing programs, use the wheel of progression to address three stages of retention that health club members should experience: integration, acceptance, and commitment. The three stages each contain two phases: introduction and instruction, involvement and achievement, and improvement and fun. Always use one program to promote another to increase retention.

## DEVELOPING A SUCCESSFUL PROGRAM

As you have seen, programs play an important role in why people join and leave your club. Programs that engage members and provide opportunities to connect with others are a critical part of the club experience. Have you ever wondered how your club came to offer the programs it does? Was there a survey of members asking what kind of programs they would like? Are your programs offered because someone thinks health clubs are supposed to run these types of programs? Did you inherit the current program mix from an earlier administration? Are your programs ones that certain staff members just love? Or are you just not sure where these programs came from? Program directors often get so wrapped up in the daily management tasks that there is precious little time to critically assess current programs or think about the creative development of new ones. The club may have stale programs that need to be updated or replaced or have programs with low attendance that lose money, or they might be missing out on the latest and hottest program trend that could bring in new members. In the absence of a planned approach to programming, club programs might be missing the mark. If you want to improve membership sales and retention, you need to be adept at programming. Successful

clubs understand this and continually monitor their programs for quality and relevancy.

The most important information on retention offered here is on the systems, agendas, checklists, parameters, promotions, marketing techniques, communication skills, agendas, evaluations, and follow-up procedures that must be followed for every program. Although not foolproof, the process for program development has been proven to work, and following it will greatly enhance your probability of developing program after program that members will love.

Many club managers and program directors don't understand how to put together a successful program. For many of them, the programming scenario goes something like this: Get a program idea; announce the program in the club brochure, website, or newsletter; establish an enrollment process; talk it up; and sit back and hope members enroll. Even great program ideas will fail with that system. The proven steps for developing a program that will attract participants and have a positive effect on your club's retention rate are as follows:

1. Define a purpose.
2. Set a goal.
3. Develop a marketing and promotion plan to reach the goal.
4. Measure the results.
5. Implement a follow-up program.

## Define a Purpose

As an example, the purpose could be to get new members to commit to an 8-week cardio and strength training program. They will meet other new members and they will gain strength, endurance, and satisfaction by completing the program. A staff member will be assigned to track participation, give recognition for performance, and promote the next program. Members will enjoy their involvement and gain a sense of belonging, a degree of personal achievement, and a comfort level to take on a new challenge.

## Set a Goal

A program can be thought of as a club project that directly affects the bottom line, and a good business doesn't undertake a project without having a clear goal in mind. The success of a program is typically measured by the number of participants.

What is a realistic number to expect if the purpose of the program is clearly beneficial to the club and to a specific group of members? Let's continue with the new-member cardio and strength training program as an example. If a club is selling an average of 50 new memberships per month, it is reasonable to think that 20 to 30% would be good candidates for this entry-level program. Conservatively, 10 of the current month's new members would enjoy the program and benefit from it. Members are considered new for the first 3 months, so new members from the previous 2 months would be good candidates for this program as well. That would be another 20 potential participants for the program. You should always set an attainable goal that is plausible to reach and possible to surpass. You must always reach the set goal. In this example, the goal is 30 participants.

## Develop a Marketing and Promotion Plan

A marketing and promotion plan should identify how a club will create initial interest in a program among new and established members. The plan should contain the strategies to be used to attract the types of members the program is designed for and result in the goal number of members needed to make the program a success. Traditionally, clubs use posters, brochures, displays, news releases, website articles, or paid advertisements to promote their programs. Because using every possible promotional tool is not feasible for most clubs, you need to identify the best strategies to reach the intended target audience for each program. As discussed in chapter 7, new digital marketing methods are available that enable fitness managers or marketers to use search engines, websites, social media, email, blogging, and mobile apps for target-specific promotional messaging. Gaining an understanding of the real-time dynamics and effects of these digital channels is paramount for success in marketing your programs. Furthermore, the **data analytics** for digital media now allow managers to evaluate the effectiveness of these new marketing tools.

The program marketing plan must resemble the sales plan for marketing to new prospects. All the program staff, fitness trainers, and instructors for the program must be able to tout the positive aspects of the program, including its features, benefits, and purpose. Second, they must be able to overcome member objections, such as "I'm too busy," "The program costs too much," and "I don't want to make a commitment right now." Third, they must ask for the sale three to five times. Asking may consist of a postcard, an email, and phone call delivering a personal invitation to the member. How often do your employees ask a member to participate in any given program?

## Measure the Results

Now that you have defined a purpose, set a goal, and developed a marketing and promotion plan, you must measure whether the result is good for the bottom line. Using our example, you could expect the following results:

- Fifty new members join the club per month.
- Ten new members (20%) get involved in the new-member program per month.
- Each member pays $50 in monthly dues ($600 per year).
- The program delivers enjoyment, accomplishment, friends, recognition, and a follow-up program.
- Each year, 120 new members who might not have renewed are retained because of their participation in the program, which delivers $72,000 in annual revenues (10 new members per month = 120 members per year; 120 members × $600 yearly dues = $72,000).

Isn't that the result you are looking for? It starts with the first program and continues only if all the participants complete the program, which will be the result of constant communication, promotion, and recognition by the program staff. The program is only as good as the way it is managed.

Also note that active, happy new members in their first year of membership are most likely to bring in 60 to 80% of your new business by word of mouth. A professionally trained program staff with a well-planned program calendar should be able to run six to eight different programs six to eight times per year. Well-managed programs keep hundreds of members enjoying themselves and using your club regularly.

## Develop Follow-Up Programs

Retention doesn't occur automatically after the first 6- to 8-week program. If you want your new members to become active club users, then timely, well-designed follow-up programs are crucial. The program calendar must include activities for everyone: men, women, youth, older adults, first-time exercisers, and experienced exercisers and athletes. The programs must include classes, training sessions, leagues, lessons, clinics, contests, seminars, and tournaments that are carefully targeted to different member groups that share similar interests. You must sell each of these programs as a new challenge or a new beginning, and always use one program to promote another to keep the retention going.

### *The Bottom Line*

Developing programs that engage members, meet their needs, and provide opportunities for them to connect with others is critical to club operational success. Take a planned approach to program development that includes critically assessing current programs and being creative in the development of new ones. Avoid letting programs become stale when they need updating or replacing, and make sure your program options include the hottest program trends to excite current members and bring in new ones.

## RECOGNIZING THE IMPORTANCE OF PROGRAM DIRECTORS

Program directors are typically responsible for coordinating all club activities, programs, and the staff involved in those services. The responsibilities of the program director are many and varied: having special events to lure back inactive and former members, recognition programs to keep new members active, competitive programs to keep dedicated exercisers interested, social programs to get members involved, and educational programs for those who need specific information on aspects of health and fitness. All this should be done in an environment that's fun and comfortable, and it should be orchestrated by a leader with good communication skills. Increasingly, the most successful clubs are those that have professional programs as outlined in this chapter.

Is a program director worthwhile in your club or organization? Many clubs debate this issue, but a look at the numbers should convince you that a program director will increase retention and decrease attrition. Let's look at what we know:

- Retention is vital to your bottom line. Industry statistics say that it costs four to six times more to get a new member than it does to keep an existing one.
- The goal of programming is retention. Programs keep members active and happy.
- Word-of-mouth referrals account for 60 to 80% of your new business. People who are regularly enjoying your programs and using your club will refer new members.
- Getting 10 new members per month involved in a program can yield $72,000 per year in membership dues.

The bottom line is clear. Can you afford *not* to have a program director? Business is measured in results. Every business needs leaders to be accountable and to keep others accountable. The program director does just that.

### *The Bottom Line*

Program directors are responsible for developing and managing programs as well as supervising staff. The program director also oversees programs that keep exercisers motivated, organizes special events and social opportunities to engage members, and offers educational programs. Program directors at successful health clubs are leaders with good communication skills and knowledge of how to run professional programs. Analysis of membership and program finances, along with attendance data and member evaluations, should be used to determine whether the program director is having a positive effect of membership retention.

## Program Development Checklist

This checklist outlines the steps and considerations necessary in developing programs that retain members. Use it to ensure a successful program. It will help you remember that you should never run a program unless it has been thoroughly planned.

1. The program leader is responsible for the event and its result.
2. Every program should have the following:
   - Purpose: Define how the program will benefit the club and the member.
   - Goal: Know the number of participants needed for success.
   - Plan: Create a written plan that includes marketing and promotional procedures, staff assignments, and deadlines to reach the goal.
   - Follow-up: Always have a follow-up program ready to promote.
3. Consider all groups of members for programs:
   - New members
   - Active members
   - Inactive members
   - Potential members
4. When introducing a program, it is a good idea to offer it during all the time frames (peak hours, off-peak hours, and weekends) to reach the most members.
5. Place each program in a phase of the wheel of logical progression.
   - Integration stage: introduction phase and instruction phase
   - Acceptance stage: involvement phase and achievement phase
   - Commitment stage: improvement phase and fun phase
6. Have introductory programs that create interest and integrate new members in the following ways:
   - Promote camaraderie.
   - Qualify skill levels.
   - Categorize personalities.
   - Recognize individual achievements.
   - Promote involvement in follow-up programs.
7. Review the 10 keys to successful programming and have a written example of each key before running the program.
8. Always use one program to promote another. Have the promotional materials, enrollment procedures, available schedules, rules, costs, and other information ready for follow-up programs.
9. Every program must have enrollment and attendance procedures for follow-up and program analysis.
10. If a program is successful, look for what worked (and what didn't) and make any necessary adjustments before running it again. Have a consistent schedule on your calendar of events to present to members.

# Key Terms

| | | |
|---|---|---|
| acceptance stage | fun phase | programming |
| achievement phase | improvement phase | reliability |
| commitment stage | instruction phase | involvement phase |
| data analytics | integration stage | wheel of logical progression |
| diversified programming | introduction phase | |

# Generating Revenue Through Profit Centers

## Learning Objectives

After studying this chapter, you will be able to

- identify different types of profit centers,
- understand the operating expenses of profit centers,
- determine profit centers with the highest net operating income,
- identify common pitfalls in the development of profitable programs, and
- appreciate the importance of hiring staff with specific competencies and technical skills.

A health club owner was concerned that membership dues accounted for nearly all the revenue for his club; with almost no other income streams, the club's profitability was limited. He learned from a colleague at another club that specialty programs and services accounted for 25% of that club's annual revenue—significantly enhancing the bottom line. As a result, the club owner met with his management team to brainstorm revenue-generating initiatives. Together, they came up with four new services that could generate additional revenues: healthy cooking, weight management, tai chi, and ballroom dancing.

After finding qualified instructors, the club produced a brochure describing the new programs and mailed it to all members. The brochure production and mailing costs were significant, but it seemed a worthwhile investment. Some exercise classes had to be moved or cancelled to make room for the new programs, causing some members to grumble. Despite the difficulties, the staff persevered because of the promise of new revenue.

Upon launching the new programs, each specialty class was offered at several times of the day to help the club find the most popular time slot. Although registration numbers were encouraging, the average class size was only three participants, resulting in high personnel costs coupled with insufficient revenue.

The addition of these new programs had not improved club profitability, and customer service complaints had increased. The owner decided to hire a program consultant to analyze the situation. After meeting with staff and reviewing the program schedule, the consultant provided a list of issues, many of which had not been considered in the initial planning:

The author acknowledges the significant contributions of Cheryl Jones to this chapter.

- Too many class times had been added to the schedule, resulting in small classes
- Instructor pay rates were above the market rate
- Additional front-desk staff had been hired to take program registrations
- Custodial hours had been increased due to the additional facility usage
- Program fees were too low to cover expenses and produce a profit
- Member cancellations had increased because some members felt their needs were being cast aside to accommodate new programming

The addition of new programs managed poorly had driven the club's expenses up significantly and not provided enough additional revenue to support them. With the consultant's guidance, the team would now devise a plan to put their program revenue on track for success.

———————————————————●———————————————————

**A** **profit center** is a subunit of a business that is responsible for both revenues and expenses. In the health club business, programs or services that carry an additional fee for members are often considered profit centers because they are responsible for both revenues and expenses and are designed to generate a surplus, or profit. By comparison, a cost center is a subunit of a business that is only responsible for its costs, or expenses. A prime example of a health club cost center are group exercise programs, which are typically included as part of the membership fee but can incur high costs, such as specialty instructors and equipment. Profit centers are usually managed by program specialists who are responsible for the planning and control of the program within a department. Managers of profit centers have to drive the revenue generation from fees, or cash inflows, and at the same time control the expenses. Good program managers treat profit centers as independent businesses within the company, because viewing a program as a distinct entity not only allows its profitability to be measured but also fosters a more businesslike treatment of the program when making decisions regarding its management.

Managed correctly, profit centers offer opportunities to significantly increase the profitability of a health club. These revenue-generating programs can enhance the club brand, improve member retention, and increase revenue per member, as well as add profit to the bottom line. In this chapter, we review the operation of five common health club profit centers: personal training, specialty group training, spa services,

youth programs, and pro shops. You will begin to understand how a new profit center can add value to your memberships and improve membership net gain. Guidelines will be provided to assist in determining what types of profit center are best for your club. Once a profit center is selected, there will be initial investment costs and ongoing expenses, and operational support will be needed, and these requirements will be reviewed. (See chapter 16 for additional information on evaluating profit centers.)

Managing a health club in any setting is a highly complex and demanding venture. No longer can club operators simply expect initiation fees and dues revenue to guarantee success and provide ample profit for the long run. With more competition in the market than ever—including commercial, not-for-profit, and community facility options—and a range of price points, the club with the lowest cost and leanest operating structure has a far greater advantage. Yet constantly competing on price leaves your business vulnerable year after year. Clubs with limited services and marginal programming will not stand out in a crowded marketplace, and their business will suffer.

Revenue from programs outside of the membership fee can make or break a club's bottom line. According to the IHRSA *Profiles of Success* report (International Health, Racquet, and Sportsclub Association 2015), clubs reported earning more than 3 out of every 10 dollars from services not included in the dues (personal and small group training, nutritional counseling, spa services, etc.). In addition to adding to a club's bottom line, nondues revenue historically has been linked to higher member retention. "The more they pay, the longer they stay" is a longtime axiom in the fitness industry. It is not uncommon for clubs to have membership attrition rates of 40%-50% in a given year. Yet the clubs from this study were retaining 7 out of 10 of their members. Hence, the quest for improved member retention may drive the decision to add profit centers. Each health club has the opportunity and financial necessity to create additional programming and services to generate profit. These profit centers will not guarantee financial success, but if run properly, they can have a positive result on the bottom line as well as differentiate your club from the competition.

# DEVELOPMENT AND ORGANIZATION OF PROFIT CENTERS

Financially, profit centers can run as separate entities within the global profit and loss statement of the health club. Operationally, most profit centers are run as separate departments within the scope of the organization. That said, intraclub awareness among management, departments, and staff (e.g., front-desk staff, membership directors, fitness instructors, and training staff) is critical to success. When introducing a new program, the ability of the facility manager to plan, organize, and communicate the purpose of the new profit center within the global organizational mission will contribute to the financial success of the operation. Large multipurpose health clubs typically have more fee-for-service offerings than smaller clubs, basing their offerings on what their members want and are willing to pay extra for. A report from IHRSA shows that in clubs with 60,000 square feet (5,574 square meters) or more, the median percentage that profit centers contribute to total revenue is 37.6%, and in clubs between 20,000 and 34,999 square feet (1,858 and 3,252 square meters), the median is 19.7%. The median percentage of profit center contribution to total revenue in clubs of all sizes is 31.6% (International Health, Racquet, and Sportsclub Association 2015). Typically, the larger clubs offer more ancillary services because they have more space available, a larger staff to teach programs,

greater financial flexibility, and more members to purchase extra services.

Developing and operating successful profit centers are demanding responsibilities for the facility manager. The types of profit centers and their daily operation can vary greatly—not only from each other but also from the general operation of the facility.

The steps to initiating a profit center are in many ways similar to the steps to planning and developing a health and fitness club. First, determine what services make the most sense for your club and your market. Beyond the value-added services the club already offers that break even in profitability yet enhance the value of the membership, consider what programs will have broad appeal and will be something people are willing to pay extra for. Make sure the proposed profit center is a good fit for your club and its membership. If it is too specialized, the operations might be too complex, the resources too scarce, and the appeal too limited in the marketplace. Find out whether other clubs charge a fee for similar services or if they include it as part of the membership fee. If it is a free commodity in other health clubs, members will feel as if the club is taking advantage of them by charging extra for the service.

Once you have decided on the right profit center, determine specific, measurable goals and objectives for each operation. After researching areas such as competition, market demand, consumer interest, income, and price considerations, develop a marketing plan with an identified target market, typically the existing membership and local community. Often a member focus group or an informal member survey can provide a great deal of information for this aspect of the business plan. Ask yourself these questions: Will members think the program is worth paying more for? Does your membership demographics tell you that the clientele can afford additional service fees, or does your club cater to lower-income segments of the community? Will you offer the program services to nonmembers? If so, what is the best strategy to reach them, and how much will the price differ from the program fee members will pay?

A management plan that considers issues such as staffing, space allocation and design, equipment needs, vendor management, operating procedures, and sales procedures is the next logical step. Finally, develop a **financial pro** forma evaluating the capital investment needs, operating expenses, tax and insurance considerations, accounting procedures, documentation, and potential profitability. Establish desired return on investment and profit margins. Many a well-intentioned club operator has implemented profit center programs with complex operational systems that generate minimal profit. A realistic evaluation is required to determine major areas for profit and to provide a road map for developing a successful profit center. Is your club a small facility with limited space and equipment? Do you have a multipurpose facility with a swimming pool and tennis, squash, or basketball courts? Can your group exercise studios be areas that can generate revenue during down time or off-peak hours? What other spaces in the club can be utilized or expanded? What types of staff training and certification are needed? Do you have access to adequate staff resources, or do you need to outsource program leadership?

## The Bottom Line

Developing a detailed business plan that defines the right profit center for your club and includes a market analysis, goals and objectives statement, marketing plan, management plan, and financial pro forma is vital for a successful venture.

Before starting a profit center, the club operator should select someone to oversee the development and operation of the endeavor; he or she may choose a member of the existing staff or hire a qualified person. Selecting someone with a background and interest in the venture relieves the already busy club manager and program director of much of the start-up burden. The person selected should have direct access to the club manager and the business plan for continued advice and direction. Link the compensation to the successful launch and operation of the profit center and create a bonus structure that drives achievement beyond 100% of the goal. The profit center manager should also be responsible for promoting the new service or product to the members and clearly articulating the differences between free and for-fee programming to the membership staff and other program instructors. Use the mar-

keting and promotion strategies identified in the marketing plan to guide this effort.

## The Bottom Line

Selecting a qualified and motivated profit center manager with great communication, program development, and sales skills will increase the potential for success.

## FIVE COMMON PROFIT CENTERS

There are various profit centers that you could implement, depending on facility space available, club location, marketplace demand, and demographics. Personal training, specialty group training, physical therapy and rehabilitation, performance training, sport instruction, youth and adult specialty programming, wellness and spa services, food and beverage, and pro shops are possible choices. Evaluate the operating model, expenses, and revenues of each option to determine which profit center will likely have the highest financial return and add the most value to the membership. This section explores five profits centers common to many health clubs: personal training, specialty group training, spa services, youth programs, and pro shops.

### Personal Training

Personal training is a significant income source for health clubs, with $9 billion in annual revenue and annual growth of 3.2% from 2012 to 2017 (IBISWorld 2017). Now a mainstream fitness program, it has come a long way from its beginnings in the early 1990s as a service mostly for the rich and famous. As it has grown and evolved, personal training is one of the most popular programs in the health club industry, a service used by people from all walks of life. As people of all generations look for professional guidance to become healthier, the need for personal training services has never been greater. After membership, income from all forms of personal training is the second largest source of revenue in leading health clubs, with operators generating a median of 8.4% of total revenues from personal training (International Health, Racquet, and Sportsclub Association 2016b). IHRSA also reports that 12%

of health club members engaged in at least one individual or one-on-one personal training session and 31% of members reported taking at least one small group personal training session in 2015. While the average fee for small group training is $20 less than personal training per session, overall training volume has increased because there are considerably more members taking advantage of the group format (International Health, Racquet, and Sportsclub Association 2016a).

Personal training can be defined as an individual fitness program designed and monitored by a certified personal training professional, conducted one-on-one or with a small group and delivered in person or via online or mobile technology. According to the 2017 International Fitness Industry Trend Report by ClubIntel—done in collaboration with the International Health, Racquet & Sportsclub Association (IHRSA), the Association of Fitness Studios (AFS), Club Industry, and others—personal training is the top program or service offered in health clubs, with 78% of clubs offering it (ClubIntel 2017). Numerous books, manuals, and training courses have been developed on the theory and practice of personal training, but in this section we will simply touch on the key elements that any health club owner or operator needs to be familiar with in order to manage a successful personal training profit center.

## *The Bottom Line*

A strong personal training program correlates to improved member retention because people who participate in personal training remain members longer.

## Location

In most facilities, personal training occurs either on the main fitness floor or in a private or semi-private personal training area. Dedicated personal training areas can be constructed separately or can be adjacent to the main fitness area, which provides some privacy and a sense of exclusivity and perceived value. Specialized equipment, including functional training equipment and free weights, can be provided for the sole use of personal training clients.

## Customers

All members are potential personal training clients, whether they are new or long-time members. People wanting to learn new techniques, needing motivation, or seeking a personalized program are all prime candidates for personal training. Personal training is a great vehicle for the new member to begin the club experience and start on a fitness program designed specifically for him or her, increasing the probability of success and retention.

Instead of assuming that all personal training clients are looking for weight loss and muscle toning, trainers must take the time to conduct a needs assessment with each new client to determine the person's personal goals. Until you understand what the member wants, you cannot provide a solution to get there. A fit member could be bored with her current routine and need some new training tools to reenergize her workout, or a new member might be looking for help to get in shape for a special event in which he will participate. The club manager should focus on building a strong team of membership sales staff and personal trainers, and an understanding of how these two roles can work together to achieve the training goals is key. Membership staff who introduce prospective members to a personal trainer create a sense of comfort and exert a favorable influence on the decision to purchase a membership. This also creates an avenue for the personal trainer to begin to establish a relationship with a new member who might become a new personal training client.

**New Customers**   There are many methods of introducing new members to personal training and all that it has to offer. One tried and true method is to give new members a taste of the product through a free initial session. A free personal training session or fitness assessment with a trainer is often included as a benefit to new members and gives the trainer the opportunity to develop a rapport with the member. Trainers can be assigned **conversion goals** for converting free sessions or assessments into personal training packages sold. Bonuses for meeting these goals can be an added incentive.

An email or phone call congratulating new members on their commitment to get fit is another way to promote personal training and start to build a relationship with the new member. Another sales strategy is to **bundle** personal training packages with different membership options, offering one or more sessions in a tiered pricing format (e.g., basic, premier, elite). Some clubs assign personal training quotas as well as membership quotas to their sales consultants in order to promote personal training at the point of a membership sale. Whatever method you choose at the point of sale, linking sales consultants' compensation to the sale of personal training is necessary to drive them to include this product sale in the often-lengthy membership sales process. If this quota process is not monitored and enforced with some rigor and the commission is too small to make an impact, sales consultants will stop selling personal training at the point of membership.

**Existing Customers**    Once a club has established a base of personal training clients, methods must be in place to retain them. Satisfied customers continue to purchase more sessions as well as recommend the service to others. Scrutinizing the delivery of the personal training product is necessary to maintain the business. Surveys of current and past clients (done by phone or email) will help the manager assess the quality of the training experience. Even if the club manager is not trained in the exercise science behind personal training, there are a number of observations the manager can make to evaluate safety and customer satisfaction.

The simplest inspection by a manager is observing whether the trainer looks engaged with the client and whether the client looks motivated. Also, every trainer should keep a written program card or computerized record to chart the progress of each client toward his or her goals. (This is not only a good safety practice but also an evaluation tool for a well-planned progressive program.) Managers should make it a practice to discuss this progressive plan with the personal trainers. What is the goal of the client, and why were these exercises selected? Trainers should be able to articulate their methodology and rationale. Are there changes in weight, equipment, or types of exercises from week to week, or do they remain the same? For the safety of the client, is every session beginning with a warm-up and ending with a cool-down?

## *The Bottom Line*

As with membership sales, there must be a constant focus on driving new personal training business and attracting new personal training clients while also concentrating on retaining and serving existing clients.

## Package and Program Types

A personal training department or profit center usually has a menu of training packages and options. Single 1-hour sessions and packages of 5, 10, and 20 sessions are common at many clubs. Sessions of 30 or 45 minutes are appealing to those clients with time constraints. For clients looking for a lower-priced alternative, small group training with up to five clients has become a popular option. Other affordable and time-efficient programs can include independent sessions that begin with an evaluation and program design by the trainer, followed by the client working out on his or her own with periodic check-ins and progress evaluations from the trainer. Solution-based programs that are tied to a specific desired result are often requested by clients. Weight loss, preparation for social events like reunions and weddings, and sport-specific performance programs for golf, tennis, triathlons, and marathons are other popular choices.

Personal trainers are being more creative in the ways that they package personal training sessions. The American College of Sports Medicine's Worldwide Survey of Fitness Trends for 2018, with input from over 4,000 industry professionals, lists personal training as number 8 out of the 20 top trends and lists group personal training as number 13 (Thompson 2017). These small group sessions involving two to five clients have grown in popularity because they offer potentially deep discounts to each member of the group and create an incentive for clients to put small groups together. Additionally a group setting improves social interaction and training efficiency. Training two or three people at the same time in a small group often makes good economic sense for both the trainer and the client. These trends point to new opportunities for driving personal training revenue through structured group formats.

Determining the needs of your customers will help identify what types of personal training options and packages you want to offer. The execution of predesigned training programs is hard to monitor, and trainers can tend to veer off course by adding variations of their own design, straying from the predesigned format. If these predesigned programs are part of your personal training business, then an ongoing staff training and review process needs to be in place. Buy-in from the trainers is critical to the successful implementation of any personal training packages or predesigned programs. Time spent coaching and working with your trainers is invaluable to this process.

## Cost of Sale, Profit Margins, and Metrics

After you complete a competitive analysis of personal training in your area, pricing can be determined. Standard overall profit margins range from 35 to 50%. Expenses include payroll and payroll taxes, commissions, and any advertising and promotion costs. Single-session pricing can vary based on the certifications and experience level of your trainers, but they are usually priced higher than multiple-session packages. The cost of a single hourly session varies based on the area's demographics and cost of living and can range from $50 to $125 a session. Specially priced introductory packages of three to five sessions can be created to entice members to try personal training.

There are of number of **industry metrics** that clubs can use to monitor the growth of the personal training business, including training revenue as a percentage of total membership revenue, personal training clients as a percentage of total membership, percentage of personal training to member usage, as well as operating cost of training per client. The number of **active clients** (unique users who have trained in the past 6 months to 1 year), percentage of new clients, and percentage of repeat clients all warrant tracking and review.

## Guidelines

After you have determined what personal training options you will offer and set prices for them, the guidelines and policies for the purchase and use of the packages need to be constructed.

Determine expiration dates for personal training sessions; expiration dates can vary from 30 days after purchase to 1 year. A tracking report or system for identifying expired sessions should be developed. Establish a cancellation, refund, and makeup policy and adhere to these policies. Sometimes trainers can be their own worst enemies when building a solid training business. In a fledgling business where their schedule is not yet in demand, they may be uncomfortable charging their clients for missed sessions or may empathize with their clients' problems and consistently allow them to cancel with less than 24 hours notice. The manager may have to enforce these policies until the trainers become more confident and self-assured.

## Equipment

The investment in equipment specifically for personal training is minimal, because the majority of training sessions use existing club equipment, such as free weights, resistance training and cardio machines, and stability balls. Trainers often utilize a number of different props for variety, to accommodate client favorites, and for specific training purposes. If certain types of workout props are popular with both trainers and the general membership, the club may need to purchase additional items to accommodate the demand.

## Operations

When structuring a personal training business in a health club, it is common to develop a mixture of free and paid services for members. The club owner first needs to decide the extent to which the club will offer members free fitness services, such as an equipment orientation and an initial assessment, which add value to membership. These free services can serve as a stepping stone to personal training, because they provide the staff with an opportunity to build a relationship with the member and discuss other services available. After free services are defined, a structure for personal training services can be developed. An independent contractor or an on-staff personal training director can be in charge of developing this structure.

If the club plans to provide a free fitness service (particularly to new members) and provide personal training for an additional fee, then several types of management support can be used. A fitness manager may be in charge of the free services, overseeing the fitness floor and the basic services helping drive personal training revenues, while a personal training director is assigned to promote and oversee personal training sales and service.

Roles, responsibilities, and priorities need to be defined, as do commission structures. Health clubs are in the business of both service and sales. How do you manage these two aspects of operation and be successful economically? Will one manager be able to handle the service in a high-usage club and still coach and hold trainers accountable for meeting their training quotas? Will members understand the difference between personal trainers and fitness floor staff? How will they know how to ask for assistance?

## Staffing

After defining your business model, you can establish staffing roles, responsibilities, job requirements, budgeted floor hours, pay rates, and commissions. Will trainers be required to work a certain number of floor service hours? Do they need to do a minimum amount of training sessions, and do they have a specific time frame in which to achieve this? Will you hire only full-time employees or have different standards for part-time employees? Pay rates for working the fitness floor usually differ from those for personal training. Commissions can be assigned for personal training sales, incentives can be used to increase the amount of sessions trained, and those with advanced certifications and continuing education can command higher pay rates. What's the right structure for your company to build this profit center and attract and retain staff? Strong short- and long-term strategies that are in line with your business goals will point you in the direction of success.

Once your structure is in place, you can define the type and number of employees you need to drive the business. Unless your top sales staff are selling all of your personal training programs, you need to find motivated, positive people with good communication and people skills and then train them on how to effectively sell personal training. Additionally, you need to hire personal trainers who understand that there is more to running a successful business than teaching exercises. A personal training certification provides knowledge in exercise science, physiology, and program design but typically does not provide practical business skills such as time management, customer service, and sales proficiencies. A trainer with great fitness knowledge does not necessarily equate to a financially productive trainer. The initial excitement and passion for fitness may wane when confronted with the realities of the club environment and struggles to attract and keep clients. Trainers need to be trained in the sales process. Successful trainers always have goals, and these goals translate to new business and repeat business objectives.

After overall budgets are finalized, all trainers need to understand their contribution to the overall sales and revenue goal. **Personal training sales** refers to the number of personal training sessions sold, and **personal training revenue** is the number of personal training sessions used. Management should meet with trainers to discuss a realistic business plan that projects sales and revenue based on repeat purchases (existing clients) and new purchases (new clients). Tracking client training patterns (e.g., one time per week, two times per month) and the number of sessions left on a client's package makes it easy to determine when and what that client will purchase next. (Trainers should always consider holidays and vacations in predicting current client usage.) Subtract repeat business from the overall sales target, and the negative variance will determine how many dollars are needed in new client sales. Trainers should be able to articulate where and how they will attract that new business. The number of sessions should be determined based on existing client training patterns and average training usage of new clients. The manager should know the sales abilities of the trainers and, after a time, create a conversion ratio (number of leads, contacts needed to create a sale) to help assign individual trainer quotas.

**Recruitment**    With top trainers in high demand, clubs are always challenged to find qualified, experienced, and outgoing personal trainers. Fitness staff with a positive attitude and passion for helping people achieve their fitness goals can be developed into trainers who fit your model. Other areas of recruitment are job websites, career fairs, personal training certification organizations, and colleges.

## *The Bottom Line*

The right personality is the most important qualification for a successful personal trainer. Technical skills are the other qualification—the person needs to have the right experience, training, and certifications.

**Certifications**   More than 300 organizations offer personal training certifications in the United States, but most of them are not independently evaluated and accredited to ensure that they adequately assess professional competency. In an effort to improve credibility and client safety, in 2006 the International Health, Racquet & Sportsclub Association (IHRSA) implemented a recommendation that it would only recognize certifications that had independent, third-party accreditation. Influenced by the IHRSA decision, most of the fitness industry followed suit.

The primary accreditation organization utilized by the fitness industry is the National Commission for Certifying Agencies (NCCA) of the Institute for Credentialing Excellence, known for its long history of establishing quality standards for certifying agencies and programs. As a result of their stance adopted in 2006, IHRSA recommends that club owners only hire personal trainers who hold at least one current certification from a certifying organization that has obtained third-party accreditation from NCCA or an equivalent organization. In addition, the American College of Sports Medicine (ACSM) and the Medical Fitness Association (MFA) have adopted similar stances recommending third-party accredited certifications. As of this writing, there are 16 accredited personal training certifications recognized by IHRSA—13 accredited by NCCA, and 3 by the Distance Education Accrediting Commission (DEAC). The following 13 organizations that offer personal training certification are accredited by NCCA:

- Academy of Applied Personal Training Education (AAPTE)
- American College of Sports Medicine (ACSM)
- American Council on Exercise (ACE)
- The Cooper Institute (CI)
- International Fitness Professionals Association (IFPA)

- National Academy of Sports Medicine (NASM)
- National Council for Certified Personal Trainers (NCCPT)
- National Council on Strength and Fitness (NCSF)
- National Exercise and Sports Trainers Association (NESTA)
- National Exercise Trainers Association (NETA)
- National Federation of Professional Trainers (NFPT)
- National Strength and Conditioning Association (NSCA)
- Training and Wellness Certification Commission (TWCC)

The Distance Education Accrediting Commission (DEAC) is another recognized accreditation organization for certification programs. However, the DEAC only accredits organizations and their education programs, not the examination. Therefore, it does not hold the same weight as NCCA accreditation in the eyes of some fitness establishments. The following organizations that offer personal training certification are accredited by DEAC:

- Athletics and Fitness Association of America (AFAA)
- International Sports Sciences Association (ISSA)
- United States Career Institute (USCI)

The average national certification costs $250 to $500 and requires current CPR and AED certification. To ensure program quality and client safety, it is strongly recommended that all personal trainers hold at least one national certification, preferably from an accredited organization, even if they have a college degree in a field related to exercise science. Specialty certifications in sport performance training, training select populations, wellness coaching, nutrition, and so on broaden a trainer's scope of practice and appeal to clients with specific needs.

Aligning your club with a narrow list of certifications or one certifying body, particularly an accredited one, can provide credibility, reassure clients regarding program safety, and create consistency in training methods on the fitness floor.

To supplement what trainers have learned through certification programs, some facilities create their own internal training programs to provide trainers with continuing education and new skills. If an internal training program is too large of an investment of time and resources for the club, the owner or program manager can recommend articles and websites for trainers to review, as well as workshops and seminars available for continuing education.

**Scope of Practice** The American Council on Exercise (ACE) has established scope of practice to guide personal trainers regarding their role and duties to the client. By following this scope of practice, personal trainers will provide effective services to personal training clients, avoid legal ramifications for practicing outside their professional scope, and protect the health and safety of clients. Client safety should be the governing principle of personal training; when it is not, the risk of harm increases. Personal training can never be effective in achieving improved physical fitness if it is not first and foremost safe for the client. Club owners should use the ACE Certified Personal Trainer Scope of Practice to ensure that program quality and the safety of club members are paramount in their personal training program.

**Retaining Staff** Time and money are invested in coaching and mentoring trainers, and a company risks losing its investment if it does not make an effort to retain these trainers. Over time, trainers may relocate, experience poor health, find new jobs, or start their own personal training business. The personal training business is entrepreneurial; successful trainers with the ability to attract and retain clients may decide to strike out on their own so they can take home all the profit and set their own schedule. (Becoming a self-employed personal trainer is fairly easy since the equipment investment is minimal and personal trainers can train out of their homes, in their clients' homes, or in a rented space.) With each new hire, you should explain all the benefits of working in a club environment: They have access to the entire

## ACE Certified Personal Trainer Scope of Practice

- Developing and implementing exercise programs that are safe, effective, and appropriate for individuals who are apparently healthy or have medical clearance to exercise
- Conducting health-history interviews and stratifying risk for cardiovascular disease with clients in order to determine the need for referral and identify contraindications for exercise
- Administering appropriate fitness assessments based on the client's health history, current fitness, lifestyle factors, and goals utilizing research-proven and published protocols
- Assisting clients in setting and achieving realistic fitness goals
- Teaching correct exercise methods and progressions through demonstration, explanation, and proper cueing and spotting techniques
- Empowering individuals to begin and adhere to their exercise programs using guidance, support, motivation, lapse-prevention strategies, and effective feedback
- Designing structured exercise programs for one-on-one and small-group personal training
- Educating clients about fitness- and health-related topics to help them in adopting healthful behaviors that facilitate exercise program success
- Protecting client confidentiality according to the Health Insurance Portability and Accountability Act (HIPAA) and related regional and national laws
- Always acting with professionalism, respect, and integrity
- Recognizing what is within the scope of practice and always referring clients to other healthcare professionals when appropriate
- Being prepared for emergency situations and responding appropriately when they occur

member base; they may receive employee benefits; the heat, lighting, rent and equipment, advertising, and promotions are paid for; and they get to network and learn from their peers. This conversation is time well spent since the company needs a solid team of trainers. Time, appreciation, and recognition build a loyal professional. Knowing your trainers is an important part of maintaining a loyal workforce.

## *The Bottom Line*

A solid personal training business cannot be built on the skills and performance of only a few trainers.

**Advertising and Promotion**    Creating awareness and attracting attention will benefit your club's personal training business. Market positioning to show members how personal training will satisfy their specific needs is a smart business initiative. New-member trial sessions, package discounts to new members and new clients, and client reward programs are good methods to foster awareness of the personal training offerings and cultivate loyalty among clients. Brochures, posters, email, social media web sites, direct mail, referral programs, trainer biography boards, and business cards are other ways to promote your program.

## Specialty Group Training

Specialty group training programs are those for which members pay an additional fee, typically because of high operating expenses like specialized equipment and advanced instructor training requirements. Specialty group programs are distinguished from the more common group exercise programs that are usually included at no extra cost for members. New programs may fall into the specialty category when first introduced because of the high start-up costs of marketing, instructor training, and equipment purchases. Some prime examples of this are programs like spinning, yoga, and Zumba, which are initially rolled out in clubs with an added fee but over time became mature programs viewed as a membership commodity. Though specialty offerings are typically the lifeblood of boutique fitness studios, large clubs too can build significant

profit centers by adding one or more specialty training program.

Operators of boutique or niche exercise facilities such as barre, Pilates, boxing, martial arts, high-intensity training, cycling, and yoga studios are able to get up to several hundred dollars from each member each month. What these club operators have discovered is that people are willing to pay more for a favorite program or activity if it is held in a specialty facility. About 41% of Americans over the age of 6 were members of a boutique fitness studio, according to the 2017 Health Club Consumer Report from IHRSA (International Health, Racquet, and Sportsclub Association 2017). The report also found that 87% of boutique facility members also belong to another facility, often a traditional health club. Clients at the niche facilities may pay monthly for their standard health club membership and also pay per class or in class bundles for the boutique facility program. Although boutique studios offer a certain ambiance or cachet not found in a large health club, there might be an opportunity to grow revenue at a health club by expanding your program options and adding some of the same specialty programs that boutique studios offer.

When promoting specialty programs, remember that most members will understand and accept that there is an additional expense for programs that require specialized equipment and specially trained instructors. Specialty group training programs such as these can easily be delivered in a health club's existing group exercise studio, but the profit from them may be limited due to not having significant amounts of time available on the schedule, particularly during peak hours. Because of this limitation, clubs often create a dedicated space for a profit center program to maximize the financial gains. To show an example of a specialty group training program profit center, the rest of this section will discuss Pilates programs in a health club.

Pilates is a prime example of a specialty training program that can be a profit center for a health club. Fitness enthusiasts from professional athletes to older adults have embraced Pilates, a form of resistance training that strengthens muscles and reduces tightness through precise, demanding exercises and movements performed on mats and elaborate equipment. Pilates has become one of the most popular fitness activities in the country, especially among women, who account for over

80% of Pilates participants (IDEA 2015). Pilates is also popular among those with exercise- or sport-related injuries. It is estimated that 8.9 million people participated in Pilates in 2016 (Sports & Fitness Industry Association 2016).

According to an industry survey conducted by the IDEA Health and Fitness Association, 74% of responding health club program directors offer Pilates and 50% offer Pilates-yoga fusion programs (IDEA 2015). The 40 million female baby boomers, who tend to place a priority on staying healthy and looking good, will control two-thirds of all consumer wealth over the next decade (Landers 2018); a profit center that appeals to their sensibilities has the potential to be a significant revenue source. Beyond appealing to that market, Pilates exercises are versatile and can be modified to meet the needs of every demographic in your club, from older adults and pregnant women to athletes wanting to increase their performance. At health clubs across the country, there are popular specialty classes for specific sports, including the following:

- Pilates for golfers
- Pilates for tennis players
- Pilates for runners
- Pilates for equestrians
- Pilates for cyclists

Survey your members. What are they interested in? Then create Pilates classes to meet those needs.

Pilates mat classes are often free for members at many clubs and can act as feeder programs into more specific and intense Pilates training programs. When specialized equipment (e.g., reformers, towers, and Cadillac systems) is involved, the need for an additional fee is understood and accepted because of the perceived value of the equipment. Growth in mat and equipment-based Pilates programs continues in health clubs of all sizes. An IDEA (2015) survey lists Pilates among the top 11 group fitness trends, stating that

*"the rise of Pilates and its message of injury prevention through strengthening the body's core*

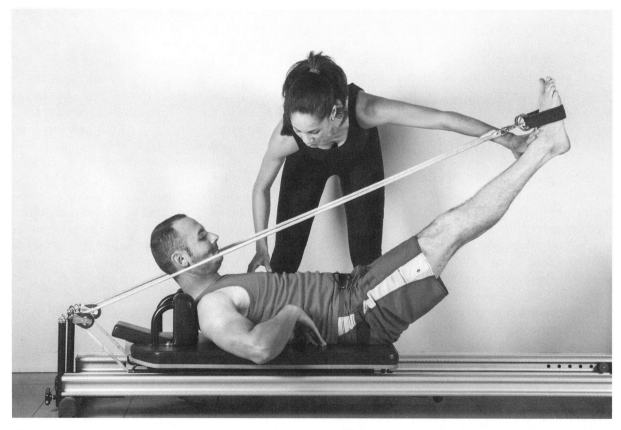

Pilates is one of the most popular specialty programs in the fitness industry. The consumer's perceived value of the specialized equipment and instructor expertise make the additional fee understandable and acceptable to participants.

poco_bw/fotolia.com

*musculature has fueled the growth of core-themed classes in health clubs. Fitness professionals have learned a great deal about connections and interactions among core muscles, fascial lines and movement, and the general population is benefiting from this knowledge."*

Pilates programs can progressively train participants to reach specific performance goals.

## Location

As previously mentioned, the growth of a profit center program may be limited due to insufficient time scheduled in the exercise studio. A dedicated space for a fee-based program allows the program to be offered during peak hours in the club, which will generate higher revenues. An increasing number of clubs are creating dedicated studios for Pilates, mind–body, and yoga programs. A space that is 800 to 1,100 square feet (74-102 square meters) typically can operate as a stand-alone profit center that generates revenues from specialized training.

To help promote an equipment-based mind–body program, the studio is best located where it is visible to the members. Though visible to club traffic, the studio must be soundproof, with limited visibility into the studio (preferably diffused viewing) and its own heating, air-conditioning, and sound systems. Light dimmers, ceiling fans, and built-in spaces for participants' shoes and gym bags help create a comfortable environment similar to a small boutique studio and are appreciated by participants.

## The Bottom Line

In order to increase revenue, a space for profit centers such as Pilates must be available during peak hours. Having a dedicated space for such programs eliminates the scheduling restraint.

## Operations

Private one-on-one sessions and semiprivate sessions for two to four clients are standard studio offerings. In order to maximize participation, schedule group classes during peak hours and schedule more one-on-one and semiprivate sessions during off-peak hours. Hiring a studio coordinator who teaches the majority of classes and has a lower hourly rate for administrative and marketing duties is typically a successful strategy. Because finding qualified and certified instructors can be challenging, this part-time manager may be able to grow the business and train new instructors so they can assume more teaching hours. One caveat: Be cautious about building a business around one top-notch trainer or instructor. That trainer or instructor may become sick, get injured, leave the fitness field, or decide to open a new business, taking the club's customers. Make sure the trainer's contract includes an exclusivity clause and a noncompete agreement (with a distance restriction for operating a similar business) and continually develop a team of certified instructors.

## The Bottom Line

Small-group training sessions make personal training more affordable than one-on-one sessions and can be held in a dedicated studio simultaneously to increase your profit per class hour.

## Cost of Sales and Profitability

Typically, a certified Pilates instructor commands a higher rate than a group exercise instructor, so you may not be able to run a class with fewer than three people and remain profitable. If such a class is initially too small to be profitable, there may be marketing potential in running the small class in an attempt to build the class, so club managers must use their judgment to determine whether the expense is outweighed by the marketing benefit. Bonus incentives based on class participation are good motivators for instructors to build their classes. Because many participants in mind–body studios aren't health club users, both member and nonmember pricing for this specialty program should established. The member pricing should be significantly lower than the nonmember pricing to show the advantages of membership. Do not price your nonmember rate above the standard rates of competing stand-alone studios, however, or you will price yourself out of the market. Introductory offers, single sessions, and packages should be priced using a methodology similar to that for personal training packages. The bundled class option allows members to buy 10 or 12 classes and take those at their convenience over a period of weeks or months, perhaps adding one Pilates session per week to their routine. This strategy can pay off if a club offers other specialty program options as well. After a few months of Pilates sessions, members may want to try something else, like barre or boxing. Not being locked in for a long-term commitment allows members to move from one new specialty program to another, bonding with a whole new group of people each time and still providing new revenue to the club.

Pilate mat classes are usually free with club membership, while specialty and private Pilates sessions are usually priced similarly to personal training ($50 to $100 per session). Group reformer classes can make equipment-based Pilates much more affordable, typically priced at $15 to $30 a class. Many clubs offer a multiple-session package that greatly reduces the cost per class and attracts more members. In addition, group reformer sessions for 4 to 10 participants feel like semiprivate classes because participants get plenty of individual attention from the instructor. Research what other clubs in your market charge and what services they offer, then price your services competitively.

## The Bottom Line

When determining pricing, you should know what the minimum class size must be in order to remain profitable.

## Equipment Costs for Pilates Programs

A reformer program for four to six participants, with the use of economical equipment like Allegro, is a great choice for health clubs. If the program includes classes with and without equipment, then stackable or collapsible equipment is recommended. Types of equipment and props include the following:

- *Mats.* The most basic and essential Pilates apparatus used in free Pilates mat classes; a quality mat has a textured nonslip surface and antiskid grip on the bottom to prevent injuries.
- *Magic circle.* A flexible isometric ring with handles that can be used as a prop in any Pilates class, this tool is used to firm the muscles of the upper arms, neck, and thighs. Magic circles cost approximately $35.
- *Reformers.* These are the most popular equipment for group classes. Portable and stackable equipment is available. The reformer has a gliding platform on which you can sit, kneel, stand, or lie on the front, back, or side. It is equipped with springs, straps, and pulleys and is designed to promote torso stability and proper alignment. Reformers can range from $2,000 (stackable) to $3,500 (studio).
- *Towers.* These upright units can be attached to a reformer to add more exercise variations. Tower attachments for Allegro reformers are $1,100.
- *Chairs.* Commonly known as *wunda chairs* or *stability chairs*, these resemble a stool. Most exercises are performed while seated on top and pressing down on the step with the feet, but the chair can be also used lying while on the floor, standing up, or lunging forward. The cost ranges from $750 to $1,300.
- *Cadillac.* Also called a *rack* or *trapeze table,* the Cadillac is a raised horizontal table with a four-post frame affixed with a variety of bars, straps, springs, and levers. Cadillacs cost from $1,300 in a wall system to $5,500.
- *Barrels.* These specialized pieces of equipment are shaped like a barrel and enhance breathing, work the spine to correct posture, and help develop the arms and legs. Semicircle barrels cost $200, whereas high ladder barrels cost $900.

Equipment can be purchased or leased. For a fully equipped studio system, expect to pay anywhere from $25,000 to $40,000.

## Advertising and Promotion

Make sure that your front-desk staff and all fitness instructors are knowledgeable about your Pilates program. Meet regularly with your Pilates instructors to discuss ways to improve and promote the program. Encourage all staff members to attend demonstration classes and gain a better understanding of the benefits of Pilates. Promote classes to your members. If you offer a specialty class like Pilates for triathletes, make sure your triathlete members know about it. Offering a free class gives participants a taste of the product before they commit to the purchase. As in an introductory personal training session, a great experience and a motivating instructor are sure ways to close a sale. Even instructors who are uncomfortable with the selling process can easily demonstrate the benefits of training with them. Packaging a free group class with a massage or fitness assessment is another way to expose customers to your product. Inviting nonmembers to an open house that features free classes and demonstrations is another marketing tactic, as are newsletter articles, emails, flyers posted in the club, direct mail, and direct community outreach. For example, your instructors can lead a warm-up at a running or cycling event and talk about the benefits of Pilates and core strength to improve overall performance.

## Training and Development

Well-trained instructors are expected to know anatomy, exercise physiology, human movement, and individual specialties of the discipline. Some certifications require a weekend-long course; others require months or years of study, or even an apprenticeship, before instruction is permitted.

Pilates certifications can be divided into two parts—mat certification and equipment (apparatus) certification. Certification programs range from a weekend to a year, with some certifications requesting apprentice hours. Costs range from $2,000 to $4,500. Certification companies include the following:

- Pilates Method Alliance
- Power Pilates
- Stott Pilates
- Peak Pilates
- Polestar Pilates Education
- Balanced Body
- BASI Pilates

# Spa Services

A spa is a business specializing in professional wellness services that enhance health and well-being, beauty, and relaxation. The types of personal care treatments typically found in spas include massage therapy, skin and body treatments, hair and nail salon services, and facials. Spas that are located within or adjacent to health clubs usually include areas such as sauna, steam, massage, meditation, and treatment rooms; whirlpool baths; and hot tubs. There are many types of spas besides health club spas—including stand-alone day spas, mineral spas, hotel and resort spas, medical spas, and cruise spas—each with their own specialty or focus. Spas may offer wellness services that include diet, life coaching, meditation, and other programs. As the use of spas has become increasingly popular and the demand for services has grown, a number of health clubs have incorporated spa facilities and treatments to provide members with a place to relax and reduce stress and to be a significant profit center for the club.

## Spa Industry Trends

At one time thought to be for only the rich and famous, spa services are becoming an integral part of many people's lifestyles because of the relaxation and stress reduction these services provide. There are an estimated 21,260 spa locations throughout the United States, with the largest category being day spas (79.6%). The International Spa Association (2017) reports that approximately 184 million spa visits were made in the United States in 2016, with an average revenue per visit of $91. Industry trends reported in the 2017 *ISPA Spa Industry Study* include express treatments, more frequent visits to spas by clients choosing shorter treatments, the use of natural and organic products, partnerships with local organizations as a way for spas to give back to the community, the use of social media outlets for promotion of services and online booking, and consumer perception of spa visits as a staple of a healthy lifestyle. ISPA also reports that survey respondents believe the next trend to shape the industry will be related to wellness, health, and fitness. Consumer visits to spas are driven by one or more of the following:

- Indulgence (i.e., pleasure, fun, appealing to the senses)
- Escape (i.e., relief from pressures of daily life)
- Work (i.e., individual work, largely related to self-improvement on some aspect of one's emotional state or long-term spiritual and personal dispositions)

The investment in a full-fledged day spa can be significant, and the scheduling component can be complex, so many health clubs opt for individual treatment rooms that offer bread-and-butter services like facials, pedicures, manicures, and, massages, which are particularly popular among health club members for stress reduction, muscle soreness, and injury rehabilitation.

## Menu of Services

The list of possible services a fitness or wellness center could offer its members is restricted only by the amount of space, facilities, and creativity available. Body care services include Swedish, sports, aromatherapy, and shiatsu massage; reflexology; herbal wraps; and loofah scrubs. Examples of skin care services include aromatherapy facials, glycolic acid peels, moisturizing facials, cleansing facials, and waxing services for the lip, brow, back, bikini area, and legs. The following are descriptions of body and skin services.

### BODY THERAPIES

- *Aromatherapy massage.* Combining the sense of smell with touch, this light, rhythmic massage uses essential oils to balance and restore energy levels. Different types of essential oils produce different results (i.e., relaxation versus stimulation).
- *Fango.* The word *fango* is Italian for "mud," and this service involves a highly mineralized mud mixed with oil or water and applied over the body as a heat pack to detoxify, soothe the muscles, and stimulate circulation.
- *Herbal wrap.* A body wrap made of strips of cloth is soaked in a heated herbal solution and wrapped around the body, followed by a period of rest. Herbal wraps are used to eliminate impurities and detoxify, as well as for relaxation.
- *Hydrotherapy.* Hydrotherapy includes underwater jet massage, showers, jet sprays, and mineral baths.

- *Loofah scrub.* A full-body scrub with a loofah sponge exfoliates the skin and stimulates circulation.
- *Reflexology.* This ancient Chinese technique uses pressure points, usually on the feet but sometimes on the hands and ears, to restore the flow of energy throughout the body.
- *Salt glow.* The body is rubbed with a coarse salt, sometimes in combination with fragrant oils, to remove the outer layer of dead skin and stimulate circulation.
- *Shiatsu massage.* This traditional Japanese massage is typically performed on a *tatami* (floor mat) with no oil. This acupressure massage applies pressure to specific points in the body to stimulate and unblock meridians, or pathways in the body through which life energy flows.
- *Swedish massage.* This classical European massage technique uses gentle manipulation of the muscles using massage oils. It is used to improve circulation, ease muscle aches and tension, improve flexibility, and create relaxation. This is the most common form of massage performed in the United States.
- *Sports massage.* Performed with or without oil, this massage uses strokes similar to those used in Swedish massage but typically with much deeper pressure. This massage enhances circulation and reduces pre-exercise muscle tightness or postexercise muscle soreness.
- *Thalassotherapy.* These treatments use the therapeutic benefits of the sea and seawater products. Seaweed and algae wraps and seawater hydrotherapy treatments are common.

### SKIN CARE THERAPIES

- *Aromatherapy facial.* Essential oils are used to moisturize, cleanse, and increase circulation to the face. Fragrant essential oils enhance relaxation.
- *Glycolic acid peel.* Low-level glycolic acids are used to remove the outer layer of dead facial skin and cleanse and moisturize the face. Peels are typically done in a series of 6 to 10 treatments.
- *Moisturizing facial.* This facial is ideal for those who suffer from dry skin or who are exposed to harsh environmental conditions. It uses masks, massage, and cleansing to rehydrate the skin and enhance circulation.

In addition, many salon services such as hair care and nail care can be offered by spas. Facilities that venture into salon services make a larger financial and spatial commitment to the spa concept and have the opportunity to reap the financial benefits of these services.

## Facility Requirements

Most facilities that are contemplating adding spa services begin by offering massage services. Whether the facility offers only massage or a menu of body, skin, and salon services, the facility setup is crucial to the success of the operation. The environment must create a sensory refuge from the hustle and bustle of everyday life.

Spa services should offer a luxury experience in a quiet and relaxing atmosphere. Careful consideration should be done before renovating an existing space for spa services—although adding services such as massage won't require a great deal of space, the location of the space is crucial. The ideal spa treatment room is located in a quiet area away from the normal traffic patterns of the club. Place the rooms where they are accessible from the locker rooms or provide convenient dressing facilities close by. The decor and lighting of the rooms and surrounding areas should be soft and indirect to create an ambiance of relaxation and stillness. Equip the treatment rooms with a sink and electrical outlets. Play relaxing music in the treatment rooms and surrounding areas. The ventilation of the treatment areas is crucial. Although the treatment room is typically kept warmer (70 to 76 degrees Fahrenheit, or 21 to 24 degrees Celsius) than the health club environment, the room must never feel stuffy or hot. The space requirement for each treatment room is approximately 120 square feet (11 square meters).

Creating a private, luxurious treatment room and surroundings will enhance relaxation, project a positive image for the facility, and encourage repeat business.

## Equipment Requirements

Equipment requirements for spa services vary depending on the type of services the club offers and the personal preferences of the technicians hired to perform the services. Equipping a massage room will cost approximately $1,500 to $3,000. Additional operating supplies such as linens, oils, towels, and so on will cost approximately $500 to $1,000, depending on the volume of traffic and the quality of the supplies. Facial rooms will cost approximately $7,000 to $10,000 to equip. Operating supplies will necessitate an additional investment of $500 to $1,500. Retail sale of facial products enhances the profitability of the spa by providing revenue with little overhead. An initial investment in this retail inventory can range from $500 to several thousand dollars. You can equip nail care stations for $1,000 to $5,000, depending on the types of equipment.

The necessary equipment for each spa treatment room is listed in the Spa Equipment and Operational Supply Lists sidebar later in this chapter. These lists are intended to be thorough, but they are not exhaustive. The preferences of the therapist you hire should determine the equipment and supplies you order. Depending on the type of treatment room, it is important to purchase the best equipment available. The equipment used in most services will dramatically affect the overall service delivery. Use a spa consultant or ask the service provider you have hired before selecting and purchasing any spa equipment.

## Operations

The operation of a spa facility is much different from that of a fitness facility. The types of products needed and the services delivered differ dramatically. The club manager should consider using an experienced spa consultant or hiring experienced treatment professionals to increase the probability of success.

## Marketing

Marketing spa services within the fitness operations can enhance the professional image of the facility. Careful consideration of the marketing aspects of the spa services can improve member retention and enhance the profile of the facility within the community.

Before offering spa services, the club operator should perform a market survey to analyze the need and desire for the services to be offered. The increasing demand for spa services nationwide should provide the club operator with a reasonable sense of security in offering these services. Local examination of the demand for these services, however, is always warranted. Once the need for spa services has been confirmed, the club operator should determine the target market for the services, then evaluate the competition and their pricing structures.

Determining the target market is an important consideration. Will services be available to members only or will nonmembers also have access to these services? Will members receive discounts on products and services? Will you allow nonmembers who frequent the spa to join the fitness facility at discounted prices? Several opportunities exist for creative marketing. The club operator should review what competition exists for these services, keeping in mind that many people enjoy these services only if they are convenient. Pricing should be competitive, with club members receiving discounts on services and products.

The club operator should also research all local, state, and federal codes involving delivery of spa services. Review codes and regulations as they relate to the treatment room, the treatment provider, and the facility offering spa treatments.

Once you have researched these areas and made decisions, the marketing personnel should put together a brochure explaining the benefits of spa services, the types of services offered, a brief description of the services, the rates for each service, the qualifications of the treatment

## Spa Equipment and Operational Supply Lists

### Multipurpose Treatment Room Equipment

- Clock
- Face cradle
- Floor and room heater
- Hydrocollator
- Massage and facial table (adjustable)
- Roll cushions and supports
- Therapist stool
- Towel and sheet storage cabinet

### Facial Equipment

- Double-pot wax melter
- Electric warming booties
- Electric warming mitts
- Facial bed with arm set
- Facial chair with back support
- Galvanic machine, high-frequency machine, brush and suction machine (all in one)
- Heating pad
- Hot towel cabinet
- Lucas mist spray
- Magnifying lamp with stand
- Paraffin wax unit
- Steamer with ozone and stand
- Three-tiered trolley with drawer
- UV sterilizer (dry)
- Wet sterilizer kit

### Manicure Equipment

- Client chair
- Manicure table
- Manicurist chair

### Pedicure Equipment

- Pedicure tub (requires water hookup and drain)
- Pedicure accessory cart
- Pedicurist chair

### Nail Care Equipment

- Cotton dish for pedicure station
- Finger bowls
- Large sanitizer jar
- Locking cabinets and drawers
- Magnifying lamps
- Nail polish rack
- Paraffin wax unit (hands and feet)
- Polish dryer (hands and feet)
- Terry booties
- Terry mitts

providers, the cancellation policy, and how to schedule an appointment. Additionally, we recommend that you create a pamphlet that answers frequently asked questions about the services. Many first-time spa goers are apprehensive about the services. In this pamphlet, answer questions regarding modesty, where to go, how to pay, and how to communicate with the therapist. Enjoyment of the service will be heightened if the client knows what to expect and can fully relax.

From a digital marketing perspective, staff can create a social media calendar (as discussed in chapter 7) for posting pictures and videos to Facebook, Twitter, Pinterest, Instagram, and YouTube to promote spa services. An increasing number of spa participants book appointments online, so having user-friendly booking tools will be a requirement. A final marketing technique is having and promoting spa gift certificates. Many people have their first spa experience as a result of a gift certificate they have received. Provide gift certificates for tournament prizes, charity donations, or new-member gifts. Certificates for spa treatments and services are popular gift items for holidays or birthdays. There is a great likelihood that people will spend money on a spa service for someone they care about before spending the money on themselves. Promoting gift certificates for spa services around Valentine's Day, Mother's Day, Father's Day, and Christmas will help generate strong revenues year-round because of return business.

## The Bottom Line

An innovative marketing staff can use spa facilities to enhance the image of the organization, to increase member satisfaction and retention, and to aid in recruitment. Additionally, the use of social media channels such as Facebook and Pinterest can foster engagement with the target market.

## Staffing

The staffing of the spa facility is crucial to its success. Treatment providers must be qualified and experienced in the type of luxury service the club is marketing. Spa staff are either hired by the facility as employees or are independent contractors, who often work for a percentage of the revenue. If the goal of the spa program is to be a profit center, it may be best to have the treatment providers on staff and pay an hourly wage plus commission. If the spa services are only an amenity to enhance the professional image of the facility and profitability is not crucial, the use of outside contractors is worth considering.

Typically, treatment providers hired as staff members are paid an hourly wage for the hours they are scheduled to be available plus a commission for each hour when they have a client. This commission gives the professional a vested interest in building a regular clientele. Gratuities are customary. The gratuity can be at the discretion of the client, or you can apply a service charge and include it in the service price. Competitive compensation for treatment providers ranges from $15 to $40 per hour of service. Benefits are an optional incentive that the club can offer to treatment providers who demonstrate a commitment to the profitability of the spa. Although the treatment provider may be able to earn more per hour in a private practice, the benefits of working for an organization that pays all overhead, purchases all supplies, markets aggressively to attract clients, and perhaps offers a benefits package cannot be overestimated.

Staff members who perform spa services are typically required by local and state regulations to maintain a current license or registration. Maintain proof of these licenses and registrations in the human resources files of the organization. Regular training and continuing education classes are recommended for treatment providers to stay abreast of current standards of practice in the industry. Maintaining membership in the American Massage Therapy Association (AMTA) or another governing body will help in this process.

Any facility employing more than five treatment providers should consider appointing a department head or senior treatment provider. In addition to being an experienced technician, this person should possess the business, communication, and supervisory skills for managing all scheduling, commissions and gratuity reconciliation, product and supply ordering, and hiring, training, and discipline of staff. This person should work closely with the marketing staff and fitness staff to ensure all employees understand the benefits of spa services and to assist in marketing.

## Legal Considerations

As mentioned, a variety of local and state regulations exist regarding the operation of spa facilities. Treatment providers in many states must maintain current registration and licensure. Additionally, the facility or spa itself must be registered or licensed by the state. Particular treatment practices, such as those that deal with cleanliness or draping the client during the service, are also regulated in many states. Be sure to check with the state department of health or human services that oversees the operation of spa or salon facilities.

In addition to state registration and licensure, each therapist should be covered by a professional liability and malpractice insurance policy with a minimum coverage of $1 million dollars. Insurance is a necessity. A lawsuit filed against you or your practice can be financially devastating. This insurance policy is available to treatment professionals through membership in professional organizations such as AMTA.

## Profitability

For those facilities that have waded through the maze of renovation, organization, licensure, and registration and have opened a spa facility, the potential profits are significant. Massage services typically produce 40 to 55% profit after all wages, benefits, and operational expenses are paid. Facial and nail care services typically generate 30 to 50% profit when revenues from both treatments and retail skin care product sales are considered. Maintaining a tight control on operational spending, wages, and benefits can yield a successful profit center.

## Maintenance

The spa area should receive regular custodial cleaning, with special attention paid to the floors around the treatment table, doorknobs, light switches, and cabinet doors. These areas should be sterilized as part of a daily cleaning schedule. Linens, including pillowcases and any draping material, should be changed following each service. Spa linens should be washed separately from other club linens because they may contain oils, muds, facial products, wax, and so on. The table surface should be cleaned with alcohol between each service. All implements used in a facial or nail service, such as nail nippers or facial tweezers, must be sterilized between each use. Therapists must be required to wash their hands following each service and before working on the client's face. Alcohol can be used if water is not easily available. These sanitation rules are established to prevent the transference of skin infections or communicable diseases from one client to another. Check with local and state officials for specific rules and regulations in your area.

## Professional Organizations and Resources

Professional organizations exist to assist the club operator in developing spa facilities and treatments. You may contact the following organizations for assistance with local and state regulations and locating potential staff.

- American Massage Therapy Association (AMTA)
- International Spa Association (ISPA)
- Day Spa Association
- International Medical Spa Association
- Alternative Balance
- The health and human services department of your state government

# Youth Programs

Youth programs for fitness and personal training have been identified as an emerging trend with above average growth in health clubs. In 2017 41% of health clubs offered youth fitness programs, an increase from 34% in 2013. Additionally, 33% of health clubs offered youth personal training programs in 2017, an increase from 27% in 2013 (ClubIntel 2017). Because of an increased focus on youth and youth programming, from 2012 to 2016 the number of club members under the age of 18 has increased by 5 percent (International Health, Racquet, and Sportsclub Association 2017). A focus on youth programs is viewed by many clubs, parents, and communities as a needed response to the prevalence of inactivity among young people today.

The United States is faced with a nationwide child obesity epidemic. Youth obesity has more than tripled in the past 30 years, and it is now estimated that one third of children and adolescents are overweight or obese (Centers for Disease Control and Prevention 2015). Daily activities such as walking to school, physical education classes, after-school activities, chores, and general playing have been replaced with sedentary behaviors in front of the TV, mobile devices, and computer. In addition, unhealthy food has become much more widespread and accessible, and safety concerns often prevent children from enjoying outdoor play opportunities. Being obese or overweight is a serious health concern for children and adolescents because of the serious health consequences later in life. Data from the Centers for Disease Control and Prevention show that approximately 17% (or 12.7 million) of children and adolescents age 2 to 19 are obese. While the prevalence of obesity has remained fairly stable at 17% for the past decade, far too many children are still overweight. In addition, the CDC data indicates that obese children are more likely to become obese adults, facing a number of serious health conditions such as heart disease, diabetes, metabolic syndrome, and cancer. Statistics like these are helping to make children's recreational and fitness programs a primary focus of government, communities, businesses, and parents.

To meet the need for youth physical activity programs, health clubs have been targeting the younger market. Strategies such as lowering membership age requirements, offering family memberships, and adding youth programming have been successful in attracting kids and their families. Some clubs with a strong family focus offer an entire menu of services to their younger clientele. With new fitness classes designed specifically for children by large companies such as Zumba, Les Mills, and Beachbody, young people now have a number of exciting options for exercise. For example, dance, core, and strength-based classes are gaining popularity among teens who might not be involved with sports. Youth boot camp classes can be designed with fun elements that will appeal to kids, including sprinting drills, jump rope, body-weight exercises, mini-band workouts, and obstacle courses. Another approach that is popular with kids is the use of technology such as interactive exercise software and networked exercise equipment to engage young people in physical activity. Software programs that can be used with indoor bikes, rowers, treadmills, cross trainers, and interactive walls can get kids active and engaged in friendly competition.

Before implementing youth programming, you must determine whether your club has a family-based membership and whether the club culture and clientele are family friendly. You must determine whether the purpose of the programming is as a true profit center or as an added benefit for members who have children. Next, you should look at the available market—the percentage of children under age 15 within a 10-minute drive time to your facility.

If yours is a family-oriented club and a recreational facility as well, your ability to generate profits from youth programs significantly increases. Youth programming appeals to many nonmembers and provides an opportunity to market the benefits of membership to nonmember parents. Multipurpose clubs with swimming pools, basketball courts, volleyball courts, and recreational spaces have a greater ability to generate a large amount of revenue with high profit margins. With increasing societal focus on everyone needing to lead healthier lives, youth programming in a safe club setting will be a welcome choice for parents. Parents often prefer skill development and recreational programs over passive babysitting services, and it is well known that parents are more likely to spend money on their child than on themselves.

## Location

Youth activities or dedicated youth program spaces should be located in an area that is easily accessible to parking and strollers and handicapped access. When offering children's programs, there is a need to accommodate busy parents with multiple children of various ages. For safety and noise reduction for the sake of adult members, the location of your youth space and recreational activities should be away from main areas of the club. As the programs grow, the need to add a separate registration and point-of-sale desk may arise to eliminate congestion at the front desk. Program spaces should be visible to parents as well as other members; the space should create a positive impression so that it draws business from other members with children. In this way, the program can compete with stand-alone children's businesses.

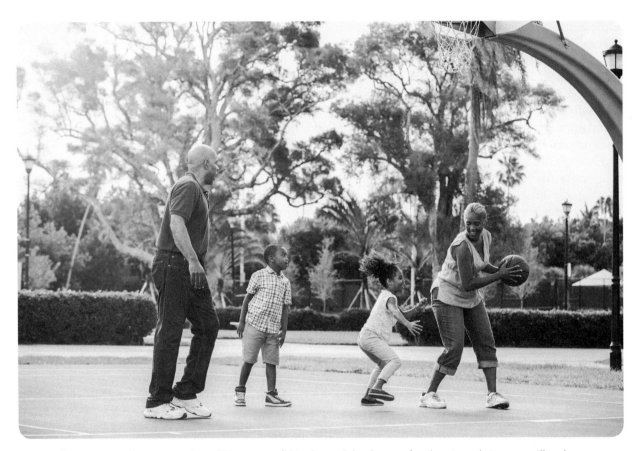

As a profit center, youth programming will be successful in those clubs that are family oriented. Parents will welcome recreational and fitness programs that provide activities for their children in a safe club setting.

bowdenimages/Getty Images/iStockphoto

## Types of Programs and Scheduling

As with any new profit center, the potential for growth and the types of programs offered are directly correlated to the size and type of facility. A strong anchor program that has proven revenue results can be the basis of your youth programs. The anchor program may be swimming lessons (a child must learn to swim to be safe around the water), summer camp (including sports camps), or special events like vacation programs and birthday party activities. Without a strong draw to the youth market, it is difficult to get the critical mass of customers necessary to build additional revenue-generating programs. Adding swimming pools and multisport areas are significant capital investments that will increase operational and facility maintenance concerns, so additional management and responsibilities should be factored into the equation. Clubs that use existing group exercise studios and fitness spaces have limited programming choices and time slots, which will limit the ability to drive significant profit.

Selecting a small cluster of two to three programs gives parents choices for their children. Offer packages in manageable 4- to 8-week sessions so as not to interfere with other extracurricular activities such as recreational leagues, church studies, and other youth programs.

Parent and child programs include aquatic instruction, tumbling, active games, and yoga for parents together with their preschool-age youngsters. These programs fit well in group exercise studios and pools at off-peak times. Preschool recreational programs such as creative rhythm and dance, gymnastics, and sports appeal to parents who are trying to identify their child's program preferences at an early stage. These types of programs will be successful in the morning and midafternoon. It is beneficial to use the group exercise class schedule and club usage as a filter to determine usage patterns by young mothers.

Programs for school-age children should be offered during after-school hours and on Saturdays. Before developing your schedule, call the local school district for the school calendar, holidays, and school start and dismissal times. Dance, youth fitness, gymnastics, swim lessons, sport skills, and martial arts are popular.

Programs that satisfy a need of the parents, such as swimming lessons and summer camps as an alternative to child care, are an instant win. Both aquatics and camp programs have licensing, certification, and safety requirements. Summer camps can be offered indoors and outdoors.

Fun and active youth events such as birthday parties are a hit with everyone from preschoolers to preteens. If you have developed some core recreational programs, use them as featured elements of the party. Swim, sport, and gymnastics parties are a great fit in a health club. A complete competitive analysis of surrounding party centers is necessary before developing pricing and party options. Some businesses include food, party favors, invitations, instruction, a personal party coordinator, and more. All of these elements must be figured into the cost of sale and overall profitability.

Special events during club hours or after hours present an opportunity to open the club to the community and generate revenue. Sports teams, Scout groups, youth groups, schools, and other community groups can take advantage of your facility offerings.

Stand-alone sport performance centers for athletic training are on the rise. These companies cater to young athletes who want to improve their speed, agility, and quickness in their sport of choice. Parents are looking for ways to help their children succeed in athletic tryouts. Prime hours of operation are weekdays after school from 4 to 9 p.m. and on Saturdays. The busiest times for sport performance programs are the in off-season (when that particular sport is not in play), during winter and summer months.

Because youth programs by nature have limited usage and times of operation, such that revenue may not offset the overhead costs, there is an increased risk of financial losses. High volume and pricing must occur in order to support a profitable structure. Club facilities with a strong membership base and available space can support a youth program if the existing management and trainers are used in a cost-effective manner. These programs can be packaged similarly to the adult personal training programs. Participants must commit to 2 to 3 days per week for a series of consecutive weeks. Measurable training results must be tracked and guaranteed, with a specific amount of training in a certain time period, in order for the program to prove valuable to the parent and athlete.

## Child Watch

Child watch services allow parents with young children to use the club without having to worry about the supervision of their children. Such a service is often provided at no cost or minimal cost. Although some consider child watch to be a headache to operate, this offering may make the difference when a prospective member is deciding between your club and a competitor. The increasing number of members with young children and the ongoing need to attract new members make child watch facilities a necessity for today's facilities. Child watch services are rarely profitable as individual entities and may actually be a cost center. One creative solution to address this potential financial drain is to expand from mere child supervision to youth program options for which parents pay a fee.

## Security

Security in the child watch (babysitting) area must be of the utmost concern. Analyze and reanalyze the security of the children to ensure their safety. The manager and organization must ensure that only an authorized parent or guardian drops off or picks up the child. Security cameras should be installed both in the child-watch facility and along the route from the main desk to the child watch space to ensure safe passage of children to the area. All staff members working with young people should be carefully screened: Check the references of potential hires and complete a criminal background check for each person who will be involved with the youth program.

## Pro Shops

Pro shops that sell a variety of club merchandise—including clothing, workout supplies, and food and beverage items—can be a great amenity for members and guests at a health club as well as a way to generate revenue and improve member retention. These on-site stores provide one-stop shopping for all of a member's workout needs, and they are a convenient source when members need supplies right away. Pro shops have come to be viewed as a necessary club service, and clubs willing to invest effort and a dedicated space for a pro shop operation will be rewarded with profitability and more satisfied members.

Treating a pro shop as a separate business entity is critical in turning it into a profit center. For a pro shop to be successful, it is essential to have a diverse set of items in stock that generate revenue. To maximize profitably, sell an assortment of products that appeal to many members. Members may need an energy bar, a bottle of water, or new workout apparel, or they may simply need a place to go when they forget their socks. Clubs with successful pro shop operations typically have put careful thought into the shop's placement, size, layout, product offerings, and management.

## Location

In setting up an attractive, inviting, and profitable pro shop, one of the first factors to consider is its placement within the club. A basic merchandise sales operation at a busy front desk, with some items in a display case and clothes hung on a wall, is not conducive to generating sales. Having a defined pro shop area or room adjacent to the main desk, where there is high traffic, is a successful strategy. Locating the shop so there is increased opportunity for members to interact with the shop's products is one of the secrets of good merchandising. The more people see the merchandise, the more likely they are to make a purchase. Think about the high visibility in a shopping mall, where it's easy to see products just by walking by the store; this product visibility helps draw people in. To increase sales, consider placing the shop where it is visible from outside the club through a street-side window, and have an entrance where people who are not club members can walk in and out easily.

## Size

Although a pro shop can generate a respectable amount of revenue, it usually does not warrant a large amount of facility space; less than 1 percent of the total club square footage is typically sufficient. Depending on the size of the club, a pro shop can usually be operated in 300 to 500 square feet of space.

## Design

A well-designed pro shop can help club operators make the most of limited space and increase store patronage. Clubs should consider hiring a professional interior designer to plan the shop layout and recommend the color scheme, lighting, and display strategies to be used. The design of the pro shop should be bright, colorful, and inviting so members and guests will want to visit the space and browse the available products.

A professional-looking display system (shelves, racks, mannequins, etc.) is the foundation upon which to build the shop's layout. A display system will effectively highlight the products for optimal visibility and also draw people into the space. Many suppliers of the display items and systems have design consultants who are skilled at setting up display areas, giving a professional look and design to the pro shop. Some larger clubs may opt for high-end modular store fixtures in their pro shops to create an area that feels like a high-end clothing boutique.

If space allows, include a dressing booth in or adjacent to the pro shop, so customers don't need to go to the locker room to try on merchandise. Finally, be sure the store design includes the capability to lock up the shop at the end of the day.

## Products

When considering what products to offer in a pro shop, begin by researching the expected market demands in the club. Find out what similar pro shops typically stock. The easiest way to learn what your members will buy is to listen to their requests. A shop's inventory must be relevant to the membership and the club's activities in order for merchandise to move off the shelves and not collect dust. Many shops start by first considering items that will be regular sellers—products like padlocks, energy bars, swim caps, socks, and bottled water—keeping in mind that many small sales every day can add up quickly. Small, inexpensive convenience items tend to be bought on impulse, and members often appreciate having these available. Small items with a high price markup can make a big difference in the shop's bottom line, particularly if they are prominently displayed to entice customers.

With more expensive products like clothing lines, there are other factors to consider. First, look at various potential product lines relative to their price and the type of membership at the club. It is not advisable to carry a high-end line of fashionable workout attire if your members would not purchase designer clothing. Basic, yet stylish, T-shirts and tank tops suffice for some clubs. Another factor to be aware of is current style trends for workout attire. This is particularly true for women's athletic clothing, because women are more likely to consider the pro shop a retail place comparable to a specialty clothing store. The types of programs that are conducted at the club is another consideration; members may be looking for clothing specific to yoga, cycling, kickboxing, or dance, for example.

Whatever the type of clothing, custom imprinting can make products in the pro shop unique by adding the club's name and logo. Imprint the logo on a variety of items such as T-shirts, tank tops, sweatshirts, warm-up suits, bags, and hats. Wearing an item that has their club's logo on it appeals to many members, and the product serves as free advertising when the member wears it outside the club. Pro shops can be powerful tools for establishing and growing a club brand when they provide branded clothing and other items that cannot be purchased anywhere else. A partnership with a brand name active clothing company such as Nike, Adidas, or Under Armour can help a health club offer both stylish and practical fitness products that carry the club's logo. Brand name apparel can be priced higher, particularly when it's a specialty piece not available elsewhere. Other items besides clothing, such as drink cups, can be branded to help make a club name more recognizable.

## Management

Many health clubs, particularly larger ones, subscribe to the theory that in order to turn a pro shop into a true profit center, they need to hire a manager for it. Asking the front-desk staff to oversee the pro shop in addition to their other responsibilities does not have the same results as having a pro shop staff. The shop manager does not have to be a full-time employee, but he or she needs to be used exclusively for the store operation. Furthermore, this person needs to understand the retail business, including effective pricing strategies, and know what the product lines are and what to buy. The retail business skills

---

## Pro Shop Products List

The products sold in a pro shop should be selected based on member need, space availability, and club programs. The following are some suggestions of items that could be stocked in a health club pro shop.

- T-shirts
- Bra tops
- Shorts
- Tights
- Bike shorts
- Socks
- Sweatshirts
- Jackets
- Sports headwear
- Headbands
- Towels
- Workout gloves
- Resistance bands and tubing

- Exercise mats
- Workout equipment for home or travel
- CDs
- DVDs
- Books
- Earphones
- Gym bags
- Bottled water
- Protein bars
- Energy drinks
- Shake drinks
- Sport balls (if programs like tennis, racquetball, and squash are offered)

- Shampoos and conditioners
- Soaps
- Skin lotion
- Pain relief sprays or lotions
- Shave cream
- Razor blades
- Combs
- Ear plugs
- Nose clips
- Swim caps
- Batteries
- Locks
- Water bottles

of inventory management, product promotion, theft prevention, and selection of product line are usually beyond the scope of a typical club owner or manager. Besides these skills, the pro shop manager must be able to do hiring and to train staff to provide great customer service by dealing with the needs of customers, answering their questions, and making recommendations.

A club that treats the pro shop as a profit center will see a high return on investment. Pro shops can be a steady revenue source for clubs, producing anywhere from $50,000 to $250,000 per year. To achieve that type of success, pro shop managers must invest in quality product, staff training, and marketing. Shop managers need to pay attention to what is selling well and what is not selling (and is taking up valuable shelf space). Regular inventory management will help the manager plan product ordering and limit the shop's losses from products that don't sell as well. Retail software that tracks sales, monitors inventory, and has sophisticated reporting functions can be helpful in monitoring the success of the operation.

Just like any business that sells products, pro shops must be protected from theft. Although a certain amount of product loss is expected in retail shops, staff need to understand which products have the highest financial loss potential if stolen and take steps to combat the theft of these items. Providing great customer service is a good way to protect against theft, because members will be less inclined to steal from people who are nice to them and provide good service. In addition, the club may want to invest in a security camera and video monitor system to protect the pro shop. Security monitors visible to anyone entering the shop will serve as effective theft deterrents.

## The Bottom Line

Health club pro shops that sell club merchandise and food and beverage items can be a great amenity for members as well as a way to generate significant revenue. For a shop to be successful, it is essential to sell a diverse array of products that appeal to many members. Clubs with successful pro shop operations put careful thought into shop placement, size, design and layout, products, and management.

## Key Terms

active clients

bundle

conversion goals

financial pro forma

industry metrics

personal training revenue

personal training sales

profit center

# PART
# III

# OPERATIONS AND FACILITY MANAGEMENT

The operations side of running a fitness business is the final area of club management covered in this book. Do not underestimate the importance of the topics covered in this part's chapters. The contributors have all seen what can happen when these areas are neglected, poorly executed, or not thoroughly understood. The most successful clubs recognize their importance and have developed systems to ensure each area is working at its best.

In chapter 12, you will learn the importance of financial management for the club manager. Understanding how to read financial statements and to build budgets is critical to the long-term success of any business. Managing expenses and collecting payments are two other important areas that should be closely scrutinized by the club manager interested in meeting financial objectives.

Next, in chapter 13, you will dive into health and safety within the fitness industry. You will learn how to identify potential hazards and to minimize their potential impact on your business.

Mistakes in this area can cost millions of dollars in lawsuits and, more importantly, can affect the lives of members, guests, and staff.

In chapter 14, you will discover the importance of facility maintenance. A well-kept facility and a preventive maintenance schedule are cornerstones of a well-run fitness center. This chapter is full of easy-to-follow steps and guidelines to ensure that your facility and the equipment within it are running at their best.

The basics of contract law are covered in chapter 15. Employment legal issues are covered, and an overview of insurance is presented. This chapter includes case studies that will help you further engage with the material, making it more accessible to you as you navigate through the content.

In the final chapter, you will learn how to properly evaluate your fitness business. Stepping back and taking the time to properly evaluate your business is often forgotten as managers get caught up in the daily operation of the business. Evaluation is a critical task that a fitness club manager needs to perform in order for the business to be successful.

# CHAPTER 12

# Understanding Financial Management

## Learning Objectives

After studying this chapter, you will be able to

- identify the key components of the income statement, balance sheet, and statement of cash flows and understand the differences between these financial statements;

- understand the various types of budgets and the steps involved in preparing a budget;

- recognize the importance of managing expenses; and

- appreciate the impact that taxes have on financial planning and decision making.

Perhaps one of the most important tasks of a manager in a commercial health club is financial management. Managers need to be able to examine financial ratios such as profit margin, EBITDA (earnings before interest, taxes, depreciation, and amortization) margin, and return on assets. In addition, managers need to examine the company's pro forma financial statements, such as the balance sheet and income statement. Managers should also know the company's sustainable growth rate. If all of this sounds like a foreign language, you're not alone. The starting point to understanding financial management begins with the accounting terminology and financial principles. Now, get set to learn about the true business of fitness—financial management!

**A**s the fitness industry has matured over the past decade, the strongest have survived and the weakest are no longer in business. Although there may be multiple reasons a club fails, one of them is often a lack of attention to the financial aspects of the business. This may mean a complete lack of knowledge about the financials or the inability to make the right decisions. The best managers review key metrics on a daily or weekly basis, and their key staff all have a knowledge of their responsibilities as they relate to the financial success of the fitness business.

A manager needs to be able to answer the following questions:

- Is the business generating enough cash flow to pay its bills?
- Does the business have strong systems in place to collect on overdue accounts?
- Is the club properly budgeting staff hours based on the ups and downs of the business?
- What benchmarks do the best clubs in the business use to determine their success? How can I use these benchmarks in my club?
- Are there clear, established procedures for purchasing supplies?
- Does the staff know the sales goals for the upcoming month?
- Is the not-for-profit status (if applicable) of the organization being properly maintained?
- Will the club have enough money to acquire new equipment when it's needed?

Whether you are operating a single club, multiclub chain, city recreation center, or not-for-profit center, the financial principles in this chapter are critical to the long-term success of your business.

## CASH VERSUS ACCRUAL ACCOUNTING

Managers need to determine which system of **accounting**—cash or accrual—they will use when recording revenues and expenses. **Cash accounting** involves recording business transactions only when the business receives or pays cash. In a cash-based system, you record the revenue when it is received, regardless of when goods are sold or services rendered. When you sell merchandise or render services in one month and collect cash

the following month, cash-based accounting recognizes the revenue only when you receive the cash. Similarly, accounting for expenses means that when you make a cash payment, you record the amount as an expense. For example, if a utility bill is incurred in June (because that was the month that you actually used the electricity, water, or gas) but not paid until July, the expense is not recorded until the month in which it is paid.

**Accrual accounting** records transactions when they occur rather than when cash is received or paid. In this type of accounting, you record revenues when you earn them regardless of whether you have received payment, and you record expenses when they occur as opposed to when you pay them. The utility bill from the previous example would be recorded in June rather than in July.

There are advantages and disadvantages to both systems. Although a cash-based system is simple to implement, it is difficult to determine an accurate net worth because unpaid revenue and expenses are not reflected. Also, organizations that offer prepaid annual memberships will appear financially solvent when cash is received, but if funds are not properly managed in the remaining 11 months of the year, a cash shortage could occur. For example, if a member prepays a year's membership for $900, the cash-based system recognizes all $900 in the month in which the cash is received. In the accrual system, $75 ($900 divided by 12 months) is recognized each month as member revenue.

Although it is not uncommon for a club to adopt a mix of the cash and accrual methods, the preferred system for commercial health and fitness settings is accrual-based accounting because it provides a more accurate understanding of operations. There are three reasons accrual accounting is preferred among club operators (Grantham et al. 1998):

- Accrual accounting allows for better cash management because all prepaid memberships received are recorded as 1/12 of the dues for each month of the year.
- Accrual accounting provides a more realistic picture of the financial status of the business by including all unpaid expenses and unpaid revenues that are due.
- You can report the net worth of a club with accrual accounting but not with a cash-based

system. This is especially important if a club is attempting to obtain a loan or solicit investors.

A well-organized accounting system entails several functions, all designed to record, track, protect, and analyze the financial transactions of a business. A series of checks and balances should always be in place to account for every transaction that goes in and out of the organization. In addition, the process by which you accumulate financial information to prepare financial statements is integral to the accounting system. Fried (2004) says that the purpose of any accounting system is to provide information for the following purposes:

- Making decisions concerning the use of limited resources, including the identification of crucial decisions and determination of objectives and goals
- Effectively directing and controlling human and material resources
- Maintaining and reporting on the custodianship of resources
- Contributing to the overall effectiveness of the organization

## *The Bottom Line*

Most fitness clubs use accrual accounting and record revenue when the money was actually earned.

## FINANCIAL STATEMENTS

The purpose of financial statements is to provide a financial summary of the current status of the fitness organization. Generally, an in-house or outside accountant prepares financial statements from the accounting records of the company and completes the statements in a timely and accurate fashion. The preparation of financial statements depends on an organized bookkeeping system that tracks every transaction from its inception until it becomes part of the financial statement. These statements are then used within the company for budget analysis, internal controls, and short- and long-term planning. Financial statements also have external uses: They provide the requested financial information when refinancing or securing a loan for renovating or expanding the facility.

The **balance sheet** shows a company's assets, liabilities, and owners' equity at a specific point in time. For example, on October 31, 2018, Club ABC had the balance sheet seen in figure 12.1.

## Balance Sheet

The basic formula used for all balance sheets is as follows:

$$assets = liabilities + owners' equity$$

For a balance sheet to be accurate, this formula must always hold true. Another way of looking at the formula is to express it as a function of owners' equity:

$$owner's equity = assets - liabilities$$

**Assets** are anything a business owns that has monetary value. In figure 12.1, the cash, land, exercise equipment, office equipment, inventory, and furniture are all assets. Assets are divided into two main categories: current assets and fixed assets. An accountant classifies an asset as a **current asset** if it is cash or something easily converted into cash: accounts receivable, inventory, and prepaid expenses. *Liquidity* refers to the ease and quickness with which assets can be converted into cash. The entries shown under current assets are considered the most liquid, whereas the entries shown under the fixed assets are the least liquid. **Fixed assets**—the land, building, office furniture, and fitness equipment—are the more long-lived resources owned by the business. With the exception of land, these assets are valued at book value minus depreciation.

**Liabilities** are amounts owed to creditors. Like assets, liabilities are divided into two categories: current liabilities and long-term liabilities. Current liabilities consist of notes payable, accounts payable, and accruals (such as wages or taxes payable) that are due within 1 year. Long-term liabilities are obligations to be paid beyond 1 year. An example of a long-term liability in the health and fitness industry is a loan for new outdoor tennis courts.

**Equity** (or net worth) represents the owner's claims on the assets of the business. This is a

# CLUB ABC BALANCE SHEET

## OCTOBER 31, 2018

**Assets**

Current assets

| | | | |
|---|---|---|---|
| Cash | | 185,236 | |
| Inventory | | 85,693 | |
| Total current assets | | | 270,929 |

Fixed assets

| | | | |
|---|---|---|---|
| Equipment | 1,256,756 | | |
| Furniture and fixtures | 356,458 | | |
| | 1,613,214 | | |
| Less: accumulated depreciation | 563,254 | 1,049,960 | |
| Land | | 650,000 | |
| Total fixed assets | | | 1,699,960 |

Other assets

| | | | |
|---|---|---|---|
| Loan fees | 56,000 | | |
| Security deposits | 7,500 | | |
| Total other assets | | | 63,500 |
| Total assets | | | 2,034,389 |

**Liabilities and owners' equity**

Current liabilities

| | | | |
|---|---|---|---|
| Accounts payable | | 75,896 | |
| Current portion of long-term debt | | 2,584 | |
| Payroll taxes | | 6,589 | |
| Total current liabilities | | | 85,069 |

Long-term debt

| | | | |
|---|---|---|---|
| Note payable—bank | | 953,450 | |
| Less: current portion | | 2,584 | |
| Total long-term debt | | | 950,866 |

Owners' equity

| | | | |
|---|---|---|---|
| Capital stock | | 1,000 | |
| Additional paid-in-capital | | 25,000 | |
| Current period profit (loss) | | 254,875 | |
| Retained earnings | | 717,579 | |
| Total stockholder's equity | | | 998,454 |
| Total liabilities and owners' equity | | | 2,034,389 |

**Figure 12.1**   A typical balance sheet for a fitness club.

residual claim because owners receive only what remains after all claims, including taxes, have been paid. It is important to understand that the amount of owner's equity is not the market value of the business. As is the case with any investment, what the business is worth on the open market (the amount a buyer is willing to pay for the business) is typically determined by placing a value on the future cash flow it is expected to produce. Equity shown on the balance sheet reflects the book value of the business, not the market value.

To best analyze the financial condition of a club, an owner or manager must have information about its assets, liabilities, and owners' equity. A balance sheet is a snapshot of an organization's financial status on a given date. Consequently, changes in balance sheets between two statement dates provide important information about the financial health of a club. Understanding the implication of changes in financial statements can help provide answers to questions such as the following:

- How much did the funds in accounts receivable and inventory increase or decrease relative to the change in member sales for the period?
- Has the amount of debt increased to unsatisfactory levels since the last statement date?
- Are accounts payable amounts rising too high?
- Has the club maintained a satisfactory level of cash flow from operations?

## Income Statement

The **income statement**, or the statement of profit and loss, reflects the financial results of the business operations over a specific time (month, quarter, or year). It summarizes the transactions that produced revenue for the time frame and the operating expenses and taxes the business has incurred in generating this revenue. See figure 12.2 for an example.

The two major financial categories on an income statement are revenues and expenses. Revenues are earned through selling products or providing a service. In the health and fitness industry, revenues are generated primarily through membership sales, racket sport programs, fitness programs, profit centers, and miscellaneous income (e.g., guest fees, locker rentals,

towel fees). To fully understand the concept of revenue, note the following two points:

- Although you may think the value produced by the sale of a new club membership is cash received, an accountant measures the membership by either a cash sale or a credit sale. To an accountant, a credit sale means something of value: a claim on the new member for the amount of the membership sale. This claim appears as an asset and is classified as accounts receivable. Accounts receivable have a definite value to the club, but they are not cash and may never become cash.

- In preparing an income statement, an accountant recognizes a credit sale as revenue in the time frame in which the credit sale was made. This means that the revenue figures on the income statement for a given time frame include all credit sales made during that time, even though cash from those transactions may not be received until later. There could be a significant difference between the membership sales revenue shown on the income statement and the actual amount of cash received during that time.

Comprehending these concepts is essential to interpreting an income statement and becoming familiar with cash flow.

Expenses represent the costs incurred for generating revenue and operating the fitness facility. In the health and fitness industry, expenses are typically broken down into operating expenses and fixed expenses. **Operating expenses** are the costs associated with the operation of a club, such as payroll and benefits, administration, utilities, maintenance and repairs, advertising, marketing, and program and profit-center costs. **Fixed expenses** are costs that remain constant over a designated time. Examples of fixed expenses include rent and lease payments, interest and financing charges, real estate and personal property taxes, and depreciation. The expenses recognized in a given period are matched with revenues for that time to determine the amount of profit or loss (net income or net loss).

## Statement of Cash Flows

Companies are in business to make money or at the very least to generate enough money to cover their expenses. Companies that are able to generate a positive cash flow will stay in business, whereas those with a negative cash flow will

# XYZ COMPANY INCOME STATEMENT

## FOR THE PERIOD ENDED DECEMBER 31, 2018

| Account no. | Description | 2018 | % | 2017 | % |
|---|---|---|---|---|---|
| | *Revenue* | | | | |
| 4010 | Joining fees | 145968 | 4.5 | 131371 | 4.5 |
| 4020 | Membership dues | 2415984 | 74.7 | 2174386 | 74.7 |
| | Total membership fees | 2561952 | 79.2 | 2305757 | 79.2 |
| 4100 | Random court time | 68745 | 2.1 | 61871 | 2.1 |
| 4110 | Leagues | 125698 | 3.9 | 113128 | 3.9 |
| 4120 | Tennis instruction | 254994 | 7.9 | 229495 | 7.9 |
| | Total tennis revenue | 449437 | 13.9 | 4044494 | 13.9 |
| 4155 | Personal training | 128952 | 4.0 | 116057 | 4.0 |
| 4172 | Group swim instruction | 8523 | 0.3 | 7671 | 0.3 |
| | Total fitness revenue | 137475 | 4.2 | 123728 | 4.2 |
| 4965 | Dividends and interest | 85694 | 2.6 | 77125 | 2.6 |
| 4990 | Miscellaneous | 547 | 0.0 | 492 | 0.0 |
| | Total administrative | 86241 | 2.7 | 77617 | 2.7 |
| | Total revenue | 3235105 | 100.0 | 2911596 | 100.0 |
| | *Expenses* | | | | |
| 6110 | Wages—tennis | 350558 | 10.8 | 315502 | 10.8 |
| 6340 | Wages—fitness | 330563 | 10.2 | 297507 | 10.2 |
| 7140 | Wages—accounting | 75894 | 2.3 | 68305 | 2.3 |
| | Total payroll | 757015 | 23.4 | 681314 | 23.4 |
| 9520 | Group insurance | 275854 | 8.5 | 248269 | 8.5 |
| 9530 | FICA—employer | 57912 | 1.8 | 52121 | 1.8 |
| 9540 | Federal unemployment | 46935 | 1.5 | 42242 | 1.5 |
| 9545 | State unemployment | 39845 | 1.2 | 53345 | 1.8 |
| | Total payroll and benefits | 420546 | 13.0 | 395977 | 13.6 |
| 8910 | Electricity | 134191 | 4.1 | 120772 | 4.1 |
| 8920 | Water | 21781 | 0.7 | 19603 | 0.7 |
| 8930 | Gas | 25194 | 0.8 | 22675 | 0.8 |
| | Total utilities | 181166 | 5.6 | 163050 | 5.6 |
| 8522 | Contract landscape | 41142 | 1.3 | 37028 | 1.3 |
| 8620 | Repair pool | 32568 | 1.0 | 29311 | 1.0 |
| 8720 | Supplies locker room | 75105 | 2.3 | 67595 | 2.3 |
| | Total maintenance | 148815 | 4.6 | 133934 | 4.6 |
| 7210 | Accounting fees | 50000 | 1.5 | 45000 | 1.5 |
| 7230 | Bad debt expense | 115000 | 3.6 | 103500 | 3.6 |
| 7820 | Office supplies | 35577 | 1.1 | 32019 | 1.1 |
| | Total administrative | 200577 | 6.2 | 180519 | 6.2 |

**Figure 12.2**  Sample income statement.

*(continued)*

| Account no. | Description | 2018 | % | 2017 | % |
|---|---|---|---|---|---|
| 8120 | Advertising | 42897 | 1.3 | 38607 | 1.3 |
| 8250 | Printing | 25478 | 0.8 | 22930 | 0.8 |
| 8280 | Promotions | 31913 | 1.0 | 28722 | 1.0 |
|  | Total advertising | 100288 | 3.1 | 90259 | 3.1 |
| 6150 | Supplies tennis | 31568 | 1.0 | 28411 | 1.0 |
| 6180 | Special events tennis | 24569 | 0.8 | 22112 | 0.8 |
| 6195 | Tennis balls | 27976 | 0.9 | 25178 | 0.9 |
|  | Total tennis | 84113 | 2.6 | 75701 | 2.6 |
| 6450 | Aerobics music | 10464 | 0.3 | 9418 | 0.3 |
| 6480 | Supplies fitness | 27336 | 0.8 | 24602 | 0.8 |
| 6494 | Nutrition | 4256 | 0.1 | 3830 | 0.1 |
|  | Total fitness | 42056 | 1.3 | 37850 | 1.3 |
|  | Total operating expense | 1934576 | 59.8 | 1758604 | 60.4 |
| 7450 | Insurance | 737603 | 22.8 | 663843 | 22.8 |
| 7300 | Depreciation | 213517 | 6.6 | 192165 | 6.6 |
| 7460 | Debt service | 152050 | 4.7 | 136845 | 4.7 |
|  | Total fixed expenses | 1103170 | 34.1 | 992853 | 34.1 |
|  | Total expenses | 3037746 | 93.9 | 2751457 | 94.5 |
|  | Net income | 197359 | 6.1 | 160139 | 5.5 |

**Figure 12.2**    *(continued)*

struggle to pay their bills and will most likely be forced to close their doors.

By *cash flows*, we are referring directly to the cash flowing into the business as well as the cash flowing out of the business. The **statement of cash flows** is a financial statement that reports changes in cash holding over a certain amount of time. To see the distinction between cash flows and other accounting measures of income, recall from the section on income statements that revenue is recorded at the time the transaction actually occurs, but this is not necessarily the time when cash is collected. This is most often the case when items are purchased on credit. The depreciation that is reported on an income statement, on the other hand, has no impact on the cash generated by the business, because the monetary amount reported as depreciation is not directly paid to any vendors or employees, as would be the case with other operating expenses.

Ideally, managers should project cash flow at least 3 months ahead so they know where the business is going. Unfortunately, the cash flow statement is one of the most underutilized reports in the fitness industry.

## The Bottom Line

An income statement is not an accurate reflection of a business's cash position. The cash flow statement should therefore be one of the reports a manager pays attention to.

## Financial Statement Analysis

Interpreting financial statements and applying the information to the operation of a club are primary responsibilities of every manager. Experienced managers take the time each month to review the income statement and evaluate the overall business performance. Make monthly comparisons between the income statement and the projected (budgeted) income statement. Also, analyze all departments and share the information you obtain with each department head. Either the manager or department head should investigate any significant variations between the actual and projected figures to determine the cause of the variations.

Some of the most important ways to analyze financial statements include the following:

- *Compare the current year to previous years.* It is useful to compare a specific month from the current year to the same month from the past year. It would also be common to compare the current year to date (YTD) figures to the last year to date (LTD) figures.

- *Calculate expenses as a percentage of revenue and track this from month to month and year to year.* Although it is important to track all expenses as they relate to revenue, payroll is particularly important. As a business grows, it will need to spend more money on staffing, but it is still important to make sure that staff costs are not outpacing revenue.

# BUDGETING

Now that we have an understanding of the key financial statements involved with running a business, we will apply this information to **budgeting**. All businesses rely on a **budget** to guide them throughout the year, and often budgets are a guide for 3 to 5 years. Budgets are based on the company's fiscal year (FY), which may be the same as a regular calendar year (starting on January 1 and ending on December 31) or may be specific to when the company started (e.g., starting on May 1 and ending on April 30). Companies can designate any time frame as their fiscal year as long as it is consistent from year to year and it encompasses all 12 months.

When preparing a budget, it is best to be conservative in your sales estimates and slightly more liberal in your expense estimations. It is much easier to deal with sales that are higher than expected and expenses that are lower than expected. Overestimating sales can put you in a position where you are not able to pay some of your expenses, and underestimating your expenses may mean that you do not have enough money to pay your staff and pay bills. Often managers are given guidelines to follow when preparing a budget, such as not budgeting for more than a 4% increase in marketing expenses. If these guidelines are shared from the beginning, it will make the budgeting process run much more smoothly.

# Types of Budgets

There are many types of budgets. For our purposes, we will review the most common types within the fitness industry.

## Increment–Decrement or Trend-Line Budgeting

This is probably the most popular budget used in the fitness industry. It uses the financial statements of the previous year to build the budget for the current year. It is relatively straightforward in that you use the exact numbers from the previous year and either increase or decrease them for the current year based on your knowledge of last year and your plans and goals for the coming year. The major benefit of this approach is that you are using established numbers as the starting point for your new budget. The drawback is that the numbers you are using may not be the most effective ones. For example, just because you spent $11,000 on payroll in January of the previous year does not mean you need to do the same thing the next year. That $11,000 may have been overspent, and staff may not have been needed for all of this time. Or just because you spent $2,000 on marketing in June does not mean you need to spend that same amount the following June. The results could have been poorer or better than expected. Either way, you cannot automatically assume that the numbers from the previous year were ideal.

To avoid this problem, two things need to be in place. First, good record keeping is critical; your financial records should include commentary explaining the results for a particular month or quarter. These explanations will allow the budget process for the following year to run more smoothly. Second, managers and anyone else involved in the budget process should still have to justify why they are allocating the amounts they are to specific areas. Simply rubber-stamping the numbers because they are what you used last year will not result in a club performing at its best. Good managers should always be questioning the way the organization does things. What worked last year is not necessarily going to work this year—just ask anyone who still owns music on a vinyl record or cassette tape.

## Break-Even Analysis

This approach to budgeting is based on the argument that you should always have plans in case unexpected situations arise. A break-even analysis is a budget that shows the minimum amount of revenue that must be generated in order to cover the expected costs.

## Worst-Case Scenario

Another budget that can be developed is one that shows the least desirable outcome for the business. Many businesses feel it is important to know what will happen if they miss all of their sales targets and their expenses are higher than expected. If this happens, the responsible manager will already have a plan in place to deal with it.

## Zero-Based Budgeting

This approach to budgeting involves taking an in-depth look at all areas of the business and establishing a budget based on your specific goals for that year. Though you might consider what has happened in the past, it is not a major consideration when developing this type of budget. The challenge with this approach is the time it takes to accurately predict your budgeted numbers for the year.

## Capital Budgets Versus Operating Budgets

Create two separate budgets: operating and capital. It's critical to commit to a separate capital budget, which indicates when large building and equipment purchases will be made. Often, the timing of renovations directly affects the operating revenues and expenses for the part of the club undergoing renovations. For example, if you are closing your racket courts and turning them into a cardio training area, it's going to affect your members who play racquetball or squash. These members may decide to cancel their membership or may require a change in their membership dues. Any capital expenses need to be closely monitored not only for their upfront cost but also their immediate impact on revenues and expenses.

## Budget Preparation

In order to prepare a proper budget, a business needs to follow a sequential process (Fried 2004):

1. Gathering information
2. Forecasting sales
3. Projecting profits and losses
4. Comparing against industry norms
5. Determining capital needs

## Gathering Information

Some typical questions that need to be addressed at this point include the following:

- How old is the club? Newer clubs will generally see significant sales growth in their first few years. This growth will slow down after 2 or 3 years.
- What is the competition doing? Are clubs opening, expanding, or closing in your area? How will their prices and services affect you?
- What do you need to pay your staff to ensure you are able to retain them and keep them motivated?
- Are the costs of heat and water expected to go up?
- Are you planning to offer any new services? What are the costs and expected revenues of these?

The starting point for the information-gathering phase is to collect information on the budgets and actual financial performance of previous years. This will give you a sense of what the club has done in the past. It may not always indicate what will happen in the future, but it is still a solid place to start. Financial statements from previous years should be accompanied by notes explaining the rationale for the numbers. This information will help you determine how relevant the actual numbers are for predicting future budgets. For example, if a club is in its second year of operation and you are looking at the employee costs for previous years, you may find that you were understaffed during the busier months. Overstaffing may result in excess wages being paid, and understaffing may result in missed revenue opportunities.

To obtain the information that is needed to prepare a budget, managers can look to the various trade publications of the fitness industry. IHRSA has various publications that will be helpful during this phase. Information that can be obtained from trade magazines includes industry benchmarks, future expectations for the industry, and new programs and products that your club may want to invest in. In addition to industry-specific publications, managers can use data obtained from the local chamber of commerce. Although these data may not be specific to your industry, they will tell you what the economic outlook is for your area, which may prove to be just as important as the industry-specific data. Other sources of data include various government groups, small-business associations, and companies that specialize in collecting and sharing business data.

Once all the information is collected, managers must examine it to figure out what it means to their business. For example, an industrywide slowdown in fitness club membership sales may not affect you if you are the only club in the area. On the other hand, a positive economic outlook for business in general may not help you if a local business that employed 2,000 people just closed. Astute managers are able to look at all the information and determine what is relevant to them and put aside the information that isn't relevant.

## Forecasting Sales

Forecasting is part art and part science. Rarely are businesses 100% accurate in their predictions of the future. Budget forecasting is based on experience, education, and assumptions. Although it is unlikely that businesses will be accurate in all their forecasts, the alternative is to work without a budget, which would be like going on a family vacation without a map. The more experience you have with the budgeting process, the better you will get at forecasting the future needs of your business.

To generate sales forecasts, it is always best to look at sales data from previous years. Sales can be broken down into various elements (see figure 12.3).

## Projecting Profits and Losses

This is the point at which all revenue and expense items are filled in. The information you gathered and the sales forecasts you just made are critical in determining profits and losses. Your job as the manager is to meet certain targets that the owners have determined ahead of time. For

## XYZ ATHLETIC CLUB ANNUAL MEMBERSHIP PROJECTIONS FOR FY 2019

Dues at end of current FY: $191,890

Number of members at end of current FY: 2,675

|  | Jan. | Feb. | Mar. | Apr. | May | June |
|---|---|---|---|---|---|---|
| Number of new members | 55 | 45 | 45 | 45 | 40 | 35 |
| Number of members lost | 30 | 35 | 40 | 35 | 30 | 35 |
| Net members gained | 25 | 10 | 5 | 10 | 10 | 0 |
| Total number of members | 2,700 | 2,710 | 2,715 | 2,725 | 2,735 | 2,735 |
| Attrition rate percentage | 13.33 | 15.50 | 17.68 | 15.41 | 13.16 | 15.36 |
| Joining fees | $22,000 | $18,000 | $18,000 | $18,000 | $16,000 | $14,000 |
| Monthly dues | $1,725 | $690 | $345 | $690 | $690 | $0 |
| Dues increase |  |  |  |  |  |  |
| Commissions | $6,225 | $5,025 | $5,025 | $5,025 | $4,425 | $3,825 |
| Total dues | $193,615 | $194,305 | $194,650 | $195,340 | $196,030 | $196,030 |
| Average monthly dues |  |  |  |  |  |  |

**Figure 12.3**   Sample sales forecast.

example, an owner may ask the manager for a budget that shows a $500,000 profit while maintaining marketing at the levels of the previous year, increasing payroll no more than 7%, and spending no more than $10,000 on equipment repairs. This is only one possible scenario; there are hundreds of possibilities. The key is to discuss the budget expectations ahead of time so that the person overseeing the budgeting process is able to move forward with all the necessary information.

## Club Operating Benchmarks

Benchmarks are standards that fitness centers and other businesses strive to achieve. Some standards are determined by looking at the best companies in an industry and using their numbers as the benchmark, and other numbers are more subjective and are set by the individual business itself. Some benchmarks are specific to the fitness industry, and some are more general. IHRSA is a good source for benchmark information and to learn more about other fitness centers.

# Elements of Budgeting

According to Rick Caro (1995), there are four significant elements when it comes to budgeting.

## Guidelines and Methodology

Mission and value statements provide a general context for financial decisions, as do a company's 3- to 5-year plan with goals. But for annual budgeting, guidelines are needed. Often you need to define an overall company goal, such as an increased bottom line of 10% over the previous year. This will force staff to take a closer look at the overall picture and not simply tweak the previous year's numbers. A goal this ambitious may require the company to operate differently, such as by creating new profit centers, significantly increasing prices, or decreasing expenses.

You can formally start the budget process by planning a meeting or a training session for key staff. Set deadlines, communicate goals and guidelines, and organize first drafts and reviews. (The process often requires several versions before a final budget is accepted.) The key is to have a final budget created and accepted before the start of the fiscal year.

## Documented Assumptions

Create detailed departmental budgets by month with specific assumptions for each line item. This way, the head of each department (e.g., sales, front desk, fitness, child care) can remember how the budget number was created and explain any differences that occur during the year. For example, the fitness department may have budgeted for an increase in wages during the months of January and February due to an expected increase in new memberships. The club manager and fitness department need to understand the reasons for this increase and the overall expectations and limitations of this change. Senior managers should feel comfortable giving feedback on the assumptions and forecasts in the budget. Many of these people actually know their department better than you do, so it would be wise to listen to their concerns.

In the ideal situation, all budgets would be zero based and not simply a revision of the previous year's numbers. In reality, most clubs will look at the numbers of the previous year and simply increase or decrease them based on the financial performance and expected sales and upcoming expenses of the previous year. Once the budget is created, it should not be changed throughout the year unless a major, unexpected event occurs that forces you to take action. If staff members feel that they can change the budget throughout the year based on department needs, there is no point in setting goals and going through the budgeting process.

## Staff Involvement

The best people to read trends and understand your business are those closest to each of the club areas: the department heads. They should create their own department budgets to meet your predetermined guidelines. If you simply dictate these budgets to them, they'll see their role in the budget process as an academic exercise and they'll never commit to meeting the bottom line.

## Incentives and Monitoring

Ideally, if your department heads exceed their bottom lines, they should be rewarded. This could be in the form of financial compensation or something else that you know will make the person feel special, like a day off, gift certificate, massage, and so on. Consider offering partial rewards during the course of the year, perhaps quarterly, with the majority tied to year-end results.

## INCOME MANAGEMENT

The health club industry in the U.S. generated $27.6 billion in revenue in 2016 compared to $25.8 billion in 2015, an increase of 7%. In fact, since 2004 when revenues equaled $14.8 billion, industry revenue has increased 86.5% (International Health, Racquet, and Sportsclub Association 2017). The cause of this consistent growth rate has been attributed to three factors: increasing new-member growth, decreasing member attrition, and increasing average revenue derived per member. Managers have discovered that focusing on new-member sales is only a portion of the success equation. They must place additional emphasis on retaining existing members, becoming as efficient as possible with use of space, and implementing creative programming that produces new revenue.

Membership dues and joining or initiation fees continue to drive the revenue that supports commercial, community, corporate, and clinical health club settings. Without a strong membership base, many facilities cannot provide the necessary revenue to offset operating costs. According to an industry survey, 69% of the total revenue generated by multipurpose commercial fitness centers comes from initiation fees and monthly membership dues (International Health, Racquet, and Sportsclub Association 2017). The remaining 31% of revenue is from nondues programs and services sources, with the top five profit centers being personal training (8.4% of total revenue), racquet sports (4.8%), food and beverage (2.8%), spa services (2.4%), and children and youth programs (2.0%).

Although membership fees have traditionally been the backbone of industry revenues and need to remain strong, today's fitness managers are paying more attention to nondues revenue sources as the key for future profits. Some experts believe that improving nondues revenue is one of the keys to improving attrition rates.

Organizations with additional sources of revenue have less need to raise membership fees and may even lower the price of dues. As the industry continues to expand into all markets, the ability to be flexible with membership rates provides a strong competitive edge over dues-driven facilities. In addition, club managers have found that they can expand their target market by implementing programs and adding profit centers that attract new members from outside the regular membership. For example, some clubs have found that by renovating a racquetball or tennis court into a youth fitness center, they can attract the family market, thus expanding their revenue base. You can learn more about nondues revenue profit centers in chapter 11.

## *The Bottom Line*

Health and fitness facilities that continue to rely on member dues for 80% or more of their revenue and ignore developing lucrative nondues profit centers may soon find themselves at a competitive disadvantage.

Once you have identified the income sources for a particular setting, organizing an internal system for receiving funds for services rendered is the next component of the accounting process. Identifying, tracking, and monitoring accounts receivable is a standard accounting practice used in all businesses.

## ACCOUNTS RECEIVABLE

**Accounts receivable** refers to an amount that is owed to a business, usually by one of its customers or members, as a result of the ordinary extension of credit. Accounts receivable in a fitness business are generated primarily from membership fees and dues, programming and service fees, and profit centers. Being able to control the funds invested in accounts receivable is an important component of income management. In addition, the system you create for tracking accounts receivable plays a major role in establishing your credit policy. A credit policy involves decisions on how to collect, manage, and control receivables.

### Accounts Receivable Management

At any given time, a percentage of a club's proceeds is in accounts receivables because they

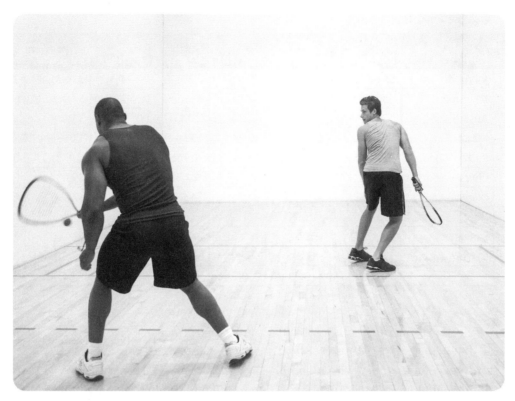

A manager concerned with the efficient use of space might consider turning a racquetball court into a youth fitness center, thereby attracting new members.

Andersen Ross/Digital Vision/Getty Images

are credit sales or unpaid membership dues. A continuing problem for organizations that obtain revenue from membership and initiation fees is collecting these funds. Typically, the club mails a bill to a member before his or her anniversary date (monthly, quarterly, biannually, or annually). Cash-flow problems occur when there is too much time between sending the bill and receiving payment. Until the point of collection, an unpaid account represents a drain on financial resources. To achieve effective management of accounts receivable, it is necessary to incorporate the three following tools.

## Aged Trial Balance

It is important to stay informed regarding the length of time individual accounts have been outstanding. You can accomplish this by generating an aged trial balance, which lists the total of all outstanding balances falling into established past due categories. Generally, the past-due categories are 1 to 30 days, 31 to 60 days, and 61 to 90 days. From this report a manager can determine which

accounts are past due and which accounts exceed established credit limits. A sample aged trial balance is shown in table 12.1.

## Credit Policy

You must establish and enforce a sound collection policy and effective procedures for dealing with delinquent accounts. The policy should provide a balance between generating the pressure needed to obtain payment from delinquent accounts and not jeopardizing future business by offending members. Unfortunately, there are no industry standards or rules that guarantee an acceptable approach to collections. However, health and fitness organizations follow certain guidelines that provide a nucleus for an effective collection policy.

1. Base your collection policy on clear, effective communication between the organization and the member.

2. Establish specific procedures to follow for delinquent accounts that reach 30, 60, and 90 days.

**Table 12.1**   Sample Aged Trial Balance

| Member number | Name | Phone no. | Last payment | Current | 30 days | 60 days | 90 days | Net due |
|---|---|---|---|---|---|---|---|---|
| 6317 | John Doe | 555-3433 | 2/09/18 | 2.39 | 2.36 | 2.34 | 236.31 | 243.40 |
| 3227 | Jane Doe | 555-6590 | 11/08/18 | 17.76 | 87.81 | 54.53 | 521.12 | 681.22 |
| 5946 | Austin Jones | 555-7117 | 12/01/18 | 13.84 | 0.04 | 0 | 3.96 | 17.84 |
| 9658 | Martin Smith | 555-0053 | 4/02/18 | 10.54 | 10.54 | 0 | 1,053.64 | 1,074.72 |
| 6211 | Becky Wilson | 555-2365 | 6/06/18 | 105.17 | 104.15 | 672.65 | 106.21 | 988.18 |
| 8076 | Jim Jacobs | 555-6347 | 1/06/18 | 102.38 | 101.38 | 100.39 | 293.54 | 597.69 |
| 9776 | Mary Walter | 555-9521 | 1/06/18 | 87.81 | 54.53 | 521.12 | 17.76 | 681.22 |
| 1205 | George Perkins | 555-7782 | 5/22/18 | 751.17 | 0.03 | 0 | 3.45 | 754.65 |
| 3499 | Samuel Johnson | 555-7811 | 1/19/18 | 190.51 | 97.33 | 102.12 | 331.17 | 721.13 |
| 5674 | Daniel Patrick | 555-3603 | 5/08/18 | 65.89 | 65.03 | 79.88 | 79.91 | 290.71 |
| Final total | | | | 1,347.46 | 523.20 | 1,533.03 | 2,647.07 | 6,050.76 |

3. Secure a collection agency to handle problem accounts that management cannot rectify.

4. Have staff prevent a member with a delinquent account from using the facility.

## Electronic Funds Transfer

To improve the collection of accounts receivable, **electronic funds transfer (EFT)** can be used to make payment easier for members while expediting the collection of funds for the business. This alternative billing method is the system predominately used in the health and fitness industry for collecting receivables.

When a business uses EFT, the customer's checking, savings, or credit card account is debited for the payment of monthly fees. Members authorize a predetermined deduction for membership fees or other incidental charges, which are then automatically withdrawn from their account or credit card on an established date. You can deposit collected funds in the club account in 5 days or within a 24-hour period if necessary.

Four recommended EFT methods are available to club managers:

- *EFT provider.* A manager contracts with an EFT provider, who keys in all member data from hard-copy membership forms sent by the business. The service provider updates all member files, performs the billing service, and credits the organization's account. Although this is considered a labor-saving

method for personnel, it is generally an expensive form of EFT service.

- *Software-supported EFT.* With this service, the organization is responsible for keying in all member information and bank account or credit card numbers. This information is then downloaded to the EFT provider. The EFT provider debits the members' accounts, minus the provider's service fee, and credits the organization's account. Software-supported EFT is the most widely used service in the health and fitness industry.

- *Bank as EFT provider.* A bank can perform all the services that an EFT provides. Although this method is the least expensive, it does not provide certain customized reports or other customer service options available through an EFT provider.

- *Do it yourself.* Depending on the size of operation, some club operators have taken on the role of EFT provider via an internal computer system. The amount of internal administration and communication with various banks makes this option difficult to administer and more costly than hiring an EFT provider.

## SALES ANALYSIS

It is effective to produce a regular sales analysis that breaks down the total sales figures into components so you can evaluate the performance for each. By tracing sales revenue to the individual

## Advantages and Disadvantages of EFT

### Advantages

- The cost of paper billing (e.g., monthly statements and coupon books) represents 12% of the total billing cost, whereas EFT transactions range from 4 to 7%.
- Payments are automatically deposited into the account within a matter of days, thus securing a predictable cash flow for the facility.
- It is an easier process for members to pay monthly fees, consequently increasing member adherence.
- Administration and collection fees are reduced.

### Disadvantages

- Members may have a negative perception of having fees deducted from their account each month.
- It takes time to correct clerical errors.
- Proper communication of member terminations is required so drafts can be stopped on time.

category, management can identify trouble spots and take action before trouble arises. Table 12.2 provides a sample sales analysis that categorizes membership types and the amount billed for each payment cycle.

## EXPENSE MANAGEMENT

Understanding expense management is an important component of financial management. Traditionally, managers have focused on income concerns such as advertising, marketing, and new-member sales as a means to increase overall profits. The health and fitness industry has always been a market-driven business, emphasizing increased revenue more than controlled spending. However, over the years, managers have realized that cutting costs is more predictable and reliable than estimating member sales. Unnecessary expenditures result when managers do not do the following:

- Provide proper accounting controls and security
- Obtain bids and negotiate with vendors
- Question every expense as though it were coming out of your own pocket
- Perform internal maintenance to reduce equipment costs

Controlling expenses starts with categorizing all costs associated with operating the business.

Then divide each expense into subheadings that represent standard industry expense categories. Table 12.3 provides an expense model of a commercial fitness setting with examples of these categories. Expense categories are separated into operated department expenses (based on the specific department), undistributed operating expenses (shared among all areas of the club), and fixed charges that will not change based on facility usage.

Another aspect of expense management is becoming familiar with all costs associated with operating the business. Knowing each vendor, what is being supplied, and the charge for each item is a prerequisite for good expense control. Review and scrutinize each invoice as though you were paying it from a personal account. Take steps to ensure consistency and predictability from one month to the next. Question monthly variances, determine the reason for each variance, and take actions to minimize excessive variances.

Health and fitness professionals must understand the effect that expense management can have on business profitability. For example, credit card processing fees can average 2 to 3 percent per transaction, a considerable expense for a club with a significant number of card payments. By increasing payments via credit card (or reducing a credit card discount) by 3% and credit card sales for the year are $1 million, you would immediately notice an expense reduction of $30,000. Changes you

**Table 12.2**  Sample Sales Analysis

| Member type | Active | Susp. | Term | Del. | Total | Last month | Change | Joined this month | Estimated dues | Last month dues | Change |
|---|---|---|---|---|---|---|---|---|---|---|---|
| 20-Ind. annual | 173 | 1 | 1 | 0 | 173 | 170 | 3 | 3 | 110 | 0 | 110 |
| 21-Family annual | 362 | 0 | 0 | 0 | 364 | 362 | 0 | 4 | 0 | 0 | 0 |
| 22-Ind. midday ann. | 8 | 0 | 0 | 0 | 8 | 7 | 1 | 1 | 0 | 0 | 0 |
| 23-Fam. mid. ann. | 5 | 0 | 0 | 0 | 5 | 5 | 0 | 0 | 0 | 0 | 0 |
| 24-Sr. ind. annual | 12 | 0 | 0 | 0 | 12 | 10 | 2 | 0 | 43 | 31 | 12 |
| 25-Sr. fam. ann. | 20 | 0 | 0 | 0 | 20 | 20 | 0 | 0 | 89 | 89 | 0 |
| 26-Cor. ind. ann. TE | 53 | 0 | 0 | 0 | 53 | 54 | −1 | 0 | 29 | 29 | 0 |
| 28-Yng. adult ann. | 1 | 0 | 0 | 0 | 1 | 1 | 0 | 0 | 0 | 0 | 0 |
| 29-Cor. fam. ann. | 11 | 0 | 0 | 0 | 11 | 12 | −1 | 0 | 0 | 0 | 0 |
| 30-Ind. semiann. | 8 | 0 | 0 | 0 | 8 | 8 | 0 | 0 | 0 | 0 | 0 |
| 31-Fam. semiann. | 4 | 0 | 0 | — | 4 | 4 | 0 | 0 | 0 | 0 | 0 |
| 40-Individual | 719 | 10 | 0 | 1 | 730 | 715 | 4 | 21 | 45,511.97 | 45,256.97 | 255 |
| 41-Family | 964 | 6 | 0 | 0 | 970 | 950 | 14 | 18 | 83,946.30 | 82,698.30 | 1,248 |
| 60-Midday ind. | 60 | 1 | 0 | 0 | 61 | 52 | 8 | 5 | 2,100 | 1,820 | 280 |
| 61 Midday fam. | 15 | 1 | 0 | 0 | 16 | 15 | 0 | 0 | 750 | 750 | 0 |
| 70-Corp. individual | 39 | 0 | 0 | 0 | 39 | 40 | −1 | 1 | 2,420 | 2,485 | −65 |
| 71-Corp. family | 40 | 0 | 0 | 0 | 40 | 39 | 1 | 1 | 3,469.20 | 3,377.20 | 92 |
| 75-Individual TE | 30 | 0 | 0 | 0 | 30 | 29 | 1 | 0 | 1,881 | 1,816 | 65 |
| 76-Family TE | 48 | 0 | 0 | 0 | 48 | 48 | 0 | 1 | 3,601 | 3,606 | −5 |
| 80-Nonresident | 13 | 0 | 0 | 0 | 13 | 13 | 0 | 0 | 499 | 499 | 0 |
| 81-Nonres. family | 20 | 0 | 0 | 0 | 20 | 20 | 0 | 0 | 801 | 801 | 0 |
| 90-Senior individual | 41 | 0 | 0 | 0 | 41 | 42 | −1 | 0 | 1,962 | 2,014 | −52 |
| 91-Senior family | 51 | 1 | 0 | 0 | 52 | 52 | −1 | 0 | 3,321 | 3,394 | −73 |
| 93-Leave medical | 4 | 8 | 0 | 0 | 12 | 4 | 0 | 0 | 0 | 0 | 0 |
| 94-Leave other | 4 | 15 | 0 | 0 | 19 | 4 | 0 | 0 | 0 | 0 | 0 |
| 95-Drop | 6 | 1 | 32 | 267 | 306 | 6 | 0 | 0 | 0 | 0 | 0 |
| 96-Employee ind. | 107 | 0 | 0 | 0 | 107 | 103 | 4 | 4 | 0 | 0 | 0 |
| 97-Employee fam. | 26 | 0 | 0 | 0 | 26 | 26 | 0 | 0 | 275 | 275 | 0 |
| 98-Corporate | 28 | 0 | 0 | 0 | 28 | 28 | 0 | 0 | 20 | 20 | 0 |
| 99-Nonpay | 34 | 0 | 0 | 0 | 34 | 33 | 1 | 2 | 0 | 0 | 0 |
| Subtotal | 2,906 | 44 | 33 | 268 | 3,251 | 2,872 | 34 | 62 | 150,828.47 | 148,961.47 | 1,867 |
| 02-Family member | 3,353 | 10 | 92 | 28 | 3,483 | 3,403 | −50 | 68 | 2168 | 2,118 | 50 |
| Totals | 6,259 | 54 | 125 | 296 | 6,749 | 6,275 | −15 | 130 | 152,996.47 | 151,079.47 | 1,917 |
| Average dues | | | | | | | | | 24.46 | 24.09 | 0.37 |

**Table 12.3** Revenue and Expenses: Fitness-Only Clubs

| | Mean | Median | Middle range |
|---|---|---|---|
| **Total revenue (thousands)** | **$1,927.00** | **$1,117.40** | **$698.50-$2,144.60** |
| Membership dues and fees | 75.50% | 79.20% | 66.6-88.0 |
| Racket sports | 0.20% | 0.00% | 0.0-0.0 |
| Fitness | 9.70% | 5.50% | 0.3-12.2 |
| Spa | 2.40% | 0.00% | 0.0-2.4 |
| Health care | 0.40% | 0.00% | 0.0-0.0 |
| Pro shop/retail shop | 1.80% | 0.50% | 0.1-2.7 |
| Food and beverage | 3.20% | 1.40% | 0.0-2.7 |
| Children's programs | 2.50% | 0.20% | 0.0-1.4 |
| Other income | 4.40% | 2.00% | 0.0-6.3 |
| Total revenue | 100.0% | 100.00% | 100.0-100.0 |
| OPERATED DEPARTMENTS EXPENSES | | | |
| Racket sports | 0.10% | 0.00% | 0.0-0.0 |
| Fitness | 10.80% | 9.00% | 0.1-17.0 |
| Spa | 1.70% | 0.00% | 0.0-1.5 |
| Health care | 0.40% | 0.00% | 0.0-0.0 |
| Pro shop/retail shop | 1.20% | 0.50% | 0.0-1.4 |
| Food and beverage | 2.40% | 0.80% | 0.0 - 1.8 |
| Children's programs | 1.90% | 0.00% | 0.0-1.9 |
| Total operated departments expense | 18.40% | 16.70% | 3.2-33.9 |
| Earnings before undistributed operating expenses | 81.60% | 83.40% | 66.1-96.8 |
| UNDISTRIBUTED OPERATING EXPENSES | | | |
| Member services | 6.10% | 3.30% | 0.0-6.5 |
| Sales and marketing | 7.10% | 5.70% | 3.2-8.6 |
| Repairs and maintenance | 3.50% | 2.90% | 1.4-5.0 |
| Housekeeping | 3.00% | 2.00% | 0.4-3.9 |
| Utilities | 6.90% | 5.60% | 3.9-8.6 |
| General and administrative | 15.50% | 9.90% | 4.3-20.9 |
| Total undistributed operating expenses | 42.00% | 44.10% | 23.2-56.2 |
| Earnings before fixed charges | 39.60% | 33.70% | 29.5-52.1 |
| FIXED CHARGES | | | |
| Insurance | 2.50% | 2.30% | 1.2-3.0 |
| Management fees | 1.90% | 0.00% | 0.0 - 2.4 |
| Real estate/personal property taxes | 1.60% | 0.80% | 0.0-2.5 |
| Rent: land and building | 16.90% | 16.00% | 7.8-23.1 |
| Rent: equipment | 1.60% | 0.00% | 0.0-0.4 |
| Total fixed charges | 24.50% | 21.50% | 15.0-29.8 |
| Earnings before interest, depreciation and amortization, and income taxes | 15.60% | 13.10% | 2.7-25.4 |
| Interest expense | 4.10% | 1.00% | 0.0-3.6 |
| Depreciation and amortization | 6.90% | 5.10% | 0.0-10.5 |
| Income before income taxes | 4.50% | 5.20% | −9-11.8 |

*(continued)*

**Table 12.3**    *(continued)*

| INCOME TAXES | | | |
|---|---|---|---|
| Current taxes | 0.50% | 0.00% | 0.0-0.0 |
| Deferred taxes | 0.20% | 0.00% | 0.0-0.0 |
| Total income taxes | 0.70% | 0.00% | 0.0-0.0 |
| Income after taxes | 3.90% | 4.40% | −9-11.3 |
| SUMMARY BALANCE SHEET (% TOTAL ASSETS) | | | |
| Current assets | 27.10% | 12.60% | 5.2-38.2 |
| Noncurrent assets | 72.90% | 87.40% | 61.9-94.8 |
| Total assets | 100.00% | 100.00% | 100.0-100.0 |
| Current liabilities | 29.20% | 17.80% | 5.3-36.5 |
| Long-term debt net of current maturities | 60.60% | 52.70% | 22.0-91.0 |
| Total liabilities | 89.80% | 86.20% | 45.5 - 113.9 |
| Owner's equity | 10.20% | 13.80% | −13.9-54.5 |
| Total liabilities and owner's equity | 100.00% | 100.00% | 100.0-100.0 |

Reprinted by permission from IHRSA, *Profiles of Success* (Boston: IHRSA, 2006), 41-42.

make that increase revenue are much less predictable—nobody can anticipate the financial outcome of the next marketing campaign or how many new members will join a facility in the next month.

## The Bottom Line

Managing expenses provides a more tangible method of controlling costs than trying to generate additional revenue.

## Depreciation

A term often seen on financial statements is **depreciation**, the process of allocating the cost of an asset to the periods of time benefited. To fully comprehend depreciation, understand that the original cost of a new piece of exercise equipment or building represents its value as an asset. If a fitness center purchases a new treadmill, this machine is an asset, because it represents potential value to the organization. Depreciation is the allocation of the cost of a long-term asset over the estimated useful life of that asset. As members use the treadmill, this asset suffers wear and tear and thus loses value. This wear and tear is represented with a depreciation expense in each accounting period.

Depreciation is technically a noncash expense, but it is a good guideline for the allocation of funds to cover the annual wear and tear of buildings and property. Health and fitness centers should expect to spend funds equivalent to the depreciation indicated on financial statements for repairs and replacement costs for the year.

Before you can determine depreciation, you need two important estimations:

- *Estimate of the useful life of the asset.* The expected useful life represents how long the business plans to receive benefits from the asset. For example, the useful life for most fitness equipment has been estimated at 5 to 7 years. In the United States, the IRS has its own guidelines for useful life for different categories of assets for which a depreciation deduction is allowed.

- *Estimate of expected salvage value of the asset.* The salvage value is the amount that the business can reasonably expect to receive from selling the asset at the end of its useful life. In the open market, fully depreciated fitness equipment yields 10 to 40% of original purchase prices.

Although we recommend that you have an accountant help prepare these estimates, the

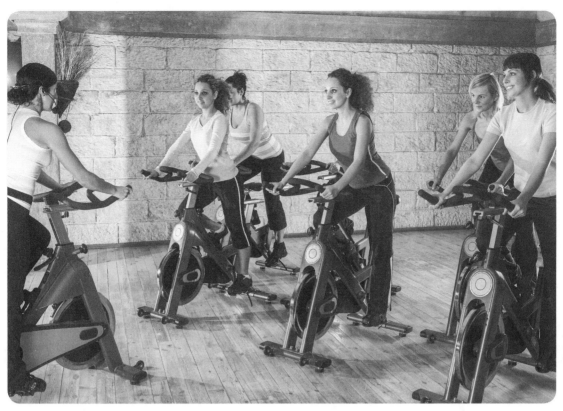

The depreciation of equipment is a noncash expense that should be reflected in the regular expense category in an income statement.

Tomasz Trojanowski/fotolia.com

manager's knowledge is required to help with determinations. Remember that depreciation rules change from year to year; however, the rule that was in effect when you purchased an asset is the rule that you use to determine the time frame for the write-off.

## Tools for Expense Management

Learning to control the expenses of a facility should be the goal of every manager. To date, there is no comprehensive method for completely controlling the expenses of any business. However, there are industry standards and management procedures that provide a gauge for expense management. A financial profile comparing the most profitable commercial health and fitness centers will typically indicate that the most successful clubs are better at controlling expenses.

### *The Bottom Line*

By being creative and embracing change, managers can have a positive effect on the bottom line of their organization. Closely evaluating and identifying cost-saving opportunities while implementing ways to control costs are factors for ensuring higher net income for the future.

## TAX CONSIDERATIONS

To understand the full nature of financial management, it is important to consider the tax environment within which the health and fitness center operates. Taxes affect the financial planning and decision making of every business. It is essential for managers to understand the tax system and its connection with financial planning in order to successfully function in the business world today.

Because tax laws are complex and revisions are frequent, we recommend assistance from an accountant or the IRS to complete tax forms and maintain record keeping. The ever-present possibility of an IRS audit is incentive enough to keep good accounting records and receipts of all bills.

## The Bottom Line

When a facility becomes operational, it is taxed under the three levels of government: federal, state, and local.

# Federal Taxes

The legal form of ownership chosen by the business has a major impact on the way tax regulations—especially income tax regulations—apply. The federal income taxation for sole proprietorships, partnerships, corporations, and S corporations is discussed next.

## Sole Proprietorship

The profits from a sole proprietorship are taxed as personal income to the owner.

- Legally, the owner and the business activity are inseparable. The owner is also treated as an employee and is responsible for his or her own payroll tax.
- A sole proprietor is expected to estimate income tax each year and pay estimated quarterly taxes.

## Partnership

As with the sole proprietorship, tax liability is only assessed for the incomes of the individual partners and not against the business.

- Partners file a separate form, noting their distributive shares of the profits.
- A report of the business must be submitted to the IRS each year. This is only an information report; no tax payment accompanies its submission.
- As with the sole proprietorship, each partner also makes estimated tax payments.

## Corporation

Tax reporting becomes more elaborate and complicated with this form of ownership.

- As an employee of the corporation, you report annual income and company dividends to the IRS.
- As a separate entity, the corporation must also file a return to the IRS.
- The corporation must make estimated tax payments.

## S Corporation

S corporations are corporations that pass their income, losses, deductions, and credits through to their shareholders for federal tax purposes. The main requirements to qualify as an S corporation are as follows:

- The company must have no more than 100 stockholders and no more than one class of stock.
- The company must be a domestic corporation and must not be affiliated with any group eligible to file consolidated tax returns.
- The corporation may not derive more than 25% of its gross receipts from royalties, rents, dividends, interest, annuities, and gains on sales of securities.

# Regional and Local Taxes

The rates for state and local taxes on health and fitness facilities vary from region to region. Common among these taxes are the taxes on gross income; sales on retail goods, food, and services; and membership fees, which some regions consider an amusement or entertainment tax.

An additional local tax assessed against every for-profit facility is a property tax or, in some areas, both property and personal property taxes. City tax assessors calculate property taxes in three ways:

- *Cost approach.* The value of the property is the selling price of the land plus the cost to construct the building and minus depreciation caused by facility wear. Regions that tax personal property also include the value of the equipment, furniture, and fixtures.
- *Income approach.* The value of the club property is the value of its earning potential. In

this approach you could use the gross income of the club or, if the facility were being rented, the rental value.

- *Market or comparable sales approach.* The value of the club is predicated on the selling price of other land and similar businesses in the area. This approach is not used as often as the two previously mentioned because most city assessors do not have realistic information on club sales.

The manager of a for-profit health and fitness center should monitor property tax assessments closely. On average, up to 5% of gross revenues are paid annually for property taxes. For example, consider the average commercial club that grosses $1.5 million in revenues. From this amount, $45,000 would be paid in property taxes. Every owner or manager has the right to appeal property taxes. You can obtain assistance for questioning or appealing property taxes by contacting an accountant or by inquiring with a representative from your local city assessor's office.

This section on tax considerations is only a brief review of certain tax codes as they relate to the health and fitness industry. You can obtain further information on these codes from an accountant or local tax office.

## The Bottom Line

In the fitness business, appealing a property tax assessment is one of the few ways to cut costs without affecting member service, staff morale, or facility upkeep.

## Key Terms

| | | |
|---|---|---|
| accounting | budgeting | fixed assets |
| accounts receivable | cash accounting | fixed expenses |
| accrual accounting | current asset | income statement |
| assets | depreciation | liabilities |
| balance sheet | electronic funds transfer (EFT) | operating expenses |
| budget | equity | statement of cash flows |

# Risk Management: Addressing Health and Safety Concerns

*Anthony Abbott and Mike Greenwood*

## Learning Objectives

After studying this chapter, you will be able to

- recognize potential safety violations and risks,
- identify appropriate qualifications to ensure competency of staff, and
- develop a comprehensive emergency response plan for untoward events.

"Emery. Emery. Report to the outdoor running track!" This directive from the public address (PA) system alerted all staff members within the facility to a life-threatening emergency to which staff members needed to respond immediately. By using the code word *Emery* (which stood for "emergency") rather than *code blue*, with which most people are familiar, staff were advised of the critical incident without alarming members and creating confusion by attracting curious onlookers to the scene.

The facility was well prepared to respond to any emergency not only throughout the building but also in the outdoor locations where physical activities took place. This capability was greatly enhanced by a buzzer system that had been installed throughout the facility and grounds. All rooms within the building, the pool area, and all outdoor sites were fitted with a buzzer that was wired to the main office. When a life-threatening incident occurred, the staff member providing supervision had only to press a button and one of many bulbs on a light board within the main office would be illuminated, indicating exactly where the emergency was located. When the light board was activated, it was accompanied by a tone that immediately caught the attention of office personnel. Then one of the office staffers would activate the emergency medical system while another would announce over the PA system that "Emery" was to report to that location.

Upon hearing the announcement, staff and instructors throughout the facility would report to the scene to fulfill their various roles and responsibilities as outlined in the facility emergency response plan. The emergency response plan was a written document that all new employees were require to carefully read and then sign to indicate that they had read and understood the plan. All supervisors were responsible for quizzing new employees to ensure that they knew their roles during emergencies. Additionally, supervisors had to verify that the employees for whom they were responsible had been maintaining their first aid, CPR, and AED skills, as well as keeping their certification cards current. Skill checks were conducted through both announced and unannounced emergency drills as well as through individual rehearsals in which fitness instructors were presented with a manikin and told to respond to a given scenario.

The facility staff responded professionally to the emergency on the outdoor track, thanks to the facility's well-thought-out emergency response plan, the superior training, and the actions of each and every employee who did their job that day. The runner who had suffered cardiac arrest was saved, and the facility received numerous letters of commendation for its emergency response. Members stated that they felt more secure working out in a facility that had demonstrated concern for the health and safety of its membership through the establishment of an effective emergency plan.

———————————————●———————————————

Without a comprehensive and well-rehearsed emergency plan, the incident described in the opening scenario could not only have undermined membership confidence in the facility but also have led to possible litigation. Hopefully, you will never find yourself or your facility named as a defendant in a lawsuit. However, in a society that is becoming increasingly litigious with every passing year, fitness facility managers are finding themselves more frequently embroiled in litigation. It would appear that the current escalation of litigation is a reflection of a serious industry problem regarding member expectations and service delivery.

It is not uncommon for a facility to advertise that the health and safety of its membership is its top priority. If this is truly the case, it will be reflected not only in the facility's documented screening program, safety plan, and emergency procedures but also in a conscientious commitment to enact them. Unfortunately, many facilities lack even rudimentary screening and testing of members, staff awareness of basic safety concerns, and the ability to respond to emergencies in a timely and effective manner.

Accidents and injuries are inevitable in an environment in which people are moving at a rapid pace, pushing their physical limits, and competing against others as well as themselves. How you handle these unexpected events can literally mean the difference between life and death. The death of a member is possible, and so is the death (financial ruin) of the facility if it is unprepared for such untoward events.

The prudent fitness manager knows that it is not a matter of *whether* an incident or medical emergency will occur but rather *when* it will occur. Well-formulated safety plans and emergency procedures allow trained staff to respond to adverse events and potential danger with confidence rather than to react with confusion (see figure 13.1). This chapter evaluates the components of a well-defined **health and safety plan** in addition to the elements of a well-designed **emergency response plan**. It also analyzes various dangers that exist in different health and fitness programs, how to avoid them, and emergency plan modifications for these settings.

Health and safety codes, industry standards, and professional guidelines must be reviewed to ensure that staff members are not only suitably qualified but also properly prepared to conduct their duties. Sample documents in this and the following two chapters are provided to help protect the facility from adverse events besides potential litigation in the eventuality of a serious emergency. To ensure that the health and fitness facility is prepared to successfully handle any exigency, the facility must review the qualifications of first responders as well as any necessary emergency equipment and supply lists.

## CREATING A SAFE ENVIRONMENT

A safe club environment for exercising members is a given. In spite of the fact that club management is aware of this necessity, many facilities still do not incorporate even basic health and safety practices into their daily operations. Compounding this problem are the irresponsible or ignorant actions of careless members. The best policies and

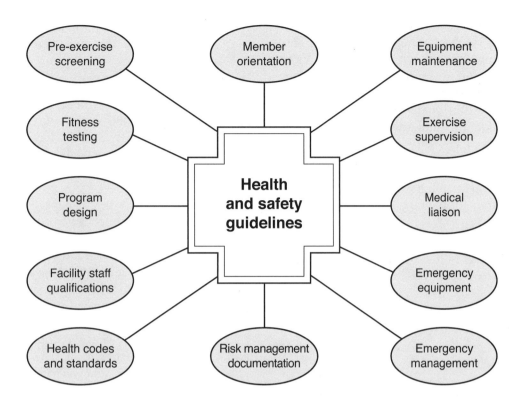

**Figure 13.1** Health and safety guidelines.

procedures for ensuring member safety are often ignored by members. Only an educated and alert staff coupled with a well-planned and maintained facility can overcome these obstacles. Ongoing training of staff and immediate correction of potentially dangerous situations, such as unsafe equipment (as addressed in chapter 14), must be a consistent practice in all facilities.

## Facility

The ongoing implementation of health and safety practices enables health and fitness managers to maintain a safe club environment. This execution must start during the initial planning phase. Facility design and development techniques along with compliance with city, state, and federal health codes can build the foundation for a safe environment. Professional consultants can help evaluate the club for safety factors while the physical structure is still in the design stage in order to eliminate potential problems long before the first member enters the club. A well-designed facility combined with ongoing staff training,

compliance with health codes, and observance of industry standards and guidelines will lead to the safest possible club environment.

## Signage

Health codes are unique in each city and state, so managers must determine what regulations are applicable for their specific location and type of operation. To protect members from potential injury or death as well as safeguard the business from frivolous lawsuits, health and safety information must be communicated. Use appropriate **signage** throughout the facility to assist staff in providing this important information to facility users.

Signage should be used to provide directions, indicate points of entry and exit, issue instructional or safety information, and communicate ongoing or upcoming club events. For signage to be effective, however, it must have a clear and concise message, be easily read from a distance, and be properly located within the facility. Local, state, or federal guidelines may specify details relating to message content, design format, or placement of signage, along with requirements for the posting of documents such as licenses or certifications. Managers should consult the proper local authorities before designing and purchasing club signage. Additional recommendations for signage include the following:

- *Use basic terminology.* The use of layman's phraseology will be better understood by the general membership. Use terminology appropriate for the target audience.

- *Use signs that can be easily read.* Select type styles that are easily read from a distance of 10 to 15 feet (3.0-4.5 meters) and place the signs 5 to 7 feet (1.5-2.0 meters) from the ground.

- *Determine the message.* Use as few words and symbols as possible, and show the wording to different people in order to test the accuracy and effectiveness of the message.

## Blood-Borne Pathogens Standard

Health codes relating to **blood-borne pathogens** offer a substantial challenge to the facility manager. Blood-borne viruses that are of primary concern to the health and fitness industry include HIV and hepatitis B and C. The facility manager is responsible for recognizing and understanding the threat inherent with regular fitness center operations, potential exposure of staff or members, and the necessary techniques for prevention of such viruses.

Managers must become familiar with the guidelines published by OSHA, which provide information on the training and record-keeping procedures related to avoiding and handling blood-borne pathogens. To adequately protect staff and members, it is important that facility managers know

- what the blood-borne pathogens are,

- what is meant by *occupational exposure* to blood-borne pathogens,

- what potential infectious materials are and how to prevent exposure to them,

- what the possible methods of transmission are and how to control them, and

- what protective equipment is required to safeguard the first responder in an emergency situation.

This information is available from OSHA, which has regional offices throughout the country that can assist managers in meeting their responsibilities. Additionally, IHRSA has prepared a briefing paper for member facilities regarding the OSHA blood-borne pathogens standard. Managers should avail themselves of the information provided within this briefing paper.

In addition to blood-borne pathogens, employees and members of fitness facilities may be exposed to potentially hazardous chemical agents and toxic materials. It is therefore essential that all employees and independent contractors are advised—by means of posted placards, notices, and memoranda—of potentially harmful materials other than blood-borne pathogens. To this end, the ACSM's fourth edition of *ACSM's Health/Fitness Facility Standards and Guidelines* (2012, 70) advises that a facility operator must "post warning signage for hazardous chemicals and blood-borne pathogens if the member or user may be exposed to either."

## *The Bottom Line*

The facility manager is responsible for the existence of a written system that advises members, employees, and independent contractors about potentially hazardous materials.

## Personnel

The key to the health and safety of facility members is the availability of knowledgeable and conscientious personnel capable of establishing a safe exercise environment. This requires that staff members at all levels be appropriately qualified to carry out their respective duties as well as sufficiently motivated to do the job to the best of their abilities.

### Management

Most health and fitness facilities are managed by people lacking appropriate training and credentials. A troubling number of managers are unqualified to oversee and direct the safe and effective operation of facilities. It is typical for managers to have a business background, which is essential for the fiscal health of the facility, but to have no exercise experience, which is essential for the physical health of the members. Managers need not have a degree in exercise physiology, but they must have working knowledge of exercise science to understand what constitutes appropriately qualified instructors as well as safe and effective exercise programming.

In regard to personnel competence (for both management and exercise instruction), the fitness industry is totally unregulated. According to the U.S. Bureau of Labor Statistics (2009), there is no state or national standard to gain employment in the fitness industry based on a specific college degree or major field of study. And as pointed out by Carnevale, Smith, and Strohl (2011), college graduates usually receive considerably higher wages than less skilled workers. Therefore, fitness facility owners and managers often choose to hire uneducated but aspiring fitness instructors and personal trainers, rather than true professionals, in order to improve their bottom line.

This lead author has spent over 45 years in the fitness industry and has been retained as an expert witness in numerous facility litigations (of which over 40 have been death cases) and can verify that time has led to little improvement regarding management's understanding of the field of exercise science. Because managers are rarely well versed in this area of expertise, they are often incapable of determining what is necessary to establish safe and effective fitness programming for their members. And they're often unable to discern the difference between the various fitness instructor and personal trainer certifications. Of particular concern is the current lack of adequate screening of new members and facilities' inadequate preparation to handle emergencies.

Despite a joint position statement in 1998 by the American Heart Association (AHA) and the ACSM that addressed recommendations for cardiovascular screening, staffing, and emergency policies (American Heart Association 1998), the fitness industry has failed to respond in the years since. In 2001, a study of fitness facilities in the state of Ohio indicated that older adults and people with heart disease (occult or known) are exercising at facilities that, more often than not, lack adequate cardiovascular screening and emergency procedures (McInnis et al. 2001), a serious problem that has seen little improvement over the years.

In addition to their lack of training in exercise science, managers often disregard good administrative procedures. The inability to provide leadership, professional supervision, and suitable staff development plagues most health and fitness facilities. The typical high turnover of personnel within fitness facilities is a reflection of staff disappointment not only with their salaries but also with their management. A well-run operation promotes an atmosphere leading to employee contentment and job satisfaction. The mark of a truly successful facility is not only membership retention but also staff retention as well.

It is common knowledge that too many facilities are sales oriented rather than service oriented. A large percentage of facilities even rely on client failure for their financial success. Many facilities have so many inactive members that if a substantial number of their total membership showed up 3 days a week for an hour of exercise, they would probably violate every ordinance in the book for overcrowding. The facility that fails to prioritize its members' success typically also fails to provide a safe training environment.

## Fitness Staff

Many health care professionals and fitness authorities are deeply concerned about the lack of qualifications on the part of fitness instructors and personal trainers. Physical education and exercise science professionalism have been bypassed in the growth of the fitness industry and, as a result, quality instruction and training have been generally ignored. In an effort to keep their overhead down, facility owners and managers frequently hire minimum-wage instructors while dismissing college-educated applicants as overqualified. It would appear that many facility entrepreneurs have jumped on the fitness bandwagon for financial gain at the expense of their members' health and safety.

## Certification

The same entrepreneurial fever and greed that have led to the hiring of untrained staff within the fitness industry have also led to inadequate fitness instructor and personal trainer **certifications**. A survey conducted by the National Board of Fitness Examiners (NBFE) determined that there are more than 75 national certification programs; these certifications and those being offered by college and university divisions of continuing education combine to make up approximately 200 certification programs available to the public. Based on 30 certification exams this author has taken, as well as his research related to the knowledge base of commercial fitness instructors, he has determined that most national certification programs are offered by self-appointed fitness authorities who have either limited training in exercise science themselves or an inability to develop a meaningful exam process. It must be remembered that a certificate is no more valuable than the training behind it as well as the standards used for awarding such a credential. In short, being certified does not equate with being qualified (Abbott 2009).

Becoming a competent fitness instructor or personal trainer requires an in-depth knowledge of human anatomy, physiology, kinesiology, and exercise science combined with practical training and experience. This cannot be achieved through weekend cram courses and certification programs during which students are primed for specific questions to which they regurgitate the answers on examination. The pseudo-professional associations that offer these certifications often forward candidates study materials in advance, but there is never sufficient time for practical training and testing to ensure candidates are capable of safe and effective exercise programming for the public. Nor can distance learning vocational programs provide the practical experience that is essential for developing the skills and ability to be a competent fitness instructor or personal trainer. Although most academic concepts can be conveyed through online or home-study programs, extremely important technical skills and safety proficiency cannot be delivered through this type of learning experience.

In order to develop the knowledge, skills, and abilities of a competent fitness instructor or personal trainer, one must undergo formal instruction in exercise science through an accredited university or a credible vocational program that provides comprehensive theoretical education and extensive practical training taught by degreed exercise physiologists with field experience. Upon completion of academic instruction coupled with substantial practical training in the areas of health assessment, fitness testing, performance evaluation, program design, and client supervision, serious and knowledgeable students will seek certification through not-for-profit professional associations such as ACSM or the National Strength and Conditioning Association (NSCA). Graduates of an athletic training program from an accredited university usually seek certification through the National Athletic Trainers' Association (NATA).

Research conducted in 1988 revealed that when facility instructors were administered a nationally validated survey test examining knowledge in exercise science, those instructors with ACSM certification scored significantly higher than those who possessed other certifications, excluding NSCA certification (Abbott 1989). This study also found that formal education, not experience, was the most significant factor correlating with a sound knowledge base, including an understanding of exercise safety. Thirty years later, the author is repeating this study; and at the time of this writing, it appears that there has been little improvement in the knowledge base of commercial fitness instructors. Additionally, it appears that those personal trainers certified by ACSM and NSCA score significantly higher on both written testing and skill testing than trainers certified by other organizations.

In 2002, a similar study conducted at UCLA reflected this importance in formal education as well as the disparity between different personal trainer certifications. This study concluded that formal education in exercise science as well as certification from either ACSM or NSCA were strong predictors of a personal trainer's exercise science knowledge, whereas years of experience were not related to such knowledge (Malek et al. 2002).

**Accreditation**    IHRSA has recommended that its member clubs hire only personal trainers holding at least one current certification from a certifying organization whose certification is accredited by an independent, experienced, and nationally recognized accrediting body. At the time of this writing, IHRSA has identified the National Commission for Certifying Agencies (NCCA) and the Distance Education Accrediting

Commission (DEAC) as acceptable accrediting organizations. To date, IHRSA has recognized 17 personal trainer certifications that have achieved **accreditation** from one of these two accrediting bodies.

Unfortunately, not all accredited certifications are a guarantee that the recipient has the knowledge, skills, and ability to be a competent fitness instructor or personal trainer. Accreditation decisions rely on the ability of a credentialing organization to assess a particular job description and then test practitioners' knowledge in specific areas related to job responsibility. This requires role delineation, task analysis, item development, psychometric review, and securely proctored exams. When the credentialing organization demonstrates that it has followed the proper steps in examination development as outlined by the accrediting body, it has increased the likelihood that it will develop a valid and reliable exam. However, to create a valid and reliable examination that discriminates between truly qualified and unqualified candidates, exam questions must not only be directed at identified content areas but also must be presented at an appropriate level of difficulty.

To be a valid indicator of competency, exam questions must possess a sufficiently high degree of difficulty to challenge an individual's depth of knowledge. Unfortunately, most accredited certifications use exams that only scratch the surface of important content areas as the questions are cursory and simplistic. The majority of accredited personal trainer certification exams are primarily composed of recall questions, and there are few application and analysis questions (Abbott 2009). The ability to identify people who are proficient in exercise science requires that exams also be based on the behavioral objectives and high standards promulgated by truly professional associations like ACSM and NSCA. Facility managers must be able to differentiate between the many fly-by-night and substandard certification programs and those that truly validate the depth of a candidate's knowledge base and skill level.

## The Bottom Line

Not all certified personal trainers are qualified personal trainers.

## Litigation

In years past, people injured at fitness facilities would accept the blame and rarely hold others responsible. The injured would attribute their strained muscles and tendons, sprained ligaments, and low back pain to just being out of shape and therefore would feel embarrassed to bring their injuries to anyone's attention other than their doctor's (Alter 1983).

Today, however, the public is beginning to hold health facilities, fitness instructors, and personal trainers accountable for unsafe instruction and inadequate supervision. Even with the deterrent of waivers and releases, the public appears more willing to take their grievances to court. Consequently, there has been an upsurge in the number of personal injury lawsuits against facilities, instructors, and trainers. This increase in **litigation** has been accompanied by a rise in liability insurance.

To lessen the possibility of litigation, facility personnel must be capable of thoroughly screening potential members, providing suitable fitness tests, evaluating health assessments and fitness profiles, designing appropriate exercise programs, and attentively supervising member activities. Additionally, staff should constantly be aware of potentially dangerous situations. Staff should be empowered with responsibility for immediately correcting hazardous conditions and should be held accountable for addressing dangers.

When health and fitness facilities become thoroughly prepared and truly committed to providing the most effective exercise programs and the safest training environments, then this industry will be recognized and applauded by the allied health care field. However, to achieve such recognition and success, managers of facilities must adhere to the well-documented STEPS to success (see figure 13.2). *Screening* members through **health risk appraisals** and **risk stratification** will determine whether they are ready for fitness testing and the stress of exercise or whether **medical clearance** is needed. *Testing* members' physical fitness with a battery of tests and establishing a **fitness profile** better enable trainers to assess their clients' current capacities for exercise. *Evaluating* health appraisals along with fitness profiles allows trainers to get an even better picture of the members' capability to

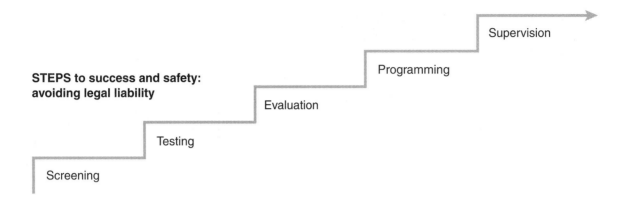

**STEPS to success and safety: avoiding legal liability**

Screening

Testing

Evaluation

Programming

Supervision

**Figure 13.2** STEPS to success.

exercise safely and what type of programs would be best suited for them. *Programming* based on appraisals, profiles, and member goals permits trainers to design the most effective and safest programs that meet members' needs. *Supervision* ensures that members' programs are being conducted effectively and safely while providing the necessary motivation. These steps will lessen the potential for litigation.

Increased litigation in the fitness industry is partly due to the failure of managers to mandate proficiency in emergency cardiac care and basic life support. Certification and mastery of first aid, CPR, and AED use must not only be a prerequisite for hiring but also be an integral part of ongoing staff training. A safe exercise setting requires highly qualified personnel who are not hesitant to implement and enforce safety standards as well as to activate emergency procedures with the appropriate equipment.

## SCREENING BEFORE ACTIVITY

The primary purpose of screening members before permitting them to engage in physical activity is to determine whether they ought to have a physical exam, perhaps including a clinical stress test, and whether they need medical clearance. **Preactivity screening** is the procedure by which a facility can identify those members who are at an increased risk for experiencing exercise-related cardiovascular incidents as well as musculoskeletal problems. The present **standard of care**

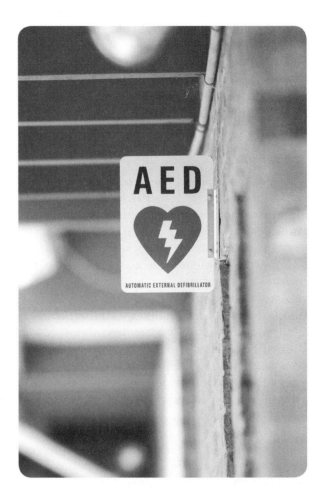

Managers who require staff to be trained in the use of an automated external defibrillator (AED) are protecting the lives of the club's members and also reducing the risk of litigation.

## Interview With Georgia Goslee

Georgia Goslee, JD, FII-CPTS, formerly certified as ACSM HFS and NSCA CPT and CSCS, has been an attorney for more than 30 years; the first 20 years were spent practicing criminal law, both as a federal prosecutor and a private defense attorney. She taught international business law in Switzerland and lectured on health and fitness in London during her European sabbatical. She practices criminal, civil, and sport law. She is a frequent author and speaker on the subject of legal aspects of sport coaching, fitness instruction, and personal training, including multiple presentations for ACSM and NSCA. She is also a media legal commentator and has made numerous appearances on CNN, CNBC, MSNBC, and Fox News.

**Interviewer:** It appears that there has been an upsurge in litigation within the fitness industry during the past decade. How would you account for this phenomenon?

**Ms. Goslee:** There are a number of reasons for this apparent anomaly where both facilities and trainers are more likely to become embroiled in litigation. There has been an obvious growth in the fitness industry that is servicing an even older clientele. We have a more educated public related to understanding their exercise needs and requirements; and when you couple this with a lack of qualified instructor personnel, personal trainers, and facility managers, it is no wonder that litigation is on the rise.

**Interviewer:** What kind of growth in the industry have we witnessed?

**Ms. Goslee:** In 2013 there were some 30,000+ fitness facilities throughout the country. Today, there are over 50 million health club members; one in six Americans have joined a fitness facility.

**Interviewer:** What do you mean by an *older clientele*?

**Ms. Goslee:** The International Health, Racquet & Sportsclub Association (IHRSA), the professional association of the health club industry, completed a research project that determined that senior citizens or baby boomers were the fastest-growing segment of the gym population. This older population is characterized by having more risk factors and, therefore, is more likely to experience problems such as cardiovascular incidents during the stress of exercise.

**Interviewer:** Why do you think the public is more educated about their fitness needs and requirements?

**Ms. Goslee:** One only has to note the abundance of health and fitness-related magazines, coupled with numerous TV shows and advertisements on this subject, to appreciate how the public is being bombarded with information about health, fitness, and consequent needs.

*(continued)*

**Interviewer:** Why do you think there is a lack of qualified instructors when facilities continually advertise the fact that they employ certified instructors?

**Ms. Goslee:** Because a fitness instructor or personal trainer is certified does not mean that he or she is qualified. Most instructors and trainers are certified by unprofessional certification programs—an individual is provided with a study manual and then attends a 1-, 2-, or 3-day workshop, during which time candidates are prepped for only those specific questions found on that program's exam. These amateurish associations never provide sufficient time for practical training and testing to ensure candidates are capable of safe and effective exercise programming for the general public.

**Interviewer:** But aren't many of these certification programs accredited?

**Ms. Goslee:** Unfortunately, accreditation has questionable value; accreditation does not require that exams really document the extensiveness of a candidate's knowledge base. Nor do exams assess practical skills by determining that a candidate can demonstrate specific skills with hands-on tests such as taking blood pressure, administering submaximal stress tests, or supervising weight training.

**Interviewer:** What is your concern with the qualification of facility managers?

**Ms. Goslee:** Most facilities managers have a business background but little or no academic training in exercise science. The average manager does not know what constitutes a qualified fitness instructor or personal trainer. Unfortunately, a large percentage of facilities are profit motivated rather than service oriented, thereby failing to provide safe and effective fitness programming for their membership. Along this line, it is interesting to note that IHRSA completed a study that revealed 67% of facility members never use their facilities. This speaks volumes about fitness facility management.

dictates that screening procedures be practiced without exception.

Any exercise programming should be initiated with a screening process that provides knowledge of a member's past and present health history as well as lifestyle considerations. Before an exercise program is undertaken, it is prudent to complete a health risk appraisal or **medical history questionnaire** to determine whether there are any medical contraindications to exercise that could necessitate a physician's clearance prior to any exercise and fitness programming.

Contraindications of primary concern are

- cardiovascular disease (heart attack, stroke, hypertension, aneurysm, claudication, and severe mitral valve prolapse),
- pulmonary disease (bronchitis, emphysema, and asthma),

- metabolic disease (diabetes mellitus, thyroid disorders, and renal complications),
- musculoskeletal problems (fractures, sprains, strains, hernias, arthritis, and structural limitations), and
- any other condition placing the exerciser at higher than normal risk.

The fitness instructor or personal trainer involved with the screening process should become familiar with the exercise-related ramifications of these conditions.

The preactivity screening process is a vital step in the health and fitness continuum. It enables trainers to begin on a safer footing as they prepare to test and create a program for the facility member. Additionally, it establishes a baseline of health parameters that serve as markers for monitoring future progress. As such, it becomes invaluable as a motivational tool. It should never be overlooked or bypassed.

Wise facility managers understand both the physiological and psychological value of comprehensive health risk appraisals. They must also understand that if trainers are to be viewed as true allied health professionals and facilities are to be recognized as safe training environments, then thorough preactivity screening is a must.

High blood pressure is a major risk factor for heart disease, stroke, and kidney failure; approximately one-third of Americans have hypertension; and almost one-third of hypertensives are unaware of having this silent killer. It therefore stands to reason that facilities must administer blood pressure testing as part of the screening process. However, managers must ensure that trainers do not go beyond their scope of practice when screening members and taking blood pressure. A blood pressure assessment only enables trainers to suspect the need for a medical diagnosis or to determine whether medical clearance is necessary.

It is essential that managers not allow personnel involved with preactivity screening to make medical diagnoses or prescribe treatment based on the data collected on health history questionnaires. Allowing them to go beyond their scope of practice in this way could lead to potential litigation related to the unauthorized practice of medicine. All states have statutes that authorize certain licensed health care professionals to diagnose and treat people. A violation of these statutes by unauthorized individuals such as facility trainers could result in criminal prosecution. Although trainers may feel that a particular diagnosis such as hypertension is likely, they may not make medical diagnoses or prescribe treatment. Managers must make sure trainers understand that they are suspecticians, not diagnosticians.

## The Bottom Line

Preactivity screening is a recognized standard that must be practiced by all fitness facilities. To ignore or treat this activity in a cavalier manner demonstrates a reckless disregard for member safety and exposes the facility to litigation.

# Health Appraisal

A health appraisal allows the trainer to better assess the suitability of exercise for members. It minimizes the risk of injury, disability, or even death while lessening the potential for litigation against the facility. It also establishes the appropriateness of the next step in this process: the fitness assessment. During the health appraisal, it is typical to acquire demographic information, complete a medical history, and administer a lifestyle questionnaire. All this information contributes to the goal of member screening, which is to classify the member in one of the following categories:

- People who should be excluded from exercise due to medical contraindications
- People with known disease conditions who require referral to a medically supervised exercise program
- People with known disease, symptoms, or risk factors that require further medical evaluation and clearance before starting an exercise program
- People with special needs for safe and effective exercise programming
- People who may begin traditional exercise programs

## Demographics

Typically, the demographics section of the health appraisal includes general information such as name, address, phone numbers, email address, age, gender, height, weight, ethnicity, marital status, nearest relative, family physician, specialty physicians, education, occupation, and other data deemed pertinent. This information is expanded on with the medical history, lifestyle questionnaire, and any other available information (such as that found within physical exam reports and laboratory test results) that may be provided to the trainer in order to generate a more complete picture of the member.

## Medical History

This section allows the trainer to better assess the health and well-being of the member. There are numerous medical history questionnaires on the market that vary in length and comprehensiveness. Recommended health history questionnaires can be found in *ACSM's Health/Fitness Facility Standards and Guidelines* (American College of Sports Medicine 2012). In general, appraisals and questionnaires include the following subjects:

- Does the member ever experience discomfort, shortness of breath, or chest pain with moderate exercise? Does the member have any known heart disorders? Is there any family history of heart disease?

- Does the member experience severe dizziness, limb numbness, or any leg cramping (claudication) with exertion? Does the member have any history of high blood pressure or vascular problems such as stroke?

- Does the member have any musculoskeletal restrictions or arthritic conditions that are aggravated with exercise? If so, what are the limitations? Has a physician ever told the member to avoid certain physical activities? Are there any physical limitations due to operations?

- Does the member have any diagnosed metabolic diseases such as diabetes mellitus, a thyroid condition, or liver or kidney complications? If so, to what extent? Is diabetes classified as type I or type II? Is it a hypothyroid or hyperthyroid condition? Is the kidney dysfunction nondebilitating or end-stage renal disease?

- Does the member have any form of chronic obstructive pulmonary disease (COPD)? Does the member suffer from chronic bronchitis or emphysema? Does the member have reactive airway disease (asthma) or exercise-induced asthma? Does moderate exercise bring on labored breathing (dyspnea)?

- Does the member currently take any medications (prescriptions as well as over-the-counter medicines)? If so, why are they being taken, how long have they been taken, how much is being taken, and who prescribed them?

- Does the member know of any physical condition or illness that might prevent participation in an exercise program? Have any such conditions or illnesses limited physical activity in the past?

If the answer is *yes* to any of the aforementioned questions, then exercise testing and programming may have to be postponed and medical clearance may be necessary. The trainer is responsible for administering a comprehensive medical history to uncover any possible dangers in exercise testing and programming. Additionally, the trainer must be aware of exercise-related complications when dealing with these physical conditions and must be able to adjust programs accordingly.

The medical history form should conclude with a statement in which members swear that the information provided is true and correct to the best of their knowledge and that they recognize that this health assessment is not the equivalent of a medical evaluation or diagnosis. The form should then be signed by the member as well as witnessed by someone other than the trainer administering the medical history.

## Lifestyle Questionnaire

The **lifestyle questionnaire** provides useful information related to the member's risk factors. Factors such as alcohol consumption, caffeine intake, tobacco use, legal and illegal drug use, nutritional habits, sleep patterns, stress and tension, driving record, recreational interests, physical activities, exercise likes and dislikes, and many other lifestyle considerations help paint a picture of the member's mental and physical health. This information along with the health history questionnaire, physical exam report, and lab test results may reflect heightened risk for heart attack, stroke, cancer, and other diseases, as well as unnecessary accidents.

Although it is impossible to change risk factors such as age, family history, and some illnesses, many other factors may be altered as the trainer addresses concerns from the health risk appraisal. More than 50% of chronic degenerative diseases are lifestyle related. Consequently, people can make a major impact on their health through lifestyle modifications. According to the AHA, the four major risk factors for coronary heart disease are smoking, high blood pressure, elevated cholesterol, and physical inactivity. In most cases, these major risk factors can be readily modified through smoking cessation, reduced intake of dietary fat and sugar, and regular exercise. Available literature indicates that such behavior modifications will not only extend the person's life but also enrich it.

## Physical Exam

Ideally, everyone should have a physical or medical exam before participating in fitness testing or an exercise program. For this reason, it is recommended that trainers encourage all members to have a physical exam, accompanied by laboratory tests. When exam reports and lab results are accessible to the trainer, there is that much more information to assist with the development of a safe and effective exercise program.

According to the ACSM, a diagnostic **clinical stress test** is a recommended screening component for older adults contemplating vigorous exercise. By ACSM standards, older adults are men age 45 years or older and women age 55 years or older, and vigorous exercise would constitute intensities above 60% of $\dot{V}O_2max$. Understandably, people at increased risk for cardiovascular events as well as those with signs or symptoms of coronary heart disease and those with known cardiac, pulmonary, or metabolic disease should also have complete physical exams with a clinical stress test before engaging in vigorous exercise.

## Laboratory Tests

Although it may not be feasible to obtain all test results from every physical exam, their availability can be most useful in the screening process; therefore, the trainer should make every effort to secure this kind of information. Of greatest importance is the blood profile, including analysis of the following variables: fasting blood glucose along with A1C, fasting triglycerides, total cholesterol, LDL cholesterol, HDL cholesterol, and ratio of total cholesterol to HDL. Classification of these blood variables can be found within *ACSM's Guidelines for Exercise Testing and Prescription*, and from such classification scales the trainer is able to better assess the member's health. It should also be noted that many physicians are looking more seriously at other variables, such as C-reactive protein as a marker of systemic inflammation and high blood concentrations of homocysteine, that appear related to occlusive heart disease.

## Use of the Health Screening Data

Managers must establish a systematic approach to ensure that the information in health risk appraisals or health history questionnaires is accurate, current, and readily available in case of an emergency. By including this form in the introductory process of membership, the club ensures that documents on all members are available and that review of the documents for potential risk is concluded before finalizing the membership agreement. Implement a process for regularly reviewing members' information to ensure health data are complete and current.

The information contained during a health screening is valuable only if it can be retrieved. A poor filing system renders the information useless and weakens the facility's legal position. Maintain the information in a computer database, keep a hard copy on file, or do both. Ensure that only authorized employees have access to the information. Set a standard that all health history questionnaires, lifestyle questionnaires, physical exam reports, laboratory test results, and any other personal health information be kept in a confidential filing system maintained by the fitness director. According to the HIPAA Privacy Act, as well as ethical standards published by ACSM, facility members have the right to expect confidentiality regarding the health and fitness information that they share with facility staff (American College of Sports Medicine 2018).

### The Bottom Line

At a minimum, a health history questionnaire coupled with a blood pressure assessment should be employed as screening devices. Require completion of a health history questionnaire and a blood pressure assessment before finalizing any membership agreement.

## Risk Classification

Many members will object to spending money for a physical exam and laboratory tests, so facilities may decide to work with some members without the benefit of this information. If a physical exam and testing have not been done, the trainer should use information from the medical history and lifestyle questionnaire to classify members as to the degree of risk in exercise testing and program participation. At this point, the trainer can make the decision to either continue with fitness testing or insist on medical clearance from the member's physician.

Guidelines for determining potential risk are outlined in the 10th edition of *ACSM's Guidelines for Exercise Testing and Prescription* (American College of Sports Medicine 2016). It is recommended that facilities adopt these guidelines. Additionally, facilities should become familiar with the fourth edition of *ACSM's Health/Fitness Facility Standards and Guidelines* (American College of Sports Medicine 2012) as well as the 1998 joint position statement by the ACSM and AHA titled *Recommendations for Cardiovascular Screening, Staffing, and Emergency Policies at Health/Fitness Facilities* (American Heart Association 1998).

Most facilities used to solely rely on the **Physical Activity Readiness Questionnaire for Everyone (PAR-Q+)** as a screening device without understanding its limitations. Typically, facilities would require that a member seek physician clearance for exercise testing and participation if he or she answers *yes* to any of the seven PAR-Q+ questions (National Strength and Conditioning Association 2012). With the release of the new PAR-Q+ form in 2014, facilities are now using this as their standard screening tool. Now, if an individual answers *yes* to one of the seven PAR-Q+ questions, they are required to fill out additional questions, which provide better guidance on whether or not physician clearance is required. Frequently trainers assume that zero *yes* answers on this questionnaire means that the member gets a clean bill of health and is cleared for vigorous exercise programs. It must be stressed that the PAR-Q+ is a minimum standard for entry into a low- to moderate-intensity exercise program and should not be the only screening device for facilities.

## Medical Clearance

People deemed high risk during the screening process and those with certain health problems should see a physician and obtain medical clearance before undertaking fitness testing or exercise programming. *ACSM's Health/Fitness Facility Standards and Guidelines* provides examples of **assumption of risk** and physician release forms for participation in physical activity programs.

Every facility should have a medical director or consultant who provides medical clearance for members or directs such individuals to their personal physician for medical clearance. With a medical director and a legal representative, fitness managers should establish a written policy for identifying high-risk individuals and those with health concerns as well as the exact process for obtaining medical clearance.

## Screening of Guests

A constant challenge facing fitness facility managers is screening procedures for guests and prospective members using the facility. Managers must develop a process of registration and **guest screening** that provides facility personnel with a level of confidence that every guest is low risk. Additionally, this process must guarantee that the guest knowingly assumes all risks related to physical activity within the facility (i.e., an assumption of risk statement). Furthermore, the staff must provide the guest with an orientation of the activity areas and equipment while stressing safety considerations.

During registration and screening, the staff should gather basic personal information in case of an incident or emergency. The information gathered can also be used as a sales tool to identify prospective members. Facilities frequently use a two-part guest registration and screening procedure. The first part is the registration form (see figure 13.3), which includes the guest's name, address, phone number, and emergency contact, as well as an assumption of risk statement. The second part is the health screening form, such as the PAR-Q+, that is also to be signed. Remember that because the PAR-Q+ is a limited screening device, guests should be restricted to low- to moderate-intensity exercise.

Managers must work with their legal counsel to determine a registration and screening procedure, to identify appropriate information that must be gathered, and to create the assumption of risk statement in order to minimize the possibility of untoward incidents and consequent liability. Regardless of whether the guest is accompanied by an existing member, participating in a spe-

## GUEST REGISTRATION

Please complete the Physical Activity Readiness Questionnaire for Everyone (PAR-Q+) and the following information prior to initiating activity.

Name: _____     Date: _____

Address: _____

_____

Telephone: (Home) _____ (Work) _____

Emergency contact: (Name) _____ (Telephone) _____

Have you visited ABC Club before? Yes _____ No _____ If yes, when? _____

I understand and acknowledge that there are inherent risks associated with exercise and the use of exercise equipment and facilities, such as those available at ABC Club, and I agree that all exercise and activities that I engage in at ABC Club will be done at my own risk. I will limit my physical activity to that of low to moderate intensity, which will be explained to me by a fitness instructor. I waive my right to any claims against ABC Club (or any affiliated agent) that may arise out of any activity, event, use of ABC Club equipment or facilities, or my presence on the premises, including personal injury, theft, and all property damage, even if caused by the negligence of any of these persons. However, I am not waiving any claims to the extent it may be based upon gross negligence or willful misconduct.

Signature: _____

**Figure 13.3**   Sample guest liability waiver.

From M. Bates, M.J. Spezzano, and G. Danhoff, *Health Fitness Management,* 3rd ed. (Champaign, IL: Human Kinetics, 2020).

cial event, or sponsored through a cooperative arrangement with a local hotel, business, or organization, the manager must recognize that the standard of care regarding preactivity screening is still in effect.

## *The Bottom Line*

All guests must undergo a screening process and should be advised to limit their exercise to a low to moderate intensity.

## ADMINISTERING PHYSICAL FITNESS ASSESSMENTS

Many health and fitness facilities routinely perform physical fitness assessments to determine level of physical fitness as it pertains to disease prevention and health promotion. Proper procedures to identify and test only appropriate individuals are as important as preactivity screening. People undergo voluntary fitness-related physical assessments for several reasons. ACSM has identified the following purposes for fitness testing:

- Provide data that are helpful in developing a program design
- Collect baseline data and follow-up data that allow for the evaluation of progress by the participant
- Motivate the participant by establishing reasonable and attainable fitness goals
- Educate the participant about concepts of physical fitness and individual fitness
- Stratify risk and limit potential for litigation

Regardless of the individual reasons for a fitness assessment, it is imperative that the examiner be well trained and qualified to safely administer all components of the assessment. The test technician must be able to determine the most appropriate testing protocols for all individuals based on their age, physical condition, health status, and current physical activity level. Any trainer administering a fitness assessment should have a degree in exercise science or be certified by ACSM, NSCA, or another reputable credentialing body that conforms to similar standards.

As indicated previously, the facility should initiate a member's program with a comprehensive health risk appraisal, including a medical history and lifestyle questionnaire, perhaps along with a review of physical exam reports such as blood profiles and even a clinical stress test. Once members have been thoroughly screened and cleared for exercise programming, the next step is the physical fitness assessment. Similar to preactivity screening, managers must develop, adopt, and adhere to specific pretest procedures as well as a reasonable and prudent testing format.

This initial education of members regarding their health status and fitness profile is important not only from the standpoint of program design but also from the perspective of providing members with greater confidence in their efforts to take charge of their health and fitness. As with so many areas of life, the more knowledge you have about a given endeavor, the more confident you will be and the more likely your success. The adage "The educated consumer is the best consumer" certainly holds true for club members.

The ability to provide follow-up fitness testing for members will further enhance their chances of achieving success. Follow-up assessments enable the trainer to provide members with definitive data about how they are progressing with their health and fitness programming. This positive feedback reinforces their efforts and allows them a taste of success, which is essential in maintaining motivation for ongoing training. Remember, success breeds success.

## Before the Assessments

Before members arrive for testing, they should be given written instructions regarding how to prepare for the tests. Explicit instructions are necessary to ensure testing validity and accuracy. In addition to not smoking within 3 hours of testing, members should be instructed not to ingest food, alcohol, or caffeine within this time frame. It is also important that members wear appropriate attire, be well rested, and not have exercised within the past 12 hours.

The testing environment is critical for test validity and reliability, especially concerning constancy of environment for accurate follow-up testing. It is recommended that room temperature be set between 68 and 72 degrees Fahrenheit (20-22 degrees Celsius) and that humidity be less than 60% with adequate air flow. Equally important are comfortable surroundings wherein anxiety can be minimized; privacy, therefore, is of utmost importance. Regarding privacy, steps should be taken to avoid any situations in which staff could be accused of making sexual advances; a third party acting as an assistant can help deter such allegations.

Testing procedures should be thoroughly explained beforehand, and any tendency to rush through the battery of tests should be avoided. During pretest instructions, all members should be required to read and sign an **informed consent** for exercise testing. For legal purposes, it is recommended that informed consents have specific content areas to be shared with members about to undertake fitness testing. Typically, these content areas are

- purpose and explanation of the test,
- likely risks and discomforts,
- responsibilities of the participant,
- benefits to be expected,
- participant inquiries about testing procedures,
- use of testing data and confidentiality, and
- freedom of consent to engage in testing.

In addition to being in the written document, each content area should be discussed with the member, and the trainer should ascertain that there are no questions that have not been answered satisfactorily.

The trainer should carefully review this information before proceeding with the assessments. Should either the member or the trainer feel that testing is not appropriate, or should the member ask to stop at any point during testing, the fitness assessment must be discontinued. For a detailed discussion regarding health-related fitness testing and appropriate informed consent forms for exercise testing, consult *ACSM's Guidelines for Exercise Testing and Prescription, Tenth Edition.*

Before initiating the actual physical fitness tests, preliminary testing should be done to measure resting heart rate, blood pressure, and lung function. Most trainers are unfamiliar with spirometers and therefore fail to include lung function testing as part of their assessment or as part of the preactivity screening. Consequently, trainers miss an invaluable opportunity to screen members for pulmonary diseases such as emphysema; members who perform poorly on the lung function test should be referred to physicians for further evaluation and diagnostic workup.

Again, when trainers do a lung function analysis, they do so not as diagnosticians but rather as suspecticians. Trainers should never diagnose a member as having high blood pressure or a lung function disability, because such a diagnosis is beyond their scope of practice. Trainers only screen members for the purpose of determining their suitability for exercise; if they suspect that there is a problem, they should refer the member to an appropriate health care professional.

## Assessments

The specific tests to be administered will vary from one person to another depending on the screening process and determination of the member's health status. Typically, tests assess the five components of health-related physical fitness: cardiorespiratory endurance, muscular strength, muscular endurance, flexibility, and body composition. Some facilities go beyond health-related fitness testing and even provide physical performance tests to those who are more athletically inclined, testing such components as agility, balance, coordination, power, quickness, and speed.

If all components of physical fitness are to be evaluated during the same session, then the organization and sequencing of the tests are important. The test order should be structured so that the resting measurement of body-fat percentage precedes the active measurements. Otherwise, the accuracy of skinfold testing can be adversely affected as a result of peripheral blood flow to the skin surface.

Cardiorespiratory endurance testing should precede muscular testing in order to avoid the misleading effects that muscular testing could have on heart rate response during submaximal workloads. The testing of muscular strength should precede that of muscular endurance because single maximal efforts are less likely to interfere with endurance activities, whereas endurance testing can have a significant impact on subsequent strength testing. Flexibility can most safely and effectively be measured after the member has thoroughly warmed up, which certainly would be the case after the other tests have been completed.

There is a vast menu of cardiorespiratory, muscular, and flexibility tests that can be administered, and the professional trainer should become familiar with this array of tests in order to provide members with the most appropriate testing protocols for their needs. Numerous books on fitness testing are available, and such literature should be available within the facility's testing center. If examiners have not taken a course on how to administer fitness tests, they should be required to undergo training with local universities or vocational programs in order to learn these valuable skills and avoid some of the pitfalls that compromise testing safety.

Fitness testing is essential not only for safe and effective program design but also for establishing a baseline against which future progress will be measured. This type of feedback reinforces member behavior and maintains motivation. Probably one of the greatest reasons for membership attrition is the failure of facility managers to recognize the importance of comprehensive fitness assessments as a necessary component of exercise programming. Fitness testing should not only be strongly encouraged but also perhaps even required as part of the screening process.

## Body Composition

There are multiple methods for testing body composition. Although body composition testing with bioelectrical impedance (BIA) has improved and become more popular, it has some significant drawbacks. Of particular concern is the fact that BIA tends to overestimate body fat in lean athletes. Variations in hydration may also adversely affect body-fat predictions.

Although near-infrared interactance (NII) is used by many facilities and is a simple, quick, and noninvasive method of body composition analysis, it has significant drawbacks. The standard of error remains excessively high; therefore, this method is not considered comparable to skinfold testing, BIA, and even body-fat calculations based on girth or circumference measurements.

For years, hydrostatic weighing, which relies on water displacement, has been recognized as the gold standard in body-fat testing, but it poses many obstacles for the average fitness facility. Equipment cost, space requirements, maintenance requisites, time needed, and subject anxiety (holding one's breath underwater after exhalation) all make this method expensive, awkward, and burdensome. However, a more recent body-fat testing procedure called *plethysmography*, which relies on air displacement, has proven equally accurate and reliable as well as more convenient. It has gained popularity among body composition researchers primarily due to the less awkward test procedure and the lack of technical expertise required (in comparison to the traditional hydrostatic weighing procedure). However, like hydrostatic weighing, it is extremely expensive and usually beyond the budget of most facilities; but with effective marketing, it could become an additional source of revenue.

Body composition measurement with dual energy X-ray absorptiometry (DEXA) has been increasingly used not only for a variety of clinical and research applications but also within the fitness industry. Typically a DEXA scan requires medical supervision by a radiologist, and some professionals now consider it to be the new "gold standard" in body composition testing. Total body scans using DEXA provide accurate and precise measurements of body composition, including bone mineral content (BMC), bone mineral density (BMD), lean tissue mass, fat tissue mass, and fractional contribution of body fat. Ultrasound devices have also become more popular for measuring multicompartment body composition and as a measurement model have gained increasing support among researchers. This modality has been able to fairly accurately measure overall body composition and by scanning targeted areas, track changes in fat and muscle thickness.

Skinfold testing probably remains the most widely applied field technique for determining percentage of body fat. In addition to the minimal expense of the equipment (calipers), skinfold testing allows the client to see exactly where decreases in total body fat are occurring. When performing skinfold testing, however, it is essential that trainers not only use acceptable technique but also match their clients with suitable protocols. Although skinfold testing has limited accuracy, its real value lies in the ability to effectively monitor change and pinpoint those areas of decreasing body fat.

Along the line of body fat determination, there has been an upsurge in body surface scanning with devices that measure morphology and girth measurements. Along with girth and volume metrics, there is an ability to deduce body fat with these 3D surface scans. Furthermore, the devices include body posture analysis and wellness metrics on body shape, which may identify problems that impact mobility. However, more research is needed to fully understand the validity of such devices.

## Cardiorespiratory Endurance

Cardiorespiratory endurance testing is usually conducted by means of step tests, ergometer tests, or treadmill tests. Additionally, many trainers use field tests to assess cardiorespiratory fitness. When analyzing these tests, the trainer must take into consideration the various advantages and disadvantages of each test and how they relate to the capabilities and health status of the member.

Although treadmill testing is appropriate for most populations, the majority of trainers do not have access to calibrated treadmills dedicated to fitness assessment. For this reason, along with the fact that heart rate and blood pressure monitoring can be more difficult on the treadmill, many trainers prefer to do bicycle ergometer testing. However, due to the expense of ergometers and treadmills, space considerations, and the greater training requirements for ergometer examiners, many facilities choose to administer only step tests.

Many trainers rely on the traditional 3-minute step test on a 12-inch (30-centimeter) bench. After 24 lifts per minute, a recovery heart rate is taken while the subject remains seated. The obvious concern with this test is that it exposes the member to an immediate 7.4 metabolic equivalent (MET) level, which may be overly demanding for those who are seriously deconditioned.

The potential danger is that the trainer could be administering what is essentially a maximal stress test but without the safety net that is available in clinical settings.

There are safer ways to administer a step test than the traditional 3-minute test. The knowledgeable trainer may administer a progressively graded exercise test (GXT) while monitoring both heart rate and blood pressure at different workloads and subsequently ensuring an appropriate cool-down. Recorded heart rates for known workloads can be applied to formulas that will predict aerobic capacity or cardiorespiratory endurance.

In order to get a handle on aerobic capacity, many trainers require members to undergo field tests such as the Cooper 12-minute test and the 1.5-mile (2.5-kilometer) test for time. Although these tests can be valid predictors of cardiorespiratory endurance, a serious concern is the tendency for subjects to overextend themselves, thereby increasing the possibility of a cardiovascular complication. For this reason, the Rockport fitness walking test has gained widespread popularity because subjects are less likely to overexert and endanger themselves.

## Muscular Strength and Endurance

Numerous muscular strength and endurance tests can be found within the fitness testing literature. Again, the tests should be chosen based on an evaluation of the member's health status, capabilities, goals, and anticipated program design. The trainer should keep in mind that due to resistance to peripheral blood flow, muscular testing can place greater demands on the cardiovascular system, especially as it relates to transient blood pressure elevation.

Muscular strength can be measured with dynamometers, tensiometers, digital strength meters, and 1-repetition maximum (1RM) tests. When using static strength tests, it is advised that the member take about a second to ease into a maximal contraction and then maintain the maximal effort for no more than a couple of seconds. Although many athletes can do actual 1RM lifts with minimal risk, it is recommended that the general public avoid such lifts. Instead, they should perform multiple lifts to failure, from which the 1RM can be predicted.

Muscular endurance can be measured using traditional resistance exercise equipment such as a bench press, leg press, or dip device. Additionally, muscular endurance tests such as push-ups or timed curl-ups can be completed using only body weight. Although static endurance tests are rarely administered, there are valid tests in which members can be evaluated for their ability to maintain a constant force against a dynamometer, tensiometer, or digital strength meter for increasing periods of time.

## Flexibility

Flexibility, or range of motion (ROM), is a component of physical fitness whose evaluation is limited. Most trainers do little more than administer the traditional sit-and-reach test. Keeping in mind the principle of specificity of exercise, it should be remembered that this traditional test measures only low back and hamstring flexibility and is not an overall indicator of flexibility. Multiple static and dynamic ROM tests exist, thus enabling the trainer to acquire a more complete picture of the member's flexibility. However, the value of flexibility assessments is being seriously questioned in light of the fact that research has appeared to document that stretching per se has little impact on injury prevention and sport performance. Flexibility remains an important component of fitness, but it may be better assessed through more functional approaches rather than traditional stretching tests.

## The Bottom Line

The failure to provide (and even require) fitness testing during the screening process lessens members' chances of achieving their fitness goals, and it also may increase the chances of injuries or cardiovascular complications, which may lead to litigation.

## Test Evaluation

Upon completing the fitness assessments, the trainer must evaluate the data from the fitness tests along with the health appraisal and be prepared to share such information with the facility member. Typically, the initial evaluation of data for each test is based on classification scales for gender and age. However, the trainer must be careful not to get locked into a mere comparison to the normative data. To evaluate members strictly upon this basis is to overlook the important principle of individual differences. Failing to recognize these differences violates this basic principle: Member needs must be understood in order to design tailor-made programs that improve the chances of success without risk of injury.

There is sometimes a tendency for trainers to impersonalize the fitness testing profile. Many trainers hand the member a computer printout of the testing results. The member is then instructed to read this printed profile in order to see how he or she performed in comparison to normative data. For many people, this type of approach to a fitness evaluation is a turnoff. The trainer must remember that although there are advantages in employing technology within the testing and evaluative process, the personal touch cannot be sacrificed. The competent trainer knows how to marry *high tech* with *high touch*.

When going over testing data with a member, it is essential to conduct the process in a professional setting and in a motivational manner. In the privacy of an office or similar sanctum, the trainer establishes a relationship that reflects the air of confidentiality that must exist between trainer and member. The testing and evaluation room should not be cold and sterile like a doctor's office but rather warm and friendly (e.g., soft pastels versus white walls).

Members must see themselves and the trainer as working together in achieving program goals. They must not view the evaluation as a necessary embarrassment in which they are chastised for a lack of health and fitness. Rather, they must view the evaluative process as one in which they have the opportunity to get a better handle on their current capabilities and future potentialities. They must see this as an educational opportunity as well as a platform from which they will be launched into a program ensuring future success. The evaluative process should be a positive and motivational experience that sets the stage for the next step: program design.

The trainer accepts the responsibility of being proficient in the science of exercise programming and therefore being knowledgeable about the appropriate stresses to be applied to the member. Suitable stress that will bring about positive physiological changes (training effects) without negative physiological consequences (injury) can most effectively be determined if the trainer has access to the information found within the health appraisal and the fitness assessment.

# DESIGNING SAFE EXERCISE PROGRAMS

Although the term *exercise prescription* is frequently found within textbooks and scientific literature, it is not the most appropriate wording when dealing with the average facility member. The term *prescription* has clinical connotations, and people associate this word with sick individuals in need of medical assistance. The term *exercise prescription* may discourage some members. Additionally, the word *prescription* may make a disgruntled member more likely to pursue litigation based on the results of the trainer's recommendations. Facilities should instead discuss the trainer's recommendations in terms of **program design**.

Program design typically has five components: exercise mode, intensity, duration, frequency, and progression. These five components can be applied not only to aerobic training but also to muscular strength training, endurance training, and flexibility activities. The challenge for personnel is to ensure that these components of program design are based on the information gleaned from the health appraisal and fitness assessment.

When trying to determine the best mode of aerobic activity for a given member, trainers must be careful not to interject their own personal bias. The cardinal rule in choosing an activity is whether it meets two criteria. First, is the activity appropriate for the person regarding muscular strength and endurance, metabolic requirements, and skills? Second, is the activity one that the person is likely to enjoy? Choose a physical activity that is both appropriate and enjoyable. Note that the term *physical activity* may also be better received than the word *exercise*, which is frequently associated with sweat, discomfort, and obligation.

For new members with low fitness levels, safe program design would consist of continuous physical activities. Continuous activities allow for stable state heart rates, whereas discontinuous activities result in fluctuating heart rates with the varying exercise intensities. Discontinuous activities require better stabilization of joints due to rapid changes of direction and lateral movements such as those found in exercise dance, step classes, martial arts, basketball, and racquetball. Because beginners may want to get involved with these types of programs, such activities then become a goal to be pursued. Once an acceptable level of cardiorespiratory and muscular conditioning is achieved, the member advances to this preferred activity.

From a safety standpoint, managers and staff must recognize that the muscles, tendons, ligaments, and skeletal structure must be strengthened before undergoing the rigors of most aerobic activities. Sometimes muscular strength training is ignored in deference to aerobic conditioning, in which case the aerobic activity may have to be eventually curtailed because of inadequate joint stabilization and consequent injury. Strength training is equally important in the initial phases of conditioning and may even take priority over the aerobic training program.

When considering the initiation of aerobic conditioning, staff must appreciate the physiological concerns of bone resorption and remodeling as well as musculoskeletal weakness. Too often beginners jump into a program, doing too much too soon. There is a tendency to try to get fit overnight by engaging in an activity every day and thereby overdoing exercise stress. Although the cardiorespiratory system rapidly responds to the stress of exercise, the musculoskeletal system is slower to react. Due to initial bone resorption from new stresses upon the body, the skeletal system is temporarily weakened and thus is more susceptible to injuries such as hairline fractures. The skeletal structure needs adequate time to undergo remodeling, which will eventually enable bones to endure even greater forces. Likewise, muscles, tendons, and ligaments need gradual and progressive exposure to stress in order to avoid muscle tears, tendon strains, and ligament sprains. Consequently, it is considered advisable that beginners not engage in aerobic activity more than three times a week with at least one day of rest between each session.

Due to the standard deviation in maximal attainable heart rate (MAHR), prudent trainers do not rely on target heart rate (THR) as the sole means of determining exercise intensity. The talk test and rating of perceived exertion (RPE) must also be used to verify that members are not overstressing themselves. Members have to learn not only how to control the intensity of their physical activity but also how to determine the duration and frequency appropriate for their capacity for exercise stress. Additionally, because the instrument panels of aerobic equipment may provide feedback related to METs, it is important that staff be knowledgeable of this concept and be capable of explaining such information.

As discussed, the final component of program design is exercise progression. When planning progression, the trainer must consider factors such as the member's functional capacity, age, and health status and should factor in activity preferences and goals. Progression planning is normally divided into three stages: the initial, improvement, and maintenance stages. The initial stage is nonaggressive to maximize program safety and compliance; it is intended to minimize discomfort and muscle soreness as well as any possibility of injury. Usually the stage lasts 4 to 6 weeks, depending on member adaptation and receptiveness to escalating program demand.

A more rapid rate of progression is typically seen during the improvement stage. Intensities will be well into the moderate and even vigorous ranges, with duration as high as 30 to 40 minutes, and frequency will progress from 3 to 5 sessions per week. Again, these increases will be dictated by member adaptation and motivation. The improvement stage normally lasts for 4 to 5 months. Inevitably, there will come a time when, in order to make any further improvements, the member's efforts and time requirements would become excessively demanding. At that point, the trainer shifts to maintenance of the member's physical fitness by implementing variety within ongoing aerobic programs and other enjoyable physical pursuits to ensure adherence to the active lifestyle.

Regarding program design for strength training, the number of sets to be assigned has always been an area of confusion and controversy; however, it is generally agreed that the beginner does not need to do more than a single set of a given exercise. In the past, the ACSM's recommendation for the general public was muscular training 2 to 3 times per week, with 8 to 10 exercises at a load, allowing for 8 to 15 repetitions and only 1 set of each exercise (Feigenbaum and Pollock 1999). Currently ACSM recognizes that most individuals respond favorably with 2 to 4 sets of resistance exercises per muscle group, but the organization has also has noted that even a single set of an exercise may significantly improve muscle strength and size, particularly in novice exercisers.

Research has documented the additional benefits of multiple sets; however, the increased time required for multiple sets may lead to a further commitment that members feel they cannot afford. Trainers must question whether multiple sets are necessary for everyone; a single set can achieve good results, whereas multiple sets may discourage members who are seeking expediency in fitness programming. Another possible concern with multiple-set training is safety, because it can lead to excessive overload and potential injury.

Regarding flexibility training, it bears repeating that, according to research, stretching by itself has little effect on injury prevention, low back pain, sport performance, and delayed onset muscle soreness (DOMS). Stretching may improve postural stability and balance, especially when combined with resistance exercise. However, the people most susceptible to injury are those who are the least flexible as well as the most flexible. This, coupled with the fact that there are many potentially injurious postures found in programs such as yoga, makes it necessary to have a staff member who is extremely well versed in kinesiology and biomechanics and who can analyze programs and ensure that contraindicated exercises are being avoided. Staff should consider the advantages of achieving healthy ROM through functional approaches rather than the traditional stretching exercises found with many group programs.

Managers and staff must ensure that a member's exercise program is based on the individual's health appraisal, fitness profile, and goals. Trainers must have not only thorough knowledge of anatomy, physiology, kinesiology, and exercise science but also good social skills, enabling them to communicate effectively with members and motivate them to take charge of their health. The ability to personalize program design is both a science and an art.

## The Bottom Line

The fitness director should be an exercise physiologist with strong credentials in kinesiology and biomechanics for overseeing the soundness of all exercise programming.

# PROVIDING SAFETY ORIENTATION

Ideally all members should undergo fitness assessments and be provided a program design to meet their unique needs. However, some facilities may only offer this more extensive service as an additional expense. Therefore, managers assume the responsibility to ensure that all members receive a comprehensive orientation related to safety and effectiveness in exercise programming.

During the orientation, members should be advised about the advantages of personal training, including fitness profiling, which will enhance the chances of success. Additionally, other program offerings and their benefits can be outlined with appropriate cautionary notes regarding preparedness for some of the more demanding activities. Activities such as aerobic dance, step classes, spinning classes, boot camps, racquetball, plyometrics, functional training, and other physically challenging activities with fluctuations in heart rate, joint stress, and rapid changes of direction may not be appropriate for the beginner who needs to achieve a base level of fitness before engaging in more strenuous programs. Beginning carefully and progressing gradually must be the theme throughout the orientation.

Areas to be addressed during the orientation should include appropriate exercise clothing and footwear, because these relate not only to safety but also to facility standards. There should be a walkthrough of the facility in which both aerobic and resistance equipment are reviewed, with an emphasis on equipment operation and safety concerns. Body mechanics should be discussed regarding skeletal alignment, safe motions, and back protection during lifting, stooping, and exercise with more challenging equipment.

The ability to control aerobic exercise intensity must be learned by all members through both explanation and application of principles using the target zone, Karvonen formula, talk test, and RPE. Members must become acquainted with how to safely monitor and adjust their heart rate during exercise as well as how to recognize the symptoms of overexertion. It is important that members understand the dangers of inadequate warm-up and cool-down, especially the concept of **blood pooling** and how it may lead to fainting and cardiac arrest. In light of blood pooling and possible cardiac complications, members must be strongly cautioned about leaving class to take water breaks and departing class before the cool-down. Members need to be advised that staff have the responsibility to ensure that all members have an adequate warm-up, work at appropriate intensity levels, and complete their workout with an effective cool-down.

Safe and unsafe breathing patterns must be addressed to avoid such problems as hyperventilation, which can lead to fainting, as well as the Valsalva maneuver, which can cause syncope as well as blood pressure irregularities and hernias. Members must be cautioned that during exercise there is to be no gum, candy, or anything else within the mouth, because this could obstruct the airway. This is a safety policy that the staff must enforce and to which members must adhere.

Members must be advised as to the difference between muscle fatigue that comes from overload during strength training versus joint pain that results from unsafe activities and unhealthy contortions. Additionally, members should be instructed as to the signs and symptoms of heart attack and how to respond. Along this line, they also need to be instructed how to respond to specific crises such as fire, power outage, weather emergencies, and bomb threats.

The orientation should conclude with the distribution of a handout that reviews the essential information that was discussed. The handout may be divided into general fitness information and then primary safety precautions. There should be an emphasis on beginning carefully, progressing gradually, avoiding competition, and, most importantly, having fun.

## SUPERVISING MEMBERS

*Supervision* refers to observing and directing activities in order to ensure their success. More specifically, it refers to the staff actions required to bring about both safe and effective exercise programming. Supervision must begin with the first contact with members, continue throughout their physical activities within the club setting, and end only with the termination of their membership.

The ability to relate well to members, communicate effectively, motivate sufficiently, and move to action appropriately is the hallmark of the professional staff member. This means being able to deal with all types of personalities and encouraging members to achieve success. Consequently, managers must seek out personnel who understand not only the science of exercise but also the art of influencing human behavior. Social skills combined with a sincere concern for others, an appropriate knowledge base, exercise expertise, and a conscientious commitment to the job provide the essentials for a well-supervised facility.

Supervision also entails the facility's commitment to having adequate numbers of qualified personnel overseeing all the physical activities within the exercise setting to ensure effectiveness of training and member safety. During personal training, this would mean constant attentiveness to a client's exercise regimen and the ability to promptly recognize ineffective or unsafe movements requiring timely correction. During group classes, this would require an observant instructor and assistant instructor prepared to monitor several members at once in order to rapidly intervene and remediate such concerns as an unsafe dance step, excessive exercise intensity, or a contorted motion.

General floor supervision requires at least one qualified trainer capable of answering any member questions, instructing beginners on equipment operation, providing guidance as needed, and responding to any potential emergency situations. Staff must be alert to potentially unsafe activities. Safe floor monitoring requires that all areas be readily visible to staff personnel on duty; there must be no blind spots in which a member who is in danger could be unobserved.

Locations where supervision is frequently lacking include locker rooms and wet areas. All too often, members develop cardiovascular complications in the locker room, and the only people present, if any, are other members. Therefore, a locker room attendant should be available at all times—an attendant can be providing housekeeping services while simultaneously monitoring members and remaining available to provide an emergency response.

It is not uncommon to witness sauna, steam, and whirlpool rooms completely unattended. There are numerous reports and documentation of people being discovered dead in sauna and steam rooms or drowned in whirlpools. This author has been retained as an expert witness in death cases involving all three of these venues. Not only should these areas be under constant surveillance, but also the staff should ensure that members limit their exposure time to about 10 minutes.

## The Bottom Line

> In addition to being a source of unnecessary expense and maintenance difficulties, wet areas are a potential area for litigation.

As stated, supervision begins with the first contact and ends with membership termination. Therefore, a facility is guilty of faulty supervision if it fails to screen members for risk factors before undertaking an exercise program, fails to provide a fitness profile determining members' capacity for exercise, fails to design an exercise program befitting a member's level of health and fitness, fails to educate members about safety concerns relating to exercise, or fails to supervise activities. In addition, faulty supervision is epitomized by the lack of a well-rehearsed emergency plan that can be executed by qualified personnel in a timely manner.

## MANAGING EMERGENCIES

While in your office and working on next year's budget, a hurried and excited message comes blaring across the PA system. "Code blue, code blue, code blue. Report to the aerobics center!" (If you're a manager, these words will get your heart racing as much as if you were doing an intense workout!) When you hear this announcement, you know that a member is down and that your emergency response system is going to be put to the test.

Regarding risk management, an emergency action plan (EAP) or emergency response plan (ERP) is of paramount importance not only for the safety of members but also for the protection of the facility from litigation. An EAP or ERP is a necessity for all facilities (Eickhoff-Shemek, Herbert, and Connaughton's *Health Fitness Management* 2009), (The NSCA's *Strength and Conditioning Professional Standards and Guidelines*

## Risks of Saunas, Steam Rooms, Whirlpools, and Sauna Suits

Saunas, steam rooms, and whirlpools need signs posted to warn of potential dangers, especially to high-risk members, such as those with heart disease, diabetes, and high blood pressure. Cautionary signage to be posted include "Do not use alone," "Do not use after vigorous exercise," "Do not exercise within," and "Do not use while under the influence of alcohol, anticoagulants, antihistamines, vasoconstrictors, vasodilators, stimulants, hypnotics, narcotics tranquilizers, or other drugs that cause sleepiness, drowsiness, or raise/lower blood pressure."

Members should understand that the only benefit of saunas, steam rooms, and whirlpools is temporary relaxation. No permanent weight loss can be achieved through heat exposure, and any weight reduction is due to water loss that will be replaced after eating and drinking. Besides having no real health benefit, saunas, steam rooms, and whirlpools generate unsanitary conditions and usually turn out to be a maintenance headache. They often become a financial burden and also pose one of the highest risks to safety in facility operations (Abbott 2015).

The potential dangers in using saunas and whirlpools are also a concern with sauna suits. The use of a sauna suit limits energy expenditure and caloric burn during exercise and may lead to hyperthermia and heat-related injuries. There have been cases in which the use of a sauna suit has led to rhabdomyolysis and compartment syndrome. There is no reason for fitness facilities to make this type of apparel available to members.

2017), (ACSM's *Health/Fitness Facility Standards and Guidelines* 2012), and (IHRSA's *Guide to Club Membership Conduct* 2005)

*"An emergency response plan is a written document that details the proper procedures for caring for participants who incur injuries (cardiovascular complications) during activity. While all Strength and Conditioning facilities should have such a document, it is important to appreciate that the document itself does not save lives. Indeed, it may offer a false sense of security if it is not backed up with appropriate training and preparedness by qualified, professional staff. "* (National Strength and Conditioning Association Professional Standards and Guidelines 2017, 7)

Similar to this NSCA standard, *ACSM's Health/ Fitness Facility Standards and Guidelines* states,

*"Facility operators must have written emergency response policies and procedures, which shall be reviewed regularly and physically rehearsed at least twice annually. These policies shall enable staff to respond to basic first-aid situations and emergency events in an appropriate and timely manner."* (American College of Sports Medicine 2012, 18)

IHRSA's *Guide to Club Membership Conduct* shares a similar standard:

*"The club will respond in a timely manner to any reasonably foreseeable emergency event that threatens the health and safety of its patrons. Toward this end, the club will have an appropriate emergency plan that can be executed by qualified personnel in a timely manner"* (International Health, Racquet, and Sportsclub Association 2005, 4)

Some typical facility emergencies to be anticipated are heat-related illnesses, physical injuries, and heart attacks. An emergency plan is designed to ensure that minor problems do not escalate to major incidents and that major incidents do not become fatal events. Heat exhaustion dealt with promptly and effectively can forestall a heatstroke; a severe laceration with appropriate administration of first aid can prevent major blood loss; a myocardial infarction responded to with emergency cardiac care can avert a cardiac arrest; and a sudden cardiac arrest responded to with timely and effective CPR, coupled with a swift application of an AED, can restore the victim's heart rhythm and lead to a full recovery with no neurological damage.

In addition to these types of accidents and injuries, emergencies also come in the form of crises such as fires, floods, tornadoes, earthquakes, hurricanes, severe storms, bomb threats, and even terrorist activities. Crises could also include sexual harassment, client intoxication, hazardous spills, thievery, unruly behavior, parking lot accidents, and other health concerns or life-threatening events. Fire evacuation plans, severe weather contingencies, and even procedures for handling and ejecting disruptive patrons are important for the staff who might have to deal with such unforeseen events.

## How to Develop an Emergency Plan

Where do you begin when developing something as important as the emergency plan? If the facility is located in a large complex such as a resort, office tower, or shopping plaza, contact the building supervisor or the security department to review existing emergency plans that can be modified to meet the resources of the facility. Managers of freestanding facilities should contact city offices that deal with emergencies, such as police and fire departments, advisory physicians, and legal counsel, as well as local safety consulting firms. Even if you have access to other facilities' plans, you must remember that no single plan will accommodate all facilities. Although this chapter presents issues to be considered during the development of an emergency plan, you will need to give careful consideration to the unique requirements of your facility and its members.

All facility personnel should be involved in developing the emergency plan to ensure that it is appropriate not only for each activity area but also nonactivity areas as well. The input of staff members will lead to a more effective plan; it will also make the staff more likely to buy into the plan, because they helped develop it.

Emergency plans must be detailed but not overly complicated. The plan should be logical and written in concise terms that are easily understood by staff as well as members. Modify emergency procedures to fit both the type of emergency and the location of the emergency. For example, the response to a life-threatening medical emergency will differ from that for a fire evacuation. A medical emergency on the fitness floor should be handled differently than one in the swimming pool or child-care center.

# Components of the Emergency Plan

A well-conceived and comprehensive plan must be in written form, and all personnel involved should sign paperwork to indicate that they have read the plan and that they understand and agree to comply with all actions outlined. This plan should include the posting of emergency procedures that highlight the sequence of events to be followed and list emergency agencies and their phone numbers. These sheets can be posted at convenient and strategic locations throughout the facility, thereby permitting periodic review by staff. Knowledge of agencies and numbers is worthless, however, if phones are not readily available and rapidly operable. Whether a large multiplex or a small facility, the requirements of an emergency action plan remain the same.

Emergency plans must guarantee the fastest available access to on-site first responders, EMS, and advanced care facilities. To this end, a good plan outlines specific roles for staff members, detailing who should activate EMS (phoning 9-1-1), alert staff to the incident, attend to the victim, secure first aid equipment, assist the principal caregiver, verify EMS personnel are en route, take charge of crowd control, guide EMS to the scene, and, most importantly, take responsibility for the coordination of the overall effort. Other duties to be assigned are notifying the victim's family, securing the victim's clothing and valuables, recording the incident, writing the after-action report, and following through with remedial actions for any duties that were not handled expeditiously and correctly.

From the initial recognition of the emergency to the final report, there are numerous steps that must be followed to maximize the health and safety of the membership. Each step needs to be analyzed with regard to the uniqueness of the facility, qualifications of staff, type of membership profile, and physical and financial resources available. For example, in alerting staff to a poten-

tial cardiac arrest, would it be most advantageous to announce to all members who are present that an emergency is in progress? Perhaps not; in order to avoid curious onlookers who would only create more confusion, it might be wiser to have a code word that only the staff will understand (e.g., "Emery," as in the chapter's opening scenario). On the other hand, are there members possessing medical skills from whom you would want to enlist their help?

The following list of plan components can be used in developing or refining an emergency plan. (Information about how to plan for other types of emergencies will be discussed later in the chapter.) It is recommended that these emergency plan components be listed on a two-page sheet. The front page outlines the vital procedures a first responder should initiate and follow, and the detailed information and directions are located on the back page for quick reference by the manager on duty or assisting staff members.

• *Activation code.* Activating the emergency plan is often the most essential component. Once a potential emergency has been identified, select a method to discreetly and rapidly notify staff and management. This can be accomplished by announcing a code over a PA system, sending a code over a group paging system, or setting a pre-arranged sequence of telephone calls in motion. Direct staff members to immediately proceed to the location of the incident.

• *Telephone numbers.* Make sure several telephone numbers are readily accessible. Although most cities in the United States use the 9-1-1 emergency system, some cities may not have this service, or the plan may direct staff to call an in-house emergency department that then activates EMS. Keep numbers for emergency assistance, poison control, the general manager, and other management personnel posted by every telephone. Because telephones are known to break down, there should be a backup communication system, such as cellular phones or two-way radios (walkie-talkies).

• *Location of nearest telephone.* If there is not a telephone in an activity area, specify the exact location of the nearest phone and how to get there.

• *Location identification and accessibility.* Staff should be provided detailed instructions regarding the location of the emergency in reference to other club areas, such as the main entrance. Staff should know how to direct EMS personnel to the closest building entry. In many larger facilities, you can contact an internal department such as security or an operator. These internal departments have the responsibility to call 9-1-1, meet EMS personnel as they enter the property, and direct them to the emergency site.

• *Locked doors or gates.* If any door or gate is kept locked and could therefore hinder the entry of EMS personnel, note the location of the door or gate and the location of the key.

• *Location of emergency supplies.* Provide the location of the nearest first aid kit, emergency oxygen, AED, blood-borne pathogen kit, and blood-borne cleanup kit.

• *Information to share.* Include directions about calling 9-1-1 or another predetermined resource. When calling for assistance, the caller should identify himself or herself, where the emergency is (include the club address in the emergency plan), the phone number he or she is calling from, the type of emergency, what has happened, how many people need assistance, their genders and approximate ages, and what is currently being done to assist them. The caller should ask for estimated time of arrival of emergency support. The caller must stay calm and stay on the line until the emergency operator says to hang up.

• *Directions for personnel responsibilities.* The plan should direct the initial responder to take charge of the incident until a manager arrives and can assume responsibility. The initial responder should stay with the injured party, leaving only to activate the emergency plan or call for assistance. The initial responder will typically delegate another staff member to call 9-1-1 and secure the crash bag with needed emergency equipment. The manager should delegate additional staff members to assist with the rescue, assume responsibilities for crowd control, retrieve any health information that may be on file, meet and direct EMS to the scene, and record the names of people who are present and may have witnessed the incident.

• *Call for member assistance.* Many medical emergency plans include a call for any medically trained members (doctors, nurses, or paramedics) present in the facility to proceed to the location of the incident for assistance.

• *Incident and accident reports.* Immediately following the removal of the victim by emergency personnel, the manager on duty should direct the staff to go to a quiet place and to write down everything they can remember about the incident and the care provided, including timelines, names of witnesses, care administered, and any outstanding concerns. During this time, the manager on duty should complete an incident or accident report (see figure 13.4).

## *The Bottom Line*

A backup communication system should be available at all times in case phone lines go down.

# Implementing and Practicing the Plan

Emergency and crisis plans must be practiced and rehearsed with regularity. Ideally, mock emergencies should be conducted at least quarterly if not more often due to a high turnover of staff. Most rehearsals will be announced ahead of time to ensure maximum attendance, but some rehearsals should be unannounced to test timely responsiveness. Responsible critiques and remedial actions of such rehearsals will only improve the plan. The emergency response rehearsals should be evaluated by facility risk managers, legal advisers, and medical providers to ensure that timely and effective procedures are being followed as well as modified when needed. It is recommended that facilities enlist a medical liaison to keep the emergency plan updated and to periodically evaluate the skills and ability of all personnel as well as independent contractors.

Rehearsals allow for the practical implementation of what has been reviewed and studied within the comprehensive emergency plan. The number of rehearsals will depend on the size of the facility, the number of staff members and their level of training, the number and variety of exercise environments, the types of emergency for which there is the greatest potential, and the emergency equipment available. Rehearsals become almost meaningless unless managers ensure that all

# INCIDENT AND ACCIDENT REPORT

Date of incident/accident: _____ Time of incident: _____ a.m./p.m.

Injured member/guest: _____ Age: _____

Membership number: _____

Address: _____

_____

Telephone: (Home) _____ (Work) _____

Location of incident: _____

_____

Describe in full how the incident occurred and what actions were taken by staff. (Write everything you can remember, no matter how insignificant it may seem.)

_____

_____

_____

Describe the injury in detail and indicate the body part(s) affected.

_____

Did any medically trained members (doctors, nurses) assist?

_____

Staff members present: _____

Witnesses: _____

_____

Was the emergency plan activated? _____ Was EMS called? _____

Was the individual taken to the hospital? Yes _____ No _____

If yes, what hospital? _____

If no, did he/she refuse medical attention? _____

Was the emergency contact notified? Yes _____ No _____

Name of person contacted: _____

On the back of this page, please document any observations or comments regarding this incident you feel important.

Signed by: _____ Date: _____ Time: _____

Manager/dept. head: _____ Date: _____

Follow-up notes: _____

Contact made by: _____ Date: _____

Condition of injured member/guest: _____

**Figure 13.4** Sample incident and accident report.

From M. Bates, M.J. Spezzano, and G. Danhoff, *Health Fitness Management,* 3rd ed. (Champaign, IL: Human Kinetics, 2020).

personnel participate in drills multiple times throughout the year. Training aids such as first aid materials, emergency oxygen, resuscitation masks, AED training units, and manikins need to be available to heighten realism.

Qualified emergency professionals should be appointed to monitor all rehearsals in order to provide feedback. A critical review of the rehearsal in the form of an after-action report needs to be provided as soon as possible. Recommendations may be made regarding how staff may improve their overall emergency response, their individual actions, and their timing. Afterward, documentation of actions to remedy the shortcomings should be verified and filed along with the after-action report.

Once the emergency plan is ready to implement, instruct all facility personnel that they must be well versed in the procedural deployment of the emergency plan; remind them that their failure to act in a reasonable and prudent manner can result in serious injury, unnecessary death, and potential litigation. Emergency plans need not be memorized in their entirety. However, every staff member should memorize the code or phone number that sets the plan in motion. More specific emergency plans should be posted next to every telephone, in each area of the club, for quick reference. The staff member in charge of risk management should carefully review the completed emergency plan with local fire and police departments as well as emergency medical services (EMS) and maintain contact with these city resources during planning of training sessions and practice drills so that these departments and resources are made aware of specific facility needs.

However, just practicing the emergency response system is not enough to ensure a successful outcome with an actual event. The system can only be fine-tuned when inappropriate actions are observed, noted to management, and then corrected. After each drill, therefore, debriefings should be conducted to address shortcomings and to discuss how best to correct these deficiencies. Involve building management, maintenance personnel, and local city resources (fire, police, EMS) in all emergency drills. These trained professionals may offer additional information or ideas that will better prepare the staff for future responses. Evaluating an emergency response plays an important role in the ongoing training of staff and should never be overlooked.

## *The Bottom Line*

Every drill or rehearsal should be monitored by appropriately trained emergency personnel who can submit an after-action report to management.

# Medical Emergency Plan for Cardiovascular Complications

Medical complications due to exercise are an ever-present possibility, and of greatest concern are cardiovascular complications. It has been well documented that coronary incidents from vigorous exercise are more common than every day, spontaneous occurrences. For those free of coronary artery disease (CAD), the relative risk of exercise is extremely low, but this risk is dramatically heightened for those with CAD. Unfortunately, occult coronary artery disease is prevalent among older, sedentary people, many of whom are now availing themselves of fitness facility services. As stated in the Georgia Goslee interview, an IHRSA research project determined that the fastest-growing segment of the gym population is the baby boomer generation.

## Use of Oxygen

As previously indicated, cardiovascular complications within the fitness facility typically take the form of a **myocardial infarction (MI)** or **sudden cardiac arrest (SCA)**. In either case, facility staff must respond with emergency cardiac care. Such care requires appropriate training and equipment. When a mild to moderate MI is suspected (e.g., tightness of the chest, radiating pain), EMS activation by calling 9-1-1 is essential. In addition to making the member as comfortable and calm as possible, the trainer should immediately administer emergency oxygen.

In addition to activation of EMS, supplemental oxygen is probably the most important step that can be taken in treating the suspected MI. In addition, any victim of a potentially life-threatening illness or injury should receive emergency medical oxygen (American Red Cross 1993). It has been estimated that oxygen administration may double a person's chances of survival. Management need not worry whether oxygen may be harmful during a medical emergency; the administration of oxygen will only enhance the likelihood of a positive outcome. All emergency medical literature affirms that the immediate use of supplemental oxygen is crucial for victims of sudden life-threatening illness or injury.

Although it is true that oxygen is a drug when given in concentrations beyond that found in the air we breathe, the U.S. Food and Drug Administration (FDA), the regulating agency for medical gases, has exempted the prescriptive requirement for emergency oxygen. In order to qualify as emergency oxygen, the delivery system must provide a minimum flow rate of six liters per minute for a minimum of 15 minutes. According to the FDA, anyone properly trained in oxygen administration can provide this emergency drug. Not only should staff rescuers be familiar with the instructional materials and directions for an oxygen delivery system, but they also should undergo formal training. Such training is available from a number of organizations such as the American Red Cross and can be accomplished in just a few hours.

Oxygen administration is also important when CPR is administered. By attaching the oxygen delivery system to a resuscitation mask, the rescuer can provide the victim with an oxygen concentration well above that of normal air. This procedure will buy the victim more time while awaiting life-saving defibrillation or drug administration by EMS personnel.

## Use of Automated External Defibrillators

When SCA occurs within the fitness facility, the prognosis is poor unless an AED is available. In the United States, SCA strikes between 350,000 and 450,000 people each year outside of the hospital environment, and more than 95% die. Rapid defibrillation is the only definitive treatment. Due to the unavoidable time it takes for EMS to arrive, defibrillation by paramedics is usually too late to provide successful resuscitation. Once blood stops circulating, as with ventricular fibrillation or pulseless ventricular tachycardia, every minute without defibrillation decreases the chances of survival by approximately 7 to 10%. However, with immediate and effective CPR, the survival rate decreases by only 3 to 4% for each minute without defibrillation. Due to the delay in EMS

arrival, the only solution to this dilemma is to have an AED on the premises.

AEDs have been effectively used for over 25 years and are credited with saving thousands of lives. As a result of their proven success, the U.S. Congress passed the Cardiac Arrest Survival Act in 2000, legislation that directed the Department of Health and Human Services to develop guidelines for placing AEDs in federal buildings nationwide. This bill also established a Good Samaritan provision that protects people from liability in those states that had not already enacted such laws regarding AEDs (Abbott 2000). Presently, all states have a Good Samaritan law protecting lay rescuers.

With the publication of a 2002 joint position statement, the ACSM and the AHA urged health and fitness clubs to implement AED programs. The ACSM and AHA recommended that AEDs be part of an emergency response plan within all facilities that have memberships of 2,500 or more, have special programs for the elderly, serve members with known medical conditions, or are in locations where EMS response time (the time between recognition of the cardiac arrest and delivery of the first defibrillation shock) is likely to exceed 5 minutes (American Heart Association 2002).

It should be noted that the fourth edition of *ACSM's Health/Fitness Facility Standards and Guidelines* has published five standards relating to AEDs within their chapter on risk management and emergency policies (American College of Sports Medicine 2012, 18):

These standards state that

1. *All facilities (staffed or unstaffed) shall have as part of their written emergency response policies and procedures a public access defibrillation (PAD) program . . .*

2. *AEDs in a facility shall be located within a 1.5 minute walk to any place an AED could be potentially needed.*

3. *A skills review, practice sessions, and a practice drill with the AED shall be conducted a minimum of every six months . . .*

4. *A staffed facility shall assign at least one staff member to be on duty during all facility operating hours who is currently trained and certified in the delivery of cardiopulmonary resuscitation and in administration of an AED.*

5. *Unstaffed facilities shall have as part of their written emergency response policies and procedures a PAD program as a means by which either members and users or an external emergency responder can respond from time of collapse to defibrillation in four minutes or less.*

Adapted by permission from American College of Sports Medicine, *ACSM's Health/Fitness Facility Standards and Guidelines* (Champaign, IL: Human Kinetics, 2012), 18.

Several states and the District of Columbia have passed legislation requiring that fitness facilities have emergency plans that include AED deployment. In states that have yet to mandate AED programs within facilities, many municipalities have legislated this type of emergency preparedness.

AEDs are safe, simple, reliable, and relatively inexpensive. Considering that the cost of an AED is comparable to that of a piece of gym equipment ($1,500), it is inexcusable for any facility to not have them as part of their emergency response equipment. An AED training unit can also be purchased for a minimal amount and made available for continuing education and testing purposes. With the availability of AED instruction through the AHA, American Red Cross, National Safety Council, and equipment manufacturers, the cost of training is also reasonable. Likewise, emergency oxygen systems can be picked up for a few hundred dollars; as with AEDs, the training is neither overly time consuming nor expensive. Emergency oxygen coupled with an AED provides a winning combination that will greatly improve the chances of survival during cardiovascular complications such as an MI or SCA.

Some lawyers may argue that the use of AEDs and oxygen increases the exposure of fitness facilities to litigation because they will be held to a higher standard of care. There is little merit to this argument, especially considering the 2002 joint position statement by the AHA and ACSM. Regarding liability, an article in *Best's Review*, a leading insurance industry publication, stated, "The need for defibrillators outweighs potential liability" (*Best's Review* August 2002, 72). Additionally, the article indicated that a failure to respond to a SCA with an AED is a liability concern. The only important question to ask is, "Will the availability of oxygen and AEDs save lives?" The answer to this question is a resounding "Yes!"

When it comes to delivering emergency cardiac care, we should look to professional organizations that specialize in this field, primarily the AHA. As far back as 1999, the AHA's *Basic Life Support Manual for Healthcare Providers* stated that "because of the intrinsic simplicity of AEDs, a markedly expanded range of persons can now be trained to provide early defibrillation, including . . . supervisory personnel at exercise facilities" (American Heart Association 1999, 9-13). The AHA's newest guidelines reflect an even stronger commitment to public access defibrillation through the use of AEDs, which have been hailed as the most exciting breakthrough in CPR since the advent of mouth-to-mouth rescue breathing. It is the goal of the AHA that victims of SCA be defibrillated within 5 minutes of onset. For this reason, the AHA recommends that AEDs be placed in locations where there is a reasonable probability of one SCA occurring every 5 years. Certainly fitness facilities fall within this category.

Unfortunately, facilities have failed over the years to respond successfully during cardiovascular complications such as an MI or a SCA. Too often, members do not recognize their symptoms or do not wish to admit that their chest pain and other classic MI symptoms portend a heart attack. Victims of an MI often experience denial and think they could not be having such a medical emergency. This psychology of denial should be addressed in basic life support classes related to recognizing a victim of an MI and how to respond with emergency cardiac care (ECC).

In the AHA's *Basic Life Support for Healthcare Providers* (American Heart Association 2001), this tendency to deny is discussed from the standpoint of not only the victim but also the potential rescuer (staff member). The text states,

*"Denial is not limited to the victim—it may also persuade the rescuer. The tendency of people involved in an emergency to deny or downplay the serious nature of the presenting problem is a natural one that must be overcome to provide rapid intervention and maximize the victim's chance of survival. Denial of the serious nature of the symptoms delays treatment and increases the risk of death." (American Heart Association 2001, 29)*

Numerous death-related lawsuits against facilities have resulted when staff members failed to recognize a heart attack and didn't respond when the member regressed into a cardiac arrest. In other cases, lawsuits resulted when the response was insufficient: CPR was provided but available AEDs were not deployed.

In cases of sudden cardiac arrest, all too frequently staff members mistake agonal breathing for a respiratory problem such as asthma and fail to provide CPR and deploy an AED. The agonal gasp (snort, snore, or groan) in a nonresponsive individual is a sign of cardiac arrest to which staff must respond immediately with CPR. The AHA's Basic Life Support student manual defines *gasping* as breathing that is not regular or normal—an indicator of the heart's inability to circulate blood, which requires immediate CPR and defibrillation (American Heart Association 2016).

Why do we see such an inability of fitness facility staff to recognize an MI or a SCA? The answer is twofold. First, staff personnel are typically required to take only a short (3- to 4-hour) CPR class that does not even address the topics of signs and symptoms, denial, MI distress, and the needed emergency cardiac care (ECC). Second, this short CPR class does not sufficiently stress the concept of agonal breathing and fails to provide sufficient hands-on practice to develop the skills and confidence needed to immediately identify SCA and aggressively begin CPR with AED deployment. When inadequacy of the CPR class is combined with a lack of practice, rehearsals, and drills within facilities, it is no wonder that staff personnel are unable to respond effectively and in a timely manner. Facilities should require more extensive CPR certifications.

## The Bottom Line

In order to provide the gift of life to facility members, staff must be able to respond with emergency cardiac care, CPR, AEDs, and oxygen. Such emergency care and equipment are essential to give the victims of MI and SCA a fighting chance.

## Plans for Other Emergencies

Although medical emergencies are more likely to occur and threaten the safety of members, there

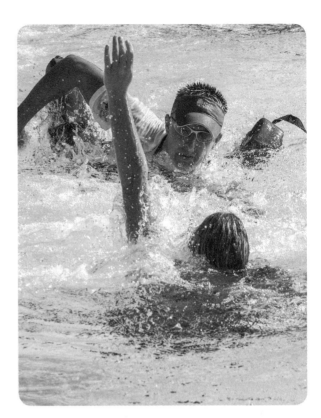

Rehearsals of the club's emergency and crisis plans must be conducted and documented regularly on file.

are other potential emergencies that managers must take into consideration. An out-of-control facility fire could become disastrous and lead to multiple injuries and deaths, as could failing to heed weather warnings. Natural disasters catch facilities unaware and can wreak death and destruction, and the threat of terrorism poses potential harm to both facility members as well as the facility itself. A poorly supervised aquatics area could result in an unnecessary drowning; likewise, a poorly supervised child-care area could result in a physical injury or a choking death. Thus, the management team must plan for a variety of potential emergencies.

### Fires

During any emergency situation, the health and safety of members and guests are the highest priority. The ability to calmly and systematically notify members of an emergency that requires immediate evacuation of the building is extremely important. Managers must establish a fire and evacuation plan that specifies procedures to effectively and efficiently clear the building. As with the medical emergency plan, the manager should obtain assistance in preparing this procedure by contacting on-site security personnel, building managers, or local departments such as fire and police. Review and practice your completed fire and evacuation plan in cooperation with these local emergency services.

## Aquatic Emergencies

A medical emergency in aquatic facilities or pool areas within a fitness facility requires special considerations. In fitness facility pool areas, supervision should only be provided by trained personnel who have demonstrated proficiency in the water as well as with emergency response procedures. In addition to emergency plan policies, specific aquatic guidelines include the following:

- If the victim is unconscious, suspect a neck injury.

- In the case of a possible neck injury, do not remove the victim from the water. Ensure all vital signs are stable. Stabilize the victim's head and body and await the arrival of emergency personnel. Use only the tools and techniques in which you are thoroughly trained and well-rehearsed.

- In the case of possible drowning, remove the victim from the pool. Turn the victim on the side to allow water to drain. Check vital signs and begin rescue breathing or CPR as necessary.

- If using an AED, ensure that the victim's chest is dry and that the victim is not in a puddle of water.

It is disheartening that many pools within fitness facilities are not monitored. Because pools that are under a certain size may not be required by law to provide lifeguards, managers sometimes try to keep overhead down by not providing pool supervision and only posting a warning sign to members that they swim at their own risk because a lifeguard is not on duty. As previously stated, the top priority of any facility should be the health and safety of its members; managers should not let revenue and profitability trump this priority.

Pools are a workout area and, therefore, should be supervised like any other workout area within a facility (Abbott 2017). IHRSA's *Guide to Club Membership Conduct* has, as Standard 9, the requirement that member clubs ensure that facilities provide credible and professional supervision of all physical activity programs and areas. Additionally, IHRSA's Code of Conduct states that member clubs must design their facilities and programs with members' safety in mind (International Health, Racquet, and Sportsclub Association 2005). The failure to monitor a pool

## Equipment and Guidelines for Pools

Aquatic emergency equipment and guidelines are required at all public pools but should be viewed as equally important for fitness facility pools. Check with local and state regulatory agencies for a complete listing of required aquatic safety and emergency equipment as well as guidelines for use. Examples of equipment needed for safety and for emergencies include the following:

- Safety and pool rules signs
- Clear depth markers on pool sides
- Pool gates that can be secured and locked when pool is closed
- AED
- Backboard
- First aid kit
- Megaphone
- Cervical collar

- Shepherd's crook
- Reaching pole
- Emergency oxygen
- First responder kits
- Resuscitation mask
- Bag-valve-mask
- Suctioning device
- Life rings and buoys
- Rescue tubes

is an obvious disregard for membership safety and could be viewed as gross negligence.

## Emergencies Involving Children

The child-care center in every facility should emphasize safety as a part of its daily operations. Even carefully supervised children will have accidents. Establish and practice safety procedures in the child-care area. The following are some guidelines to ensure a safe play environment:

- Obtain the medical history of all children.
- Obtain a signed parental directive and emergency medical authorization form. (Seek advice of legal counsel in preparing this form.)
- Set rules requiring the parent or guardian to remain on the property.
- Create a safe play environment by covering all electrical outlets, removing or padding all sharp corners, installing padded carpet to protect against falls, and purchasing only child-safe toys and equipment.
- Ensure that no items small enough to constitute a choking hazard are within children's reach.
- Maintain strict rules to ensure direct staff supervision at all times.
- Make sure a first aid kit is available.
- Ensure personnel are certified in first aid and in child and infant CPR.
- Practice emergency procedures monthly.
- If an AED is available, make sure it has pediatric pads or a dose attenuator.
- Conduct weekly safety inspections of indoor and outdoor play areas.

## Disaster Plan

Disasters can come in many forms: earthquakes, hurricanes, tornadoes, fires, floods, tsunamis, and terrorist acts as well as active shooters (a danger that has become more prevalent in recent years). Disasters endanger lives, create a costly disruption, and may cause financial ruin for the facility. As with many medical emergencies, these problems are difficult or impossible to prevent. However, being prepared may ensure the safety of members, control the extent of damage, and minimize potential liability. Managers can lessen the impact of a disaster by establishing sound emergency and evacuation procedures that are practiced, by securing complete insurance coverage that is reevaluated annually, by developing a solid risk-management program, and by maintaining strong communication channels with members, local business associates, and external agencies involved with disaster response.

The following are some guidelines that need to be considered when preparing for the possibility of implementing a disaster plan:

- Who will provide the alert for advanced disaster warnings and how
- Who will provide the alert for an immediate disaster and how
- How communication will be handled during a power outage
- Who will be in charge of command and control during disasters
- What the assigned staff roles are for each type of disaster
- What the training requirements are for the different staff roles
- How evacuations plans will differ based on the type of disaster
- Where shelters will be located within the facility or nearby grounds
- Who will direct members to safe areas and how
- What locations will be designated safe areas for each type of emergency
- Where first aid stations will be located and who will man them
- How evacuations of injured parties will be handled
- What type of communication with emergency medical services (EMS) will exist
- What type of communication with fire service and law enforcement will exist
- Who will communicate with the families of members who have been injured or killed
- Who will communicate with the media and what restrictions will be imposed regarding information disclosed
- What recovery plans may be needed after each type of disaster

## Weather Emergencies

Weather emergencies often strike with minimal warning. The geographic region where the facility is located will assist in determining the types of weather that may pose a threat. Preparation of emergency procedures when facing a tornado, hurricane, or flood will minimize liability and control damage. A weather plan should include the following:

- Television channels, radio stations, or telephone numbers to get weather advisories
- Definitions of commonly used watch and warning systems in the community
- Procedures for evacuating members who are outdoors (playgrounds, pools, athletic fields)
- A communication plan and script to follow
- The designation of an evacuation zone or shelter and procedures for transporting members to this area
- Specific actions to be taken by members, depending on the type of threatening weather

## Bomb Threat

Although most bomb threats turn out to be false alarms, they should nevertheless be taken seriously. Specific procedures and questions for gathering information from the caller should be readily available to all staff who take incoming calls. Those procedures may include recording the content of the threatening message to relay it to law enforcement personnel. Prompt but calming evacuation procedures must be instituted with the intent of getting members as far away from the building as possible.

## Events Held Off Premises

Some fitness facilities sponsor activities conducted outside of the actual facility premises, such as road races, obstacle courses, and boot camps. It is important to address potential safety concerns and have specific emergency response plans that address the unique characteristics and dangers of these events. It is equally important that managers ensure that liability insurance policies are not only limited to in-house incidents but also provide coverage for such outside events.

## Non-Life-Threatening Emergencies

Nuisance emergencies, such as power outages or accidental activation of the fire sprinkler system, can create havoc in a facility. The facility manager or chief engineer should train staff how to respond quickly and effectively when faced with such emergencies.

**Power Outage**    Power outages occur frequently in many locales. However, for those facilities in which an electrical disruption is not routine, this loss of power can frighten members and cause panic if the staff does not respond in a calm and confident manner. Ensuring members' safety is the highest priority while handling this type of emergency.

In anticipation of power outages, you should have the director of maintenance or chief engineer clearly label all breaker boxes in the electrical room so that other personnel can locate any breaker that has switched off.

Your power-outage response plan should include the steps to follow once power has been lost:

- Ensure that no one has been hurt as a result of the sudden stoppage of exercise equipment.
- By means of a battery-powered megaphone, confidently communicate that someone is looking into the problem.
- Using an authoritative tone of voice, request that all members remain where they are until emergency generator lighting or flashlights are available to assist them in moving around the club.
- In the event of an isolated power outage, have trained personnel check whether a breaker has switched off.
- In the event of a complete power outage, ask members and staff to wait patiently for a few minutes to see whether power is restored. If it is not restored quickly, ensure that emergency lighting is working in all areas and assist members in exiting the building.
- Once power is restored, check the calibration on all exercise equipment, reset time clocks and cash registers, and reboot computers.

**Accidental Activation of the Sprinkler System**

Accidental activation of the fire sprinkler system can result in severe water damage to the facility.

Flooding of a facility can ruin expensive wood flooring, such as a group exercise floor or racquetball court, as well as electrical equipment. In addition, failure to rapidly and thoroughly remove all water after such an incident can lead to mold and mildew, which can cause health concerns and can require costly indoor environmental restoration or bacterial-growth remediation. To prevent the accidental activation of the fire sprinkler system, incorporate the following suggestions into a regular maintenance checklist:

- Ensure all sprinkler heads are recessed or protected. (Most accidental activations occur when an exposed sprinkler head is knocked off or bumped loose. If heads are not recessed, the exposed structure should be covered by a cage.)
- Train enough key personnel so that there is always someone on duty who knows exactly how to shut down the system.

## Equipment

The proper handling of emergency events will often require special emergency equipment, so a first aid kit (or multiple kits, depending upon the size of the facility) must be available. It is crucial that kits be properly marked, identifiable, accessible, and easily transportable as well as stocked according to foreseeable events and the skills of responders. Kits must be checked at least once a month to verify that the contents match the list of recommended supplies. Equipment and supplies must be used according to manufacturer instructions and recognized professional guidelines. When using these materials, it is imperative that precautions for preventing disease transmission be followed as outlined by the Centers for Disease Control and Prevention (CDC) and OSHA.

Safety supplies are essential to effectively respond to an emergency. Well-stocked first aid kits provide the necessary materials in the event of a minor cut or more serious injury. First responder kits provide the staff with all the OSHA-required items as well as suggested protective barriers necessary to respond to a medical emergency in which there is the potential for contamination. Biohazard cleanup kits conveniently package all the personal protective devices and cleanup supplies needed to reduce the risk of secondary contamination following an accident in which possible infectious conditions exist.

The most serious concern likely to confront a facility manager is a cardiovascular complication such as an acute MI or SCA. To be prepared for a suspected MI or SCA, trainers need a **crash bag** that contains latex gloves, goggles, a resuscitation mask, a blood pressure unit, a pulse oximeter, and, most importantly, an AED. Accompanying the crash bag should be an emergency oxygen canister that can be attached to a nonrebreather mask for MI and resuscitation mask for SCA. Multiple crash bags that include AEDs should be available for those facilities with multiple floors or widespread areas. Additionally, AEDs should be checked daily to ensure that they are fully charged and ready for immediate use. Backup batteries should be kept on hand in order to prevent downtime while waiting for a vendor to deliver a new battery.

Additionally, flashlights and sharps containers should be kept in all first aid kits as well as in designated areas throughout the club. Flashlights can assist during a medical emergency during power outages and other situations in which seeing may be difficult. OSHA requires **sharps containers** for the proper disposal of any sharp items that may potentially cause a biohazard risk. Sharps containers prevent the accidental incision or puncture of a staff member by securing sharp items in a solid waste container. OSHA requires proper disposal of full sharps containers or any biohazard waste.

Additional equipment suggestions include the following:

- Designate a cell phone to use in the event of an emergency. This phone allows the manager to make phone calls while moving throughout the club.
- Consider having all trainers carry a resuscitation mask with inflatable cushion in a soft pack on their belts to ensure the immediate availability of a barrier device.

## Training Staff

Staff members ought to be able to respond to emergencies ranging from minor cuts to major lacerations, simple contusions to severe concussions, heat cramps to heatstroke, and mild hypoglycemia to insulin shock. The crucial question for the general manager is whether the facility personnel are well prepared so they will be able to make the difference between life and death.

Facility trainers should be certified in both first aid and CPR, including the use of an AED. Additionally, it is recommended that trainers be capable of providing emergency oxygen. Although precautionary measures, these are essential safety considerations, and a staff that lacks these credentials and skills reflects professional irresponsibility. Informal surveys show that although trainers are typically certified in CPR, most do not have certification in first aid. Of those with CPR training, many are certified only in adult CPR without training in AEDs. (And few facilities have emergency oxygen available.) It would appear that the commitment of the average fitness facility to the safety of its members is sadly lacking.

Maintaining adequate health and safety certifications among staff members is a crucial responsibility of the manager. Ideally, all facility staff, including maintenance personnel, should be required to have CPR certification as a prerequisite for employment. Trainers should have the more advanced certification with AED. Staff supervising child-care centers should have pediatric CPR as well as adult CPR certification. Although this requirement poses a challenge to facilities that experience high personnel turnover, the requirement that all personnel be CPR certified sends the message that emergency response is a high priority. Certifying long-term staff members or managers as CPR instructors is an easy and less expensive way to provide recertification courses for staff as well as complimentary or for-fee classes for members. To enhance education and testing of CPR and AED skills, the facility can purchase manikins and AED training units to practice with.

Although not all facility personnel need to have first aid certification, the number of trainers certified should be enough to ensure that at least two people with first aid certification are on duty at all times. Ideally, the facility should always have on duty one certified first responder who has undergone the requisite 60 hours of training. As with CPR, getting long-term staff and supervisors certified as first aid instructors enables in-house first aid education to be continually available to staff and members alike. If emergency oxygen is going to be available, then a sufficient number of trainers need to be certified so that appropriate administration will always be available.

Managers must educate new and existing staff members about their responsibilities in the event of an emergency. This training, which should be a priority of the supervising manager, begins with employee orientation and never ceases. The training must encompass medical, fire, aquatic, and disaster emergencies. Emergencies can occur in any location within the facility—a group exercise class, the aerobics room, the weight training area, the swimming pool, a racquetball court, a locker room, the restaurant, the child-care center, and other possible areas. Therefore, training must consist of not only reviewing written documents but also conducting hands-on drills in which staff members respond to a variety of emergency scenarios in different settings.

## RISK MANAGEMENT DOCUMENTATION

Documentation is an important component of risk management. Maintaining complete records is invaluable in the event of an accident or litigation. Documentation should include medical histories, lifestyle questionnaires, informed consents (for testing as well as programming), fitness profiles, physician releases, assumptions of risk, parental consents, maintenance checklists, after-action reports, remedial action reports, equipment checklists, restocking dates, and safety surveys. Some of these forms have been presented throughout this text; others may be found within referenced literature. It is recommended that forms be reviewed by legal counsel and a medical director.

## Maintenance Records and Safety Checklists

Regular maintenance inspections are important in preventing accidents and incidents. Maintenance inspections of flooring, exercise equipment, wet areas, mechanical equipment, and facility grounds will assist in identifying potential accident sites and injury situations. For each piece of equipment within the facility, managers should prepare an equipment history card along with a maintenance checklist. (More extensive information about the maintenance of the facility and exercise equipment is presented in chapter 14.) Proper maintenance of all club equipment and facilities provides a safer environment for the member. Proper documentation of regular maintenance practices provides the facility with a means of defense in the event of legal action.

## Manager's Safety Checklist

Health and safety concerns within a facility can demand an excessive amount of time if they are not managed properly. Therefore, managers must insist upon the awareness and action of all depart-mental supervisors and staff in this effort to offer a safe environment. Appointing specific people who can be held accountable for known health and safety concerns will assist in this important task. A weekly review of completed and incomplete tasks as well as issues demanding proactive measures will enable the busiest general manager to be aware of existing and potential health and safety concerns within the facility. A reference checklist for review by the general manager can simplify this task. Figure 13.5 provides a basic checklist that can be modified to incorporate the unique issues of each facility.

## Key Terms

accreditation

assumption of risk

blood pooling

blood-borne pathogens

certifications

clinical stress test

crash bag

emergency response plan

fitness profile

guest screening

health and safety plan

health risk appraisals

informed consent

lifestyle questionnaire

litigation

medical clearance

medical history questionnaire

myocardial infarction (MI)

Physical Activity Readiness Questionnaire for Everyone (PAR-Q+)

preactivity screening

program design

risk stratification

sharps containers

signage

standard of care

sudden cardiac arrest (SCA)

# GENERAL MANAGER'S SAFETY OVERVIEW AND CHECKLIST

| Task | Initials |
|---|---|

*Membership director*

1. Health history questionnaire completed by all new members; forms forwarded to fitness director for review          _____

2. PAR-Q+ and guest registration completed for all guests          _____

3. All reviewed health history and related forms filed properly          _____

*Fitness director (FD)*

1. All health history questionnaires reviewed by FD; medical clearance forms requested as necessary          _____

2. Equipment maintenance review and checklist complete          _____

3. Maintenance requests written as necessary          _____

4. Personnel file (to include continuing education) updated and certifications in first aid and in CPR/AED current for all fitness staff          _____

5. Emergency plan posted by all phones          _____

6. Monthly emergency plan practice session complete          _____

7. Aquatic emergency supplies in proper location          _____

*Maintenance director/chief engineer*

1. Mechanical system review and checklist complete          _____

2. Monthly test of fire warning system complete          _____

3. First aid and first responder kits fully stocked          _____

4. AEDs and emergency oxygen fully charged          _____

5. Monthly test of emergency public address system complete          _____

6. Weekly safety review and checklist of grounds complete          _____

7. All sprinkler heads protected (recessed or in cages)          _____

*Child-care director*

1. First aid and CPR/AED certifications current for all child-care staff          _____

2. Outdoor equipment safety review and checklist complete          _____

3. Parental consent forms current          _____

4. Monthly emergency evacuation practice complete          _____

To be reviewed at weekly department head meetings.

**Figure 13.5**  Sample safety overview and checklist for the general manager.

From M. Bates, M.J. Spezzano, and G. Danhoff, *Health Fitness Management*, 3rd ed. (Champaign, IL: Human Kinetics, 2020).

# Maintaining Your Facility

*Mike Greenwood and Anthony Abbott*

## Learning Objectives

After studying this chapter, you will be able to

- understand the four areas of maintenance management,
- undertake a needs assessment,
- identify goals and objectives for a facility maintenance program,
- know when to use in-house personnel and when to use outside contractors,
- understand the importance of monitoring inventory levels and controlling inventory costs, and
- evaluate a maintenance program.

After working for a few years in personal trainer and program manager positions, Sarah decided to pursue an opportunity to purchase and own an existing 16,500-square-foot health club with nearly 700 members. Although the purchase price of the club included all the assets, liabilities, and equipment, the monthly facility and fitness equipment maintenance costs seemed like a money pit. Sarah remembered from taking her undergraduate fitness management course that the starting point is to conduct a need analysis. Sarah began the process of identifying the proper goals and objectives for her facility and fitness equipment maintenance program. This process also led Sarah to take inventory of everything in the facility that requires maintenance as well as find out which items are under warranty. Once this list was identified, Sarah took careful consideration of what her in-house personnel could handle on a daily maintenance schedule and then connected with outside contractors who could perform some of the work. Finally, after a few months of committing to a monthly, weekly, and daily maintenance plan, Sarah measured the effectiveness of the plan and found that she has reduced operating costs significantly and that her now well-maintained facility has led to higher member satisfaction. Although maintaining a facility has taken considerable effort to plan, evaluate, and execute, many of the members are starting to tell others in the community about the new ownership, and Sarah's club is gaining a competitive advantage.

Establishing a maintenance program for a health and fitness organization is a vital but extremely challenging task. The success of a facility is dependent on realizing the positive impact that a safe, clean, and well-maintained facility has on prospective members and current members. An organization's success requires that managers take time to identify maintenance needs, develop and implement a plan, and regularly evaluate the plan. In today's competitive market, managers must place a high priority on areas such as client safety, housekeeping, preventative maintenance, general maintenance, equipment repairs, and renovation improvements.

This chapter addresses the steps involved in creating a facility maintenance program for the corporate, clinical, community, and commercial health and fitness sectors. The chapter also discusses the various labor options available in different fitness settings, and it concludes with how to organize and initiate a preventive maintenance program. The intent of the chapter is to present a guide for fitness professionals to follow while organizing and implementing the management of a well-designed maintenance program.

The importance of keeping a safe, clean, and well-maintained facility cannot be emphasized enough. Today's consumer is more aware of the areas to examine and evaluate when choosing a facility. Guidelines for rating health and fitness settings classify convenience as the top priority, followed by maintenance and equipment upkeep, qualified staff, program variety, and organizational management (Grantham and Patton 1998). In the eyes of a prospective member, therefore, a clean facility is nearly at the top of the list of considerations when considering the purchase of a health and fitness membership.

Maintaining a safe, clean, and well-kept facility is equally important to existing members. The results of annual member surveys have shown that facility cleanliness ranks at the top of those areas members most appreciate about a facility. It stands to reason, therefore, that cleanliness will have an impact when a member decides whether to renew.

The proper maintenance of a health and fitness facility is easy to define and evaluate. However, achieving an acceptable, consistent level of maintenance is difficult. Generally, if everything is working properly and cleanliness is apparent, members are happy, thereby allowing the facility manager to feel a sense of pride and accomplishment. Unfortunately, the fast pace of a health and fitness facility does not make this easy, and good maintenance does not occur without the concerted implementation of what is commonly referred to as the dynamics of the health and fitness industry.

We can define facility maintenance as the set of activities that, when properly managed, allow for the successful operation of a facility. These activities include decisions, work orders, and actions taken by maintenance employees. The coordinated effort of managers and the maintenance team can make or break a facility.

# MAINTENANCE ACTIVITIES

Maintenance includes activities that maintain and restore the function of the facility. Maintenance can be divided into the following categories: housekeeping, general maintenance, preventive maintenance, repair, replacement, improvement, and utilities. Place each maintenance task in one of these categories. Although the names of these categories often vary from setting to setting, the basic elements are present in every facility maintenance program.

## Housekeeping

Housekeeping comprises the daily tasks—basic cleaning, emptying trash receptacles, replacing towels and toilet paper, sweeping, mopping, and dusting—that make the facility presentable and functional. Facility staff members can be trained to perform basic daily cleaning tasks, and select contract maintenance companies can be employed (based on financial availability) to handle more extensive maintenance responsibilities before or after hours of operation. It is critical for facility administrators to evaluate the credibility and reliability of any contract maintenance company they wish to employ.

## General Maintenance

General maintenance might also be referred to as *infrequent housekeeping*. It often requires specialized equipment and specially trained individuals. Typical general maintenance activities include steam-cleaning carpets, painting walls, stripping and sealing wood floors, cleaning and waxing tile floors, changing filters on HVAC equipment, and sweeping parking lots. General maintenance improves and preserves the appearance of a facility and is performed at regular intervals based on seasonal considerations and aesthetic preferences.

## Preventive Maintenance

**Preventive maintenance** comprises a major portion of the maintenance effort in a health and fitness facility. These tasks are intended to ensure the continuous operation of all areas within the facility, with primary emphasis placed on safety and functionality. Preventive maintenance tasks are derived from manufacturer recommendations and are used to keep equipment safe and usable for as long as possible. Preventive maintenance programs are performed at regular intervals, usually by skilled employees and sometimes by contract workers.

When preventive maintenance is neglected, then dramatic, costly, and potentially dangerous failures frequently occur. For this reason, a formal preventive maintenance program should be a high priority.

## *The Bottom Line*

The difference between preventive maintenance and general maintenance is that the preventive maintenance tasks are based on manufacturer recommendations and should be followed to maintain the life of the equipment, whereas general maintenance improves and preserves the facility.

## Repairs

Repair work involves restoring to operation some component or piece of equipment after it has failed. Unfortunately, failures do not occur at convenient times and must be dealt with immediately, usually at the expense of other scheduled maintenance. In establishing objectives for repairs, it is often necessary to set priorities based on the importance of need for repair. These priorities set the maximum time required to complete repairs. As problems occur, they are classified by priority and workload. Repairs that are not immediately required (low priority) are often reclassified for future scheduling.

Ideally, equipment that needs repair should be taken off the floor and out of sight. For equipment that is too big for removal, avoid using hand-made signs; in advance, you should purchase professionally constructed "out-of-order" signs that can be used when needed. Unfortunately, some members may ignore signage and try to use damaged and potentially dangerous equipment, so it would be wise to seal off the area with the sort of tape used at crime scenes.

Excessive downtime of equipment and facility operations can be avoided with an ounce of prevention strategy. A simple approach to avoid extensive equipment usage delays, budget permitting, is to purchase back-up pulleys and cables to make repairs as quickly as possible (Feldman 1991). Anticipating maintenance needs via the needs analysis can solve many problems before they occur.

One method that has proven effective is setting aside two budgets, one for simple repairs and another for extensive repairs. This budgeting technique can prove vital because monetary concerns are often the major cause for unaddressed repairs. To minimize budgetary repair challenges, company leaders should consider the quality and functionality of the equipment and facilities purchased associated with viable manufacturer warranties and service options that are noted within the legal binding purchasing agreement. This approach can also help avoid displeased members, who can become easily frustrated when equipment is in disrepair.

## Replacement

As an element of facility management, replacement is confined to a program of planned replacement of facility and exercise equipment components. It may include such things as air-conditioning compressors, furnaces or water heaters, or generators. Replacement is performed when the equipment has reached the end of its useful life—when it can no longer perform due to internal damage or its repair is no longer cost effective.

Although replacing a piece of equipment is generally inevitable, it is not without a variety of options. Accordingly, a replacement program should be based on the costs of the equipment, installation, and maintenance. Considering these factors, maintenance managers should analyze the impact of using a different model that is perhaps more expensive initially but requires less repair or energy to operate and is not replaced as often.

For example, there are a couple of treadmill brands that have an initial cost that is two to three times as much as commonly purchased brands, but they are designed to reduce the friction and wear typical of the conventional conveyor belt treadmill. By utilizing a low-friction ball bearing system, coupled with a comfortable slat style running surface, these treadmills lessen the forces to mechanical and electrical parts, resulting in less wear, less maintenance, fewer repairs, lower energy requirements, and longer overall life.

It is always beneficial to stock common replacement parts (i.e., cables, pulleys, belts) to avoid long and frustrating out-of-order delays. Extensive repair delays that are easily correctable and not alleviated in a reasonable time frame can lead to unhappy customers and ultimately a reduction in memberships. In a competitive industry like fitness, you can't risk losing clients, particularly because of factors that can be easily avoided.

## Improvements

Improvement projects enhance the operation of a facility and can possibly reduce the operating costs. These projects may include installing an energy management system to conserve electricity, upgrading an existing pool filter system to improve water clarity, or providing security cameras for members' safety. Many professionals recommend enhancing the aesthetic quality of a facility by incorporating techniques such as landscaping, improved lighting, windows with greater scenic views, and mirrors strategically placed for appearance and training functionality, as well as remodeling lobbies for positive initial impressions. When the maintenance budget makes these aesthetic improvements possible, they can be a good investment (Feldman, 1991).

Many fitness facilities have also enhanced their offerings by adding rooms for personal training, fitness testing, and evaluation; child-care areas, concession snack areas; nutritional counseling centers; specialized aerobic and core stabilization training rooms; and retail shops in an effort to upgrade their facilities as well as provide better service to their members. Each improvement can have a positive impact if effectively implemented and maintained.

The age of the facility and the equipment already in place dictates other maintenance projects, but improvement projects are often initiated by the operations manager or general manager. Although the initial cost of an improvement project may appear high, the long-term results should always reflect a cost savings to the facility or an increased perceived value to members.

## Utilities

The maintenance areas previously discussed generally involve on-site labor. However, complex and extensive utility work often calls for skilled laborers from utility companies or independent electrical or plumbing contractors. Utilities work includes electrical power, water, gas, collection and disposal of sewage and other wastes, and disposal of storm water. These utilities should be periodically assessed, if possible, to avoid serious facility damage and personal injuries. Upgrades should be implemented to improve the safety, maintenance schedule, and function of the facility.

Municipal utility companies usually provide utilities for health and fitness settings smaller than 34,000 square feet (3,159 square meters). In this instance, the involvement of a maintenance manager is minimal. For most small to midsize facilities, utility responsibilities are limited to verifying monthly bills and calling the utility company when service is interrupted or repairs are required.

However, in settings larger than 85,000 square feet (7,897 square meters), the involvement of a full-time operations manager is a necessity. Some facilities have full electrical generating equipment, boilers for heat distribution, and even a small sewage treatment plant. Such systems become mini facilities within themselves, requiring attention around the clock. These systems are a large investment and contribute substantially to the operating cost of a facility.

## FOUR AREAS OF MAINTENANCE MANAGEMENT

When discussing maintenance management, there are four areas on which managers should focus to ensure a successful facility operation:

- *Safety.* All equipment in the facility must always be in top working order. Club managers cannot afford to take risks when their members' safety is involved. Fitness facility professionals should strictly observe and evaluate areas of potential liability (especially wet areas, weight rooms, swimming pools, the day care, and the restaurant). Preventive maintenance is the preferred method for enhancing member safety. Waiting until after an accident occurs to address a problem is expensive—and unethical.

- *Quality.* The difference between quality facilities and lesser facilities is noticeable. Consider all features of the facility from the ground up—floor surface; carpet; mirrors; heating, ventilation, and air-conditioning (HVAC) equipment; wall surfaces; lighting; decor, and so on. In addition to looking good, facilities must be durable enough to withstand the test of time. The old adage "You get what you pay for" is true where facility quality is concerned.

- *Cleanliness.* The daily maintenance of a club must be thorough and consistent. A facility maintenance program should take into account such things as after-hours cleaning, locker-room maintenance, prime-time cleaning, special events, parties, and outdoor maintenance. Each area has unique needs in terms of workers, maintenance regimens, and supplies. The maintenance program should be specific about the desired maintenance needs, communicate those needs to proper staff members, and provide adequate supervision to ensure that those needs are met.

- *Amenities.* The extras involved in serving members' needs are considered amenities. These items include towels, swimsuit plastic bags, hangers in lockers, and personal toiletries (e.g., shampoo, conditioner, shaving cream, deodorant, body lotion, hair spray). You will need to understand your members' needs to determine the appropriate level of amenities and the most cost-effective way to provide them.

Members' perception of quality is often dictated by the details. A smart manager never downplays the importance of the little things. Often these differences provide the subtle touches necessary to separate an organization from its competition.

## *The Bottom Line*

Continual review of these four areas ensures that you always maintain a level of excellence. The implementation of these four primary areas can demonstrate the values of the organization to the public and help gain a competitive advantage.

## DETERMINING MAINTENANCE NEEDS

Establishing and refining a facility maintenance program should be a goal of every manager. Because fitness facilities vary quite a bit in design, the scope of maintenance needs varies. The facility requirements for a full-service, multipurpose fitness facility differ significantly from those of a corporate club in an office building. Facilities of 10,000 square feet (929 square meters) do not have the same maintenance needs as facilities of 75,000 square feet (6,968 square meters). For example, large multipurpose facilities allocate approximately 7% of their total expenses to maintenance and repairs, whereas smaller facilities budget half of that amount. Larger facilities generally have both indoor and outdoor maintenance considerations, whereas smaller facilities have predominately indoor needs. Larger facilities typically need to use both contract workers and in-house employees, whereas smaller facilities usually rely on in-house personnel (Rice 1995).

Although there are many differences related to such size, you can apply the same process for determining the required maintenance in any setting—commercial, corporate, community, or clinical.

Developing a maintenance program starts with a **strategic plan**. Everyone would agree that a maintenance program is necessary; the question is what you are willing to commit to implement the program. How much money will it cost? Will you use additional personnel or contract labor? Should maintenance be performed after hours or only during the workday? These are questions that you must address during the early stages of organizing a maintenance program. The manager must also consider insurance risks, workforce, payroll, supplies, and facility scheduling.

Fried (2005), Ray (2000), and Patton, Grantham, Gerson, and Gettman (1989) have reinforced that an effective strategic management plan is a four-step, repetitive process that involves

1. assessing needs and interests,
2. planning the program,
3. implementing the program, and
4. evaluating the program to ensure that goals are being met.

The cycling or repetitive process is what makes this plan so effective. For example, as you implement and evaluate a maintenance program in the third and fourth stages, you collect information on how to improve for future planning. This cycling allows you to use information obtained from an initial program to design a new and improved model of maintenance. The manager then continues through the four stages of the follow-up program. The four-stage management process is illustrated in figure 14.1.

## The Bottom Line

The cycling or repetitive process yields not only effectiveness but also efficiency. The information seen in the early stages greatly enhances the fitness manager's ability to improve future planning based on a repeatable process.

## PERFORMING A NEEDS ASSESSMENT

The first stage in developing a facility maintenance program is to perform a **needs assessment** to evaluate the facility. You need a clear understanding of the size and scope of the organization in order to adequately assess maintenance needs. Greenwood and Greenwood (2000) recommend developing a professional multidisciplinary team whose members represent relevant areas of expertise to assist in strategizing and identifying specific facility assessment needs. This team could include the following experts: fitness facility administrator, architect and contractor with fitness facility experience, legal consultant, staff members, and select club members who represent various client populations (i.e., age groups, genders, fitness levels). A member of the team may also come from a service company that maintains equipment on a contractual basis and is aware of servicing problems that managers frequently overlook.

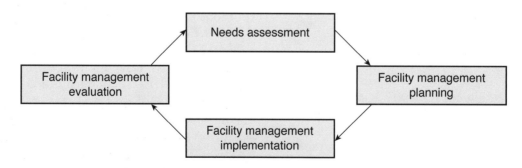

**Figure 14.1** Four-stage management process.

The needs assessment should revolve around program goals and objectives for the populations that are served; it should also take into account the future direction of the industry. Following are practical examples of pertinent questions that can be included in a facility needs analysis; answers should be derived from qualified professionals representing the multidisciplinary team.

- What is the overall size of the facility and grounds?
  - Determine the size of the facility by measuring each room and activity area in order to obtain total square footage or by referring to construction plans.
  - If outdoor maintenance is required, establish the acreage or square footage of the grounds and determine the specific uses for the area.
  - Note whether the facility is enclosed in one building or separated into multiple complexes.
- What are the hours of operation?
  - List the number of days per week the facility is open and the operating hours.
  - Indicate how holiday scheduling is handled.
  - Identify the best times of the day to perform maintenance.
  - List the times of day you consider peak usage times.
- What is the operating budget for maintenance?
  - The setting (corporate, commercial, clinical, or community) generally dictates the availability of funds.
  - If using in-house personnel, consider payroll, payroll taxes, supplies, and capital costs (maintenance equipment).
  - If contracting an outside service, obtain bids and determine a monthly charge for the service.
  - Weigh the costs of including a mix of contract labor and in-house personnel.
- How many members do you serve?
  - Determine the average number of members who use the facility daily.

- Which days of the week are the busiest?
- Indicate whether weekends are a slower time for usage than weekdays or vice versa.
- What is the availability of staff?
  - Determine whether any in-house staff can perform maintenance tasks in addition to their other job responsibilities.
  - Decide how you will divide the daytime and evening maintenance shifts.
  - If a combination of staff and outside services is being considered, decide how maintenance responsibilities will be divided.
- What are the mechanical aspects of the facility? Become familiar with the following areas:
  - Pools' mechanical areas (e.g., filters, heaters, pumps, chlorinators)
  - Spas' mechanical areas (e.g., filters, heaters, pumps, chlorinators)
  - HVAC systems
  - Boiler rooms
  - Water control systems and shut-off valves
  - Electrical panels as well as grounded electrical outlets
  - Lighting systems throughout the facility
  - Security and energy management systems
  - Emergency sprinkler and lighting systems

Whether using in-house personnel or contracting with an outside cleaning service, the next step in the needs assessment is to establish itemized cleaning and maintenance specifications for each room and activity area. Outline a detailed description of the nightly, daily, and weekly tasks for the complex. Give additional consideration to special-use areas that require specific maintenance and cleaning treatments. For example, a locker room's various cabinet finishes and floor surfaces (e.g., carpet, tile, and marble) all have certain requirements for proper cleaning. Address each area before contract workers or in-house employees begin a regular maintenance schedule. Figure 14.2 provides a sample cleaning task and checklist.

If you are considering using in-house cleaning staff, the next step after compiling the task list is to develop a list of supplies, supply vendors, and equipment (e.g., carpet cleaners, pool vacuum

# SUPERVISOR WORK ASSIGNMENT

General duties: Supervisors are responsible for seeing that all shift personnel are in proper uniform and that the uniforms are clean and worn neatly. Also, supervisors will review daily the accuracy and integrity of staff time cards.

| Position | Duties | Frequency or time |
|---|---|---|
| Laundry | 1. All equipment is clean and operating properly. | [        ] Hourly |
| | 2. Each washer is no more than 3/4 full. | [        ] Hourly |
| | 3. Each dryer is loaded to the bottom of the dryer window. | [        ] Hourly |
| | 4. Towels are folded and stacked with round ends together. | [        ] Hourly |
| | 5. Room is clean and neat. | [        ] Hourly |
| | 6. Lint traps are cleaned. | [        ] Hourly |
| | 7. Washers and dryers are never left unattended during operation. | [        ] Every 2 hours |
| Locker rooms | 1. Shelves are stacked with clean towels. | [        ] Hourly |
| | 2. Soiled towels are in bins for return to the laundry. | [        ] Every 1/2 hour |
| | 3. Vanity toiletries have been stocked; sink tops, bowls, and drains have been cleaned. | [        ] Every 1/2 hour |
| | 4. Soap and shampoo dispensers have been cleaned and filled and are working. | [        ] Hourly |
| | 5. All mirrors have been cleaned; lightbulbs are working. | [        ] Every 2 hours |
| | 6. Large and small wastebaskets are no more than 2/3 full. | [        ] Hourly |
| | 7. Carpets have been swept or vacuumed. | [        ] As needed. |
| | 8. Saunas and whirlpools have clean towels, papers, and cups. Each is set to the proper temperature. | [        ] Hourly |
| | 9. All hair dryers are clean and working. | [        ] Hourly |
| Housekeeping | 1. Large and small wastebaskets in lounge and bar have been emptied. | [        ] Hourly |
| | 2. Club manager's office and accountant's office have been vacuumed; trash has been emptied. | [        ] Before 9 a.m. |
| | 3. Exterior property is free of all trash. | [        ] Before 9 a.m. and 4 p.m. |
| | 4. Public bathrooms are clean and neat; supplies have been filled. | [        ] Hourly |
| | 5. Fourth-floor locker rooms are maintained. (See steps 1-6 in locker rooms section.) | [        ] Hourly |
| | 6. All vinyl floor surfaces are spot cleaned as needed. | [        ] Hourly |
| | 7. Lounge area is free of paper, cups; carpet is spot cleaned as needed. | [        ] Hourly |
| | 8. Stairways and walls are spot cleaned as needed. | [        ] Hourly |
| | 9. Nursery trash has been emptied and toilet cleaned. | [        ] Before end of shift |

**Figure 14.2**   Sample work assignment for supervisor.

From M. Bates, M.J. Spezzano, and G. Danhoff, *Health Fitness Management*, 3rd ed. (Champaign, IL: Human Kinetics, 2020).

systems, automatic scrubbers) that would be used. This step allows managers to become familiar with the various types of chemicals available, how they should be applied, and problematic interactions with other chemicals. This step will also introduce managers to working with supply vendors.

After completing the needs assessment, perform data analysis to define where the organization is currently and where it should be in the future. The answers you obtain from the needs assessment provide a road map to follow while implementing the program. The analysis provides answers to such questions as the following: Is the facility large enough to justify the cost of contracting for maintenance services, or should in-house personnel be used? Does the number of members served daily support both a daytime and evening housekeeping crew? Does the number of mechanical and electrical systems validate the need for a full-time operations manager? Is the operating budget large enough to support the maintenance needs of the organization?

During the needs assessment, managers must keep in mind that every facility is unique. Factors such as the existing facility layout, equipment placement, wall partitions and barriers, types of furniture and fixtures, and local and state regulatory statutes are some areas to consider when establishing a maintenance program. These factors play an important role in determining which direction to follow when assessing the various cleaning and maintenance options available.

## *The Bottom Line*

The needs assessment provides a clear path to follow when implementing the program. Also, the assessment guides the manager in making informed decisions regarding the best option or solutions available.

## PLANNING THE FACILITY MAINTENANCE PROGRAM

Maintenance planning uses the information derived from the needs assessment. Understanding the scope of cleaning and maintenance requirements for the facility allows managers the opportunity to choose the option best suited for the club. Without incorporating the needs assessment, it is difficult to establish goals and objectives for the maintenance division. Maintenance goals vary considerably depending on the intended use of the facility. See the Maintenance Goals and Objectives sidebar later in this chapter.

The goal statement defines the direction for the maintenance effort and should indicate the intensity of effort required. For example, if a goal states that the locker rooms are to consistently meet the maintenance standards established by management, then this should be emphasized to the people responsible for cleaning that area. For goals to be effective, they must be enforced with specific objectives. These objectives should address the various components of the entire maintenance program.

Housekeeping – Ensure that all locker-room facilities are cleaned at least once every 20 minutes. Fitness equipment should be cleaned and sanitized at least four to five times within operating hours and thoroughly maintained after operating hours in order to prepare for the demands of the next business day.

General maintenance – Promptly respond to and repair any discrepancies or deficiencies in facility operations.

Preventive maintenance – Establish a program of routine inspection and service of exercise equipment to prevent premature failures. Have a backup plan to avoid unnecessary breakdowns and repair delays.

Repairs – Complete 90% of all repair work within 1 to 3 weeks of notification, depending on the nature of the repair.

Replacement – Establish a program of planned replacement that replaces failing equipment with new or rebuilt components.

Improvements – Identify and conduct any improvement project that will pay back the initial investment within 3 years or less.

Utilities – Identify and immediately respond to any and all utility problems in order to avoid serious consequences and to improve the safety, maintenance schedule, and function of the facility.

## Maintenance Goals and Objectives

Following are some typical maintenance goals and objectives for fitness facilities.

### Overall Maintenance Goal

To provide economical maintenance and housekeeping services that allow the facility to be safely used for its intended purpose.

### Specific Maintenance Objectives

- Perform daily housekeeping and cleaning to maintain a presentable and attractive facility.
- Promptly respond to and repair minor deficiencies in the facility or equipment.
- Develop and implement a system of regularly scheduled maintenance to prevent premature failure of the facility, its systems, and its equipment.
- Operate the facility utilities in the most economical manner while providing necessary reliability.
- Provide rapid, easy, and complete reporting and identification of necessary repairs and maintenance work.
- Maintain proper quantities of materials and spare parts to support timely repairs.
- Accurately track and record the costs of all maintenance work.
- Perform cost bidding to ensure lowest-cost solutions to maintenance problems.
- Monitor the progress of all maintenance work.
- Maintain historical data concerning the facility, mechanical systems, and exercise equipment.

## PERSONNEL

Maintaining a safe, clean, and well-kept facility is vital for success in the fitness industry, but it is only one piece of the puzzle. One relevant area that is often overlooked is hiring staff members who are certified by reputable professional organizations. Depending upon the certification earned, this process can have many positive benefits regarding the overall professional knowledge base of qualified staff members. However, as discussed in chapter 13, it must be remembered that "certified" does not always mean "qualified!"

One benefit of hiring qualified fitness professionals is the training they often have regarding facility and equipment maintenance. According to Greenwood (2000, 2004), people who attain professional fitness certifications are often required to learn about the following areas:

- Facility layout and scheduling
- Facility design
- Equipment layout (organization, spacing, and placement)
- Staff-to-client ratios
- Maintaining, repairing, and cleaning facility equipment

## Staffing

A principal function of maintenance planning is to list the primary maintenance categories and identify whose responsibility each is. In some cases, the operating manager is responsible for all facets of the facility; in other cases, responsibility is shared with outside vendors or contract personnel. For example, in a corporate fitness setting, the housekeeping and repair work could be the responsibility of the landlord of the building or the corporation. In a commercial setting, the operations manager may be in charge of all the subdivisions. Identify responsibilities for each maintenance category before evaluating staff options or establishing job descriptions.

If given the option, managers should have on-site, qualified maintenance staff available. There is great security in knowing that a quick response is available for any maintenance problem. How-

## Interview With Dennis Jurkiewicz

Dennis Jurkiewicz has been the owner of Muscle & Wrench Fitness Equipment Service Inc. since 1990. In addition to the refurbishing and sale of exercise equipment, his company is well known for providing preventive maintenance service contracts to fitness facilities throughout the state of Florida. Each Muscle & Wrench facility owner has over 25 years of experience in the industry, and employees are factory-trained and authorized service and repair professionals for major brands of equipment such as Star Trac, Precor, Life Fitness, Cybex, Freemotion, Power Plate, Technogym, Nautilus, and Paramount. His service contracts represent agreements to conduct regularly scheduled visits to inspect, clean, calibrate, adjust, and test fitness equipment.

**Interviewer:** What kinds of fitness facilities and size facilities do you service?

**Mr. Jurkiewicz:** Approximately 90% of our work is with commercial facilities of all sizes; however, we also service community recreational facilities, corporations, hospitals, hotels, country clubs, and resorts.

**Interviewer:** What are the benefits of having a preventive maintenance agreement with a business such as yours?

**Mr. Jurkiewicz:** Most importantly to maintain the safe operation of exercise equipment; additionally, to protect an equipment's warranty by fulfilling maintenance requirements, to protect a facility's substantial investment by extending the life of the product, to prevent downtime and customer complaints, to protect the users of the equipment, to maintain a clean and safe facility and ensure a positive workout experience, to provide a detailed accounting of the history of the maintenance and repairs of equipment, and to meet the safety requirements of insurance companies.

**Interviewer:** What type of work is performed during preventive maintenance visits?

**Mr. Jurkiewicz:** With cardio equipment, which composes about 80% of our work, typically an inspection of mechanical and electrical parts along with the cleaning and adjusting of the entire product. With strength training equipment, an inspection of moving parts such as cables, belts, chains, and pulleys along with the security of pull-pins on seats and weight stacks.

**Interviewer:** What type of scheduling do you recommend for typical aerobic equipment such as treadmills, ellipticals, and exercycles? What about spinning bikes—are they exposed to more abuse and require more frequent inspections?

**Mr. Jurkiewicz:** Typically, visits are scheduled on a monthly, bimonthly, quarterly, or biannual basis, depending on the needs of the facility. Obviously, the more use, the greater the frequency of inspections and service. Most commercial facilities should have their aerobic equipment inspected and serviced on a monthly basis. Regarding spinning bikes, due to the regular and rough wear, these bikes should be inspected daily by instructors and at least monthly by a service contractor.

*(continued)*

**Interview with Dennis Jurkiewicz** (continued)

> **Interviewer:** What do you consider to be the most potentially dangerous piece of strength training equipment if not properly maintained?
>
> **Mr. Jurkiewicz:** Those pieces of equipment with which the user is pulling, such as seated rowing devices and lat pulldown machines. Probably the most frequent litigations related to strength training equipment are with the lat pulldown when frayed cables break, attachments to the weight stack become disengaged, unauthorized bars weighing more than the top weight plate are attached, and S hooks rather than gated snap hooks are used, allowing bars to fall on clients.
>
> **Interviewer:** What are the consequences of not performing regular preventive maintenance?
>
> **Mr. Jurkiewicz:** The life expectancy of equipment is minimized, thereby reducing the value of one's investment. Additionally, facility appearance will become undesirable to clients, increased downtime will create customer dissatisfaction and complaints, there will be the creation of unnecessary and preventable repairs, there will be the loss of warranty coverage, and there will be an increase in member exposure to risk of injury, heightening the possibility of litigation.
>
> **Interviewer:** What is your greatest frustration in servicing fitness facilities?
>
> **Mr. Jurkiewicz:** Probably the fact that in order to save money, many owners or managers do not schedule frequent enough inspection and service visits, which in the long run costs them more money.

ever, smaller facilities might find that financial limitations dictate that fitness staff or front-desk attendants may have to assist with maintenance responsibilities. Although not preferred, if supervised and scheduled properly, this approach can accomplish the necessary housekeeping goals. This option should always be weighed against the possible negative effect on customer service and the maintenance standards established for the facility.

Based on the needs, goals, and objectives of the facility, a maintenance program of a particular size and scope will emerge. In general, there is a correlation between the size of the facility and the size of the maintenance program, because a larger facility will have both greater maintenance needs and more resources to effectively accommodate those needs. In 2006, IHRSA conducted an industrial survey regarding size categories of commercial fitness facilities. The following information was compiled from the survey:

- Average multipurpose facility = 96,530 square feet (8,968 square meters)
- Average large facility = 140,000 square feet (13,006 square meters)
- Average small facility = 9,611 square feet (893 square meters)
- Average of all clubs = 57,355 square feet (5,328 square meters)

Because there is a great deal of variation in facility design, square footage alone may not be the best way to categorize a fitness by size. Select professional organizations such as the ACSM recommend that facility size be determined based on the membership numbers (Tharrett and Peterson 2012):

Fitness facilities = 10 square feet (0.9 square meters) to 14 square feet (1.3 square meters) per member

## Large Facilities

Large health and fitness centers often have several divisions and use full-time maintenance personnel. The operations director or facility manager is generally a skilled person with a mechanical background and previous experience in facility management. The facility manager answers directly to the manager of the club and has a support staff available for both daytime and evening maintenance. This manager's overall responsibility is to coordinate the direct effort of the maintenance division. Internal personnel, often referred to as *locker-room attendants*, handle daytime housekeeping responsibilities. Primary duties of a locker-room attendant include keeping the locker room clean and sanitized, providing general facility maintenance, and performing laundry tasks. Either a contract maintenance service or an in-house staff with a supervisor conducts evening housekeeping. In some cases, independent contract services are hired on retainer to maintain HVAC, boiler, or pool systems.

Maintenance personnel in a large setting generally have regular duties and have the workforce to perform preventive maintenance. As a result, they can prevent or quickly repair many mechanical problems. This benefit is not always available to midsize and small clubs, which may end up spending most of their days putting out fires. The maintenance portion of an organizational chart for a large fitness organization is shown in figure 14.3.

## Midsize Facilities

Although the maintenance needs are lesser in a midsize setting, the basic elements of control and execution that apply to a large facility still exist. Overall maintenance responsibilities usually belong to a maintenance supervisor who has knowledge of various mechanical systems. The maintenance supervisor is sometimes assisted by either a part-time or full-time employee who performs minor repairs and equipment upkeep. Because housekeeping is a major portion of the work, locker-room attendants or service-desk personnel are regularly scheduled to complete assigned tasks around the high-usage areas of the facility. Evening housekeeping is performed by either a contract maintenance service or an in-

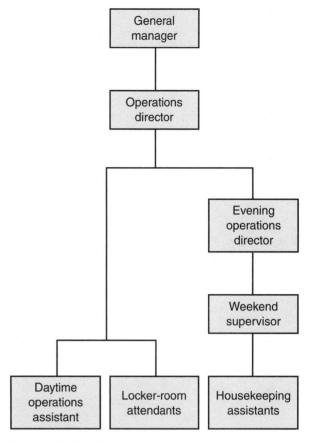

**Figure 14.3** Sample organizational chart for a large fitness facility.

house crew with a supervisor. Service contractors are brought in to perform major repairs, such as plumbing, HVAC, and electrical work.

Operations in a midsize maintenance organization are less structured than those of a large organization. More time is spent on emergency responses and repairing minor equipment problems than modifying and improving the facility. Communication is a primary consideration for midsize maintenance. Consequently, key members of the maintenance staff usually carry walkie-talkies, pagers, or cell phones to alert staff of problems in a timely fashion. Figure 14.4 illustrates the maintenance structure of a midsize facility.

## Small Facilities

In small organizations, generally only one or two people are exclusively dedicated to maintenance.

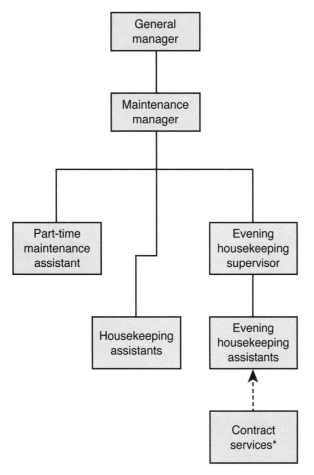

*Either contract or in-house staff

**Figure 14.4** Sample organizational chart for a midsize fitness facility.

The maintenance worker, a jack-of-all-trades, works directly for the general manager and is responsible for all maintenance duties. Housekeeping is handled internally, with personnel from across the organization involved in the daytime cleaning. In the evening, housekeeping duties are performed by the whole staff before closing, or designated employees are assigned to complete more rigorous cleaning tasks. A small facility uses contract services more than a midsize facility. In small facilities, the major system components (plumbing, HVAC, electrical) are repaired almost exclusively by service contractors. The organizational chart in figure 14.5 illustrates the maintenance for a small club.

The three classes of maintenance management (large, midsize, and small) can be adapted to fit most facility needs. The reasons for choosing to conduct maintenance internally are plentiful—better control, scheduling flexibility, ability to define specific duties, quick response to emergency maintenance tasks, and possible financial savings (Williams 1994). However, if conditions are not favorable for hiring an internal staff, consider contracting for maintenance services.

# Contracting for Maintenance Services

In the commercial health and fitness industry, **contract maintenance** is often used for services such as evening housekeeping, general repair and preventive maintenance of equipment (both exercise and mechanical), lawn care, computer maintenance, and pool maintenance. Although these services are used as needed, rarely does a facility manager contract all maintenance work to an outside service. Consequently, it is not uncommon to have a mix of in-house and contracted services. An analysis of the needs assessment and the cost comparisons of all the options suggests the best direction to follow. There are, however, several factors that may make an independent contractor more advantageous than in-house employees:

- Specialization allows higher productivity.
- Expensive servicing and diagnostic equipment would not need to be purchased.
- The contractor's spare-parts inventory can ensure quicker repair times.
- There is no need to provide employee benefits.

Make the choice between hiring in-house employees and contracting for services based on several factors:

- *Frequency of need.* Certain maintenance actions are necessary only infrequently or seasonally. For example, the routine inspection and preventive maintenance for HVAC systems requires a skilled technician; few facilities have the number of HVAC systems to justify a full-time worker. You

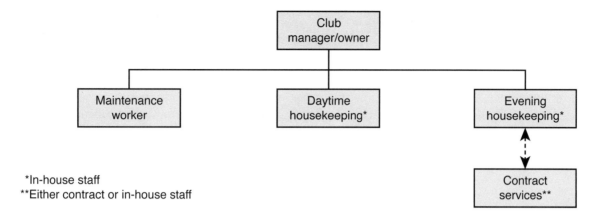

*In-house staff
**Either contract or in-house staff

**Figure 14.5** Sample organizational chart for a small fitness facility.

may reduce or control maintenance costs by identifying these infrequent maintenance activities and considering the cost of contracted services.

• *Qualifications of in-house personnel.* Depending on the complexity of the mechanical equipment, having qualified personnel may be essential. The sophistication of some systems may require the contract services of specialists. State and local regulations may require a particular level of qualification and licensing for certain work. If in-house personnel do not possess or cannot obtain such certifications, you should contract for these services.

• *Workload and staff balancing.* A dilemma occurs when some maintenance work can be performed by in-house personnel but there is only enough work to justify part-time employment. It may be possible to combine several of these tasks to justify the employment of a single maintenance person. Creating a full-time job by combining tasks provides the desired flexibility and responsiveness for emergency maintenance needs. However, you should cover overflow work with a contract service or through authorized overtime rather than adding a potentially underused employee to the payroll.

• *Other cost considerations.* Adding a maintenance employee to the payroll requires assuming the cost of providing benefits to an additional employee. These benefits commonly include health insurance, workers' compensation insur-

ance, retirement plans, bonuses, paid vacations, and several other benefits. Even if there is justification to use in-house maintenance personnel, the added cost of providing full benefits may be too expensive. In the unskilled trades (housekeeping, security, child care), the cost of contracted services is often less than the total cost of wages and benefits combined.

In a corporate fitness setting, maintenance is generally contracted through a service provided by either the building landlord or the corporation. Because the facility is housed on company grounds, this maintenance arrangement is usually the only option available. Unfortunately, this method does not always ensure a well-maintained and clean atmosphere. The maintenance standards for a fitness facility are much higher than for an office building. Regular facility usage by clients throughout the day necessitates continual housekeeping and maintenance repair. Periodic cleaning by a building maintenance crew is both impractical and inefficient. Consider identifying the areas that need emphasis and renegotiating with the company for additional maintenance services.

The maintenance arrangement for a clinical setting is similar to that for a corporate facility. If the facility is on the hospital campus, the wellness or fitness center usually contracts with the hospital maintenance staff for housekeeping and general repair. Because the cleaning standards and consistent housekeeping requirements for a

## Fitness Facility Maintenance Guidelines

Depending on the type of facility, there are usually several options offered by specialists who have expertise in maintaining a fitness facility, especially cleaning and providing preventative maintenance on the fitness equipment. Further, many leading manufacturers and service providers offer on- or off-site training for staff members who have some maintenance responsibilities. These services or training opportunities may be included in the overall purchase price, or there may be an additional maintenance fee required to continue the maintenance support and training.

hospital are much higher, this system has proven to be more effective than in the corporate setting. Facilities that are off the hospital campus have the option of entering into a contractual arrangement with an outside service or hiring personnel for maintenance and housekeeping needs.

Community fitness facilities have the same options available as commercial settings. They may choose to enter a contractual arrangement with an outside cleaning service, hire their own maintenance and housekeeping personnel, or use a combination of both options. Some community settings can contract cleaning services already being used by the city to perform evening cleaning duties. During the day most community centers use a limited maintenance staff and in-house personnel to accomplish all maintenance and housekeeping needs.

## IMPLEMENTING A MAINTENANCE PROGRAM

Implementing any program involves five steps (Fried 2005; Patton et al. 1986; Ray 2000):

1. Reviewing the planned objectives for the program
2. Reviewing the planned tasks for the staff
3. Delegating the tasks to the staff
4. Scheduling the tasks for action
5. Supervising the program implementation to ensure tasks are accomplished

This model assumes that the needs assessment has been analyzed, goals and objectives have been identified, staff or contract labor have been hired, and the maintenance plan is ready to be implemented.

An integral part of implementing a maintenance program is to identify functions that facilitate the maintenance work. These functions assist in identifying and coordinating the daily tasks and ensure that the proper level of maintenance is being sustained. Such functions include

- work identification;
- scheduling;
- purchasing, supplies, and inventory control;
- cost controls;
- equipment and mechanical histories; and
- work tracking and monitoring.

These functions may not be present in every health and fitness setting. Depending on size and scope, some managers may choose to implement only a few of the functions, whereas others may fully integrate all the functions mentioned. Regardless of the setting, management personnel should become familiar with each function and understand how to implement it if deemed necessary.

## Work Identification

All maintenance work has a point of origin. Preventive maintenance, for example, is scheduled in advance to prevent equipment breakdown or to meet seasonal needs, such as switching from heat to air conditioning. Housekeeping is a regularly scheduled activity. However, general maintenance and repair work are not scheduled until someone notices a problem and reports it to the maintenance staff. In the case of preventive maintenance and the daily rounds of equipment checks, the staff should log any problems they notice. Implement a formal reporting system to identify needed repairs. Many facilities have found that adopting a work-order request form successfully allows staff and members to report maintenance or equipment problems. (See figure 14.6 for the sample maintenance service request form.) The form should provide space for the following information:

- *What:* A concise statement of the problem. There is sometimes the tendency to request specific actions or solutions rather than stating the problem.

- *Where:* The location of the problem. Depending on the size of the facility, this may include the name of the specific area where the problem has occurred or any other necessary information to enable the maintenance worker to locate the problem.

- *Who:* The name and phone number of the member or employee making the request. (The maintenance staff uses this to obtain further information on the problem and to let the member know when work has been completed.)

- *When:* The date and time that the request was made. (The maintenance staff will later fill in follow-up information regarding when the repairs were made, who completed the repairs, and how long it took to fix. They

should also include estimated or actual repair costs to assist the bookkeeping department in tracking overall repair charges.)

These work-order forms are usually placed at strategic points (check-in desk, membership office, locker rooms) around a facility where members or employees can quickly and conveniently report any repair work needed.

# Scheduling

Because maintenance involves both planned (preventive maintenance and housekeeping) and unplanned (repairs) elements, the manager must be able to schedule maintenance accordingly. Typically, it is necessary to provide scheduled staff for the planned jobs while maintaining flexibility for unforeseen problems. Develop fixed schedules to cover such areas as preventive maintenance and housekeeping, and identify tasks with a corresponding time goal for completion. Anticipate time intervals for the unexpected repair work as well. Developing historical data for the time it takes to perform various tasks is the only way to prepare a realistic schedule. Depending on the size of the facility, the manager may use daily time logs to track work completion. Figure 14.7 provides a sample maintenance schedule.

## REQUEST FOR MAINTENANCE SERVICES

| Description of requested services | | |
|---|---|---|
| Location | Work requested by | Phone |
| Date submitted | Request priority (please circle one) | A Immediate attention<br>B Urgent attention<br>C Routine attention |
| **Below portion to be completed by maintenance division** | | |
| Special instructions | | |
| Date completed | Completed by | Time to complete |
| Remarks | | |
| Repair costs | | |

**Figure 14.6** Sample maintenance service request form.

From M. Bates, M.J. Spezzano, and G. Danhoff, *Health Fitness Management*, 3rd ed. (Champaign, IL: Human Kinetics, 2020).

## TUESDAY EVENING CLEANING SHIFT ASSIGNED TO HOUSEKEEPING SUPERVISOR

| Time | Facility area |
| --- | --- |
| 6:00 p.m. - 6:30 p.m. | Clean administrative offices, tennis entry and walk, and lower hallway |
| 6:30 p.m. - 8:00 p.m. | Continuously walk through facility to correct problem areas; provide special attention to rear hallways, employee entrance, and rear stairways |
| 8:00 p.m. - 9:00 p.m. | Clean aerobic studio and transition area |
| 9:00 p.m. - 9:30 p.m. | Clean day care |
| 9:30 p.m. - 10:00 p.m. | Meal break |
| 10:00 p.m. - 10:30 p.m. | Clean fitness and membership offices; place vacuum in pool |
| 10:30 p.m. - 12:30 a.m. | Sweep designated indoor tennis courts (see schedule) |
| 12:30 a.m. - 1:00 a.m. | Empty trash cans on all tennis courts and pick up loose trash around courts |
| 1:00 a.m. - 2:00 a.m. | Clean gymnasium floor, floor molding, backboards, and water fountains; spot clean all racquetball courts, clean glass, and dust mop all wood floors; remove vacuum from pool |
| 2:00 a.m. - 2:15 a.m. | Walk through the entire facility to check for problem areas; check and lock all entry doors; set security alarm |
| | **HOUSEKEEPING ASSISTANT EVENING SCHEDULE** |
| 8:00 p.m. - 11:00 p.m. | Walk through the entire facility to check for problem areas; check and lock all entry doors; set security alarm |
| 11:00 p.m. - 11:30 p.m. | Break time |
| 11:30 p.m. - 2:30 a.m. | Clean assigned areas per housekeeping guidelines |
| | **LAUNDRY ASSISTANT EVENING SCHEDULE** |
| 10:30 p.m. - 2:30 a.m. | Launder all soiled towels and member laundry; return clean laundry to the front desk |

**Figure 14.7**    Sample cleaning shift assigned to housekeeping supervisor.

## Work Tracking and Monitoring

It is important to ensure that all work is completed in a timely manner. Establish internal procedures to alert management or operations personnel of all maintenance problems. Use a corresponding system to ensure quick turnaround of all repairs and to inform the member of expected completion time. If you do not accomplish member-identified minor repairs in a reasonable amount of time, the member may decide that it is useless to report minor problems. If minor problems are not reported, they could lead to major problems. Consequently, the tracking system must be timely and complete.

As noted earlier, most facilities use a work-order form to track member-identified repairs or problem areas. Once the work is completed, the work-request forms are recorded and filed for future reference.

### The Bottom Line

Because forgotten preventive maintenance or neglected repair work can lead to costly repairs, facility downtime, or potential injury, use a system for tracking the source, assignment, and accomplishment of all work.

## Purchasing, Supplies, and Inventory Control

As routine maintenance work is carried out, there is a constant need for materials and supplies to sustain the work being performed. This necessitates a system for predicting needs and for purchasing and inventorying materials and supplies. Routine preventive maintenance requires a predictable type and quantity of materials. Because of their unpredictable nature, repairs may cause interruptions to facility operations if parts are not readily available.

A **purchase order system** is commonly used for ordering supplies and materials. The purpose of a purchase order system is to account for all maintenance items ordered and received. A purchase order describes what specific supplies need to be ordered, the estimated cost, what vendor you are using, bids from various vendors, who is ordering the supplies, and management authorization (see figure 14.8). Each order is given a number and

## PURCHASE ORDER

Date: _____　Date Needed: _____

Name: _____　Dept.: _____

Vendor: _____

| Item | Item no. | Quantity | Price | Page |
|------|----------|----------|-------|------|
|      |          |          |       |      |
|      |          |          |       |      |
|      |          |          |       |      |
|      |          |          |       |      |
|      |          |          |       |      |
|      |          |          |       |      |

Date ordered: _____

_____

_____

### For Office Use Only

Date Ordered: _____ PO No.: _____ Vendor No.: _____

Invoice No.: _____

| Amount | G/L code | G/L no. |
|--------|----------|---------|
|        |          |         |
|        |          |         |

Obtained from general supplies: _____ Yes _____ No

If yes, which ones? _____

**Figure 14.8**　Sample purchase order.

From M. Bates, M.J. Spezzano, and G. Danhoff, *Health Fitness Management*, 3rd ed. (Champaign, IL: Human Kinetics, 2020).

filled out in duplicate, with one copy given to the employee who initiated the order and one given to the bookkeeper or accounting department who then submits the copy order to the vendor. If the amount of the order is higher than a prearranged limit, approval must be obtained by management before initiating the order. When the supplies arrive, the purchase order and vendor invoice are matched before acceptance. Only a system of this nature can provide accountability against cost overruns and unnecessary supplies being ordered (Feldman 1991).

The level of inventory control needed depends on the size of the inventory. In most health and fitness settings, the maintenance workforce is small, the facility systems are simple, and the numbers of renovation projects are minimal. Consequently, the facility manager or maintenance person can keep a mental inventory of supplies and spare parts. More complex facilities must have a formal system for monitoring the inventory of consumables (e.g., toilet paper, facial tissues, paper towels).

You can set up this inventory manually using index cards in a file. (When an order is received, the quantity of new materials is added to the index card. When products are expended, the quantity used is subtracted from the card.) However, most inventory systems are currently handled by computers. One advantage of a computer inventory system is that it can automatically generate purchase orders for inventory items when the stock level reaches a designated low point.

If you regularly update the inventory and there is sufficient security for the stored materials, you can rely on it to depict the inventory status. Make one person responsible for issuing purchasing orders, maintaining the number entry, and verifying management's approval of the purchase.

## Cost Controls

Although most health and fitness organizations have an accounting system that monitors accounts payable and receivable (see chapter 12), it is ultimately the responsibility of the maintenance manager to identify and code all supplies and materials used. Without this interaction between accounting and maintenance, it would be difficult to do cost breakdowns for the divisions (e.g., fitness, tennis, day care, pro shop, restaurant). Main-

tenance managers must have a system (manual or computer) to account for the maintenance transactions that occurred during the day.

The purpose of cost accounting is to measure the ongoing and historical costs of each maintenance activity. From this measurement, the maintenance manager can make decisions to redirect or reallocate resources to reduce possible cost overruns. For example, excessive overtime costs might lead to hiring or reassigning additional full-time personnel. The maintenance manager also needs to monitor and manage the annual budget to meet financial goals. Consequently, timely reporting of ongoing costs is essential.

## Equipment and Mechanical Histories

To properly predict and adjust the maintenance program, the manager must have a thorough understanding of the particular facility and its components. Only with a total building history can you make proper decisions regarding the best course of maintenance for a given problem. Keep accurate documentation of all construction and renovation plans. Track major and recurring minor repairs. Record periodic inspections by the health department, OSHA, and the fire department and update them for future reference. Accurate facility records enable immediate troubleshooting and repairs.

A proper equipment history should include the make and model of the equipment, date of installation, all major repairs, any preventive maintenance, and parts replaced. You can use this equipment history to predict the need for eventual replacement or rebuilding of a unit or to diagnose an unexpected problem, which can often be traced to a recent repair. Regarding exercise equipment, there should be a filing system for all equipment manuals; both the maintenance personnel and the fitness instructors should have access to these manuals. See figure 14.9 for a sample card.

## EVALUATING FACILITY MAINTENANCE

In the implementation phase of the management process, managers ensure that the system established for maintenance care is well orga-

# EQUIPMENT HISTORY CARD

| Equipment name | | |
|---|---|---|
| Manufacturer | | Model no. |
| Equipment location | | Specific installation area |
| Date of original installation | | Installed by |
| Equipment repair history | | |
| Date | Description | Repair costs |
| | | |

**Figure 14.9** Sample history card for equipment.

From M. Bates, M.J. Spezzano, and G. Danhoff, *Health Fitness Management,* 3rd ed. (Champaign, IL: Human Kinetics, 2020).

## Advances in Monitoring and Managing Fitness Equipment

Several leading fitness equipment manufacturers now offer commercial health clubs and facilities the ability to monitor their cardiovascular equipment that is connected to the internet. This real-time equipment management system allows health club owners and managers the ability to monitor usage patterns to assist with equipment rotation to maximize the product's life. Also, the equipment management system can be used to generate customized reports that can be used to manage future purchasing decisions. One of the main features of the equipment management system is the ability to communicate via email with the service provider when the equipment needs to be serviced. Please keep in mind the weakness or disadvantage of using this management system is its inability to communicate directly with nonelectronic features, and most importantly, strength training equipment. The next time you're looking for cardiovascular equipment, check with the company representative about whether the equipment can be connected to a real-time equipment management system, because that feature just may improve your equipment maintenance program.

nized, properly staffed, and within the financial parameters authorized by management. The only way to ensure this outcome is through an internally developed set of goals and objectives. By regularly reviewing and updating these goals and objectives, facility managers will always be able to assess whether the maintenance program is producing the intended results.

Once the implementation phase is initiated, the ongoing evaluation process begins. Patton and colleagues (1989) include two steps in the evaluation phase: process evaluation and outcome evaluation. Evaluation involves analyzing the implementation tasks that were assigned to the staff to determine whether the maintenance tasks are being accomplished (process evaluation) and whether the objectives of the maintenance program are being met (outcome evaluation). Figure 14.10 summarizes the process and outcome techniques.

Schedule periodic meetings with staff to review the maintenance process and address strategies to maintain or improve current procedures. Staff should maintain careful work-order records detailing when the work was completed, how long it took to complete, what materials were used, and who performed the work. Maintenance software programs are now available to tabulate work-order data and assist in inventory management.

An innovative program called **benchmarking** has recently been introduced into the health and fitness market. Benchmarking is the process of measuring services, supplies, and practices against competitors, similar facilities, or industry standards. This practice began as a means to improve worker performance and productivity in large corporations, and only recently has it been introduced into the health and fitness market. Benchmarking involves reviewing the existing operation, looking at other operations, selecting

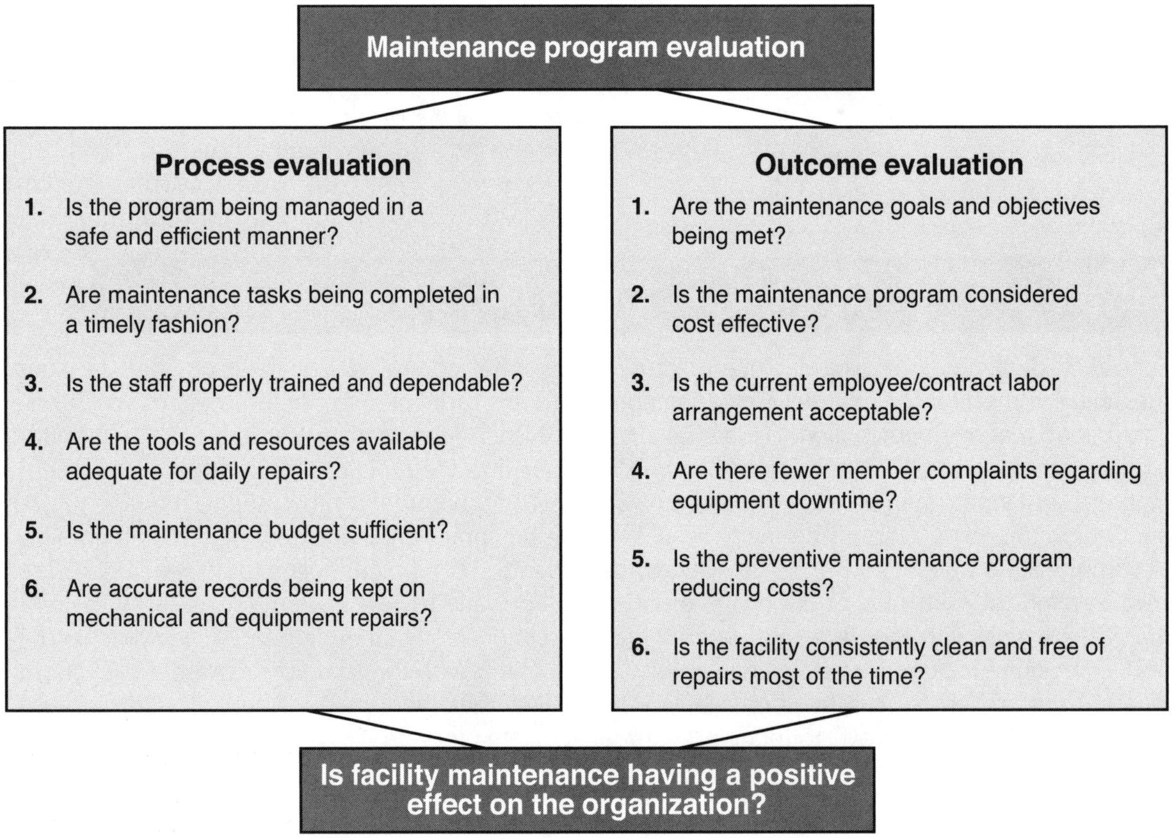

**Maintenance program evaluation**

**Process evaluation**

1. Is the program being managed in a safe and efficient manner?

2. Are maintenance tasks being completed in a timely fashion?

3. Is the staff properly trained and dependable?

4. Are the tools and resources available adequate for daily repairs?

5. Is the maintenance budget sufficient?

6. Are accurate records being kept on mechanical and equipment repairs?

**Outcome evaluation**

1. Are the maintenance goals and objectives being met?

2. Is the maintenance program considered cost effective?

3. Is the current employee/contract labor arrangement acceptable?

4. Are there fewer member complaints regarding equipment downtime?

5. Is the preventive maintenance program reducing costs?

6. Is the facility consistently clean and free of repairs most of the time?

**Is facility maintenance having a positive effect on the organization?**

**Figure 14.10** Maintenance process and outcome techniques.

the best practices, and incorporating them into the current operations.

Begin benchmarking by analyzing the existing facility and identifying areas to benchmark. Second, determine the methods of data collection. Finally, identify comparative clubs or facilities. Because benchmarking is relatively new to the health and fitness business, no industry standards exist specifically for facility maintenance. However, there are national statistics reported annually by *Cleaning and Maintenance Management* magazine and the Cleaning Management Institute for all types of facilities nationwide (e.g., hospitals, schools, hotels). You can use a number of categories from this survey to compare the average facility against an existing setting. Some areas to consider benchmarking might include the following:

- Estimated annual cleaning costs per square foot—annual cleaning budget divided by the square footage of the facility
- Wage rates—average hourly rates for shift supervisors, average cleaning worker, and starting cleaning worker
- Maintenance spending per facility—estimated costs for chemicals, paper products, powered cleaning equipment, and nonpowered equipment (e.g., mops, brooms)
- Staff time allotment for common tasks—percentage of total annual cleaning work hours spent by staff in such areas as floor care, vacuuming, other carpet cleaning, locker-room care, trash collection, dusting, and other tasks
- Total annual cleaning budget—total cleaning budget compared with similar fitness settings of the same approximate size

It is impossible to improve what you do not measure. Measuring productivity does not always have to entail a sophisticated system. You can establish categories to provide baseline parameters that communicate the overall performance of the maintenance division. These categories could include weekly towel counts, number of work orders completed each week, and number of emergency response calls completed each week.

A system of this nature provides an objective means for determining maintenance effectiveness. Many maintenance supervisors use their own judgment to decide what is best. However, this method of evaluation is too subjective and does not always provide a definitive means for measuring performance.

## The Bottom Line

Evaluating a maintenance program is different from evaluating an activity program that has a beginning and ending point. Facility maintenance is dynamic and continual and must be reviewed at regular intervals. Perform any changes or modifications to an existing maintenance program daily rather than waiting for an appropriate time. Benchmarking assists managers and maintenance personnel in evaluating overall performance and justifying time and expenses.

## DEVELOPING A PREVENTIVE MAINTENANCE PROGRAM

Once the maintenance program is operating efficiently, organize and implement a preventive maintenance program. The amount of funds invested in mechanical, electrical, and exercise equipment certainly justifies the costs of maintaining the equipment so it is safe and operational. In the health and fitness business, the cost of waiting until a system malfunctions is not worth the outcome, especially in light of increasing litigation.

Regarding litigation, an area that is frequently overlooked is the preventive maintenance of amenities such as whirlpools, steam rooms, and saunas. The previous chapter discussed the concerning lack of supervision of these areas and the resulting litigation risk. The potential for litigation may also arise when these amenities are not properly maintained. Whirlpools, steam rooms, and sauna baths are all subject to bacterial contamination that can cause numerous ailments, some of which may be life threatening.

The goal of any preventive maintenance program is to ensure the continuous operation of facility systems (HVAC, boilers, pool heaters, fire alarm, security systems) and equipment (cardiorespiratory equipment, strength equipment, computers). An organized preventive maintenance program facilitates continued operation—either through the completion of work that keeps equipment operating or through the identification of substandard performance, faulty parts, or equipment failure.

You can categorize each preventive maintenance action according to how it reduces or avoids costs to the facility operation.

- *Maintain operations.* The most obvious justification for preventive maintenance is to maintain facility operations. The continued operation of a facility directly relates to the preventive maintenance tasks performed to ensure equipment reliability. Some systems' functionality has a higher priority than other systems. For example, failure of the club's water heater could disable operations, whereas failure of a pool or spa water heater may not completely impede usage but might result in disgruntled member feedback.

- *Lengthen service life.* Many preventive maintenance procedures are designed to ensure that a piece of equipment will not fail prematurely. Most equipment is designed for a specific service life. The duration of operation depends on timely servicing throughout the use of the equipment.

- *Identify worn-out equipment.* Because exercise equipment does not always perform like new, you should implement a system to monitor its gradual deterioration. Planning specific preventive maintenance tasks to detect any subtle changes and to alert maintenance personnel to major changes in equipment performance is highly recommended. Regular preventive maintenance will reduce overall costs if you catch mechanical problems early enough to detect signs of premature equipment failure.

- *Prevent loss.* Certain installed systems exist to protect members and personnel within the facility. For example, a malfunctioning fire alarm system has no effect on the facility operation until there is a fire. Preventive maintenance performed on this equipment is justified because it prevents losses involving members, employees, and the facility.

- *Ensure personal safety.* Regularly maintain any system or piece of equipment within a club that is installed to prevent bodily injury or possible death to members. Protective systems such as exit signs, fire alarms, and emergency lighting are required by local building codes or city standards. Preventive maintenance for these systems is a necessity and the maintenance costs are unavoidable.

- *Protect facility.* Some systems are installed to protect physical property. Sprinkler systems and burglar alarms reduce the risk of property loss and reduce insurance premiums. For these reasons, the staff should perform maintenance even if the insurance policy doesn't require proof of maintenance for these systems.

- *Comply with government standards.* Numerous aspects of a facility must meet local, state, and federal standards. For example, swimming pool water must meet local health department regulations. Steam-room boilers must meet emission control standards to satisfy insurance companies. According to OSHA requirements, paint or potentially explosive materials cannot be stored next to electrical panels. In each case, the existing equipment must be maintained to perform at the levels required. Failure to comply with these ordinances will result in discipline that could range from verbal warnings to closure of the facility.

Initiating a preventive maintenance program begins with identifying those areas that have the greatest impact on the facility if not maintained. Examine each system and classify each piece of equipment as to its level of importance in facility operations. Those items that are critical to safe and continued operation of the facility receive high priority.

A primary source for identifying preventive maintenance tasks is the manufacturer recommendations. Companies that produce cardiorespiratory or strength equipment provide a user's manual specifying recommended service frequency and procedures. Any warranties provided with such equipment usually depend on completion of recommended preventive maintenance. Table 14.1 provides a preventive maintenance schedule for a StairMaster CrossRobics machine.

Once you determine the need for preventive maintenance for a system or piece of equipment, establish the procedures to provide that preventive maintenance task. Develop a **preventive maintenance order (PMO)**, a form that acts as more than just a how-to guide. Properly prepared, it describes the physical actions of performing the maintenance. The PMO is a planning document and a safety document. It provides assistance in ordering parts, and you can use it as an inspection and feedback tool. Although PMO forms have never been standardized and many variations exist, the basic components of the form are equipment data, location, tools and materials required, safety procedures, maintenance procedures, and work completion data.

**Table 14.1**    Preventive Maintenance Schedule for the StairMaster Crossrobics 1650 LE

| Part | Recommended action | Frequency | Cleaner | Lubricant |
|---|---|---|---|---|
| Plastic side cover (exterior only) | Clean | Daily | Soap and water or diluted cleaner | N/A |
| Seat | Clean | Daily | Soap and water or diluted cleaner | N/A |
| Console | Clean | Daily | Water | N/A |
| Weight stack belt and connectors | Inspect | Weekly or every 70 hours | N/A | N/A |
| Pedal arm return springs | Inspect, clean, and relubricate | Weekly or every 70 hours | Degreaser | Oil-dampened rag |
| Alternator and drive belts | Check tension and inspect for wear | Weekly or every 70 hours | Degreaser | 30W motor oil |
| | Remove, clean, and lubricate | Every 3 months or 900 hours | Degreaser | 30W motor oil |
| Guide rods | Clean and lubricate | Weekly or every 70 hours | Window cleaner | Silicone spray |
| Drive shaft and hub assembly | Grease | Every 3 months or 900 hours | N/A | Heavy multipurpose grease |
| Bottom stop sprint | Wipe clean and grease | Every 3 months or 900 hours | N/A | Heavy multipurpose grease |

Each time preventive maintenance is to be performed on a system or piece of equipment, staff should prepare a PMO and forward it to the person administering the job. Once the work is completed, return the PMO to either the club manager or the maintenance supervisor. Pay close attention to any comments the worker makes that might initiate further investigation. File the completed order and establish a date for the next PMO for that piece of equipment. Record the date of the next scheduled preventive maintenance either manually or in a computer database (Tatum 1995). Figure 14.11 shows a completed PMO.

Periodically evaluate the preventive maintenance program to determine its effectiveness. Measure the effectiveness by the performance of the facility and equipment and by the cost of the program. Address the following questions:

- Is the program running efficiently, or is preventive maintenance being forgotten or ignored?
- Has the number of maintenance request orders been reduced on those items receiving preventive maintenance?
- Have parts and equipment supply costs been reduced?

- Have there been fewer calls for outside repair workers?
- Have any equipment failures been the result of inadequate preventive maintenance?

## The Bottom Line

Preventive maintenance tasks are performed whenever the financial impact of failure to perform the activity exceeds the cost of its performance. For example, the cost of maintaining an air-conditioning system often outweighs the cost of periodically replacing condensers or complete systems. As membership surveys have shown, member satisfaction—and thus the success of the facility—relies heavily on the numerous components of a maintenance program and how it is managed. When the four-step strategic plan of assessment, program planning, implementation, and evaluation is understood and practiced, member satisfaction is almost always guaranteed.

## COMPLETED PREVENTIVE MAINTENANCE ORDER FORM

| Equipment name | Model no. | Serial no. | Manufacturer |
|---|---|---|---|
| _Concept II Rower_ | _None_ | _16897523_ | _Concept II Inc._ |

| Frequency:    daily    weekly    monthly    quarterly    annual | | | |
|---|---|---|---|

| Location | Other location information | | |
|---|---|---|---|
| _Cardio room_ | _Unit next to window_ | | |

| Tools required | _Wrench_ | | |
|---|---|---|---|
| | _Screwdriver_ | | |
| | _Pliers_ | | |

| Materials required | _1 lubricant tube_ | | |
|---|---|---|---|
| | _1 nonabrasive scouring pad_ | | |
| | _1 set of foot straps_ | | |

| Safety procedures | _Watch tension on chain after cleaning_ | | |
|---|---|---|---|

| Maintenance procedures | _Clean monorail with nonabrasive scouring pad—daily_ | | |
|---|---|---|---|
| | _Clean and lubricate chain—weekly_ | | |
| | _Check cord tension—weekly_ | | |
| | _Check chain for stiff links—monthly_ | | |
| | _Check tightness of all nuts and bolts—monthly_ | | |

| Date completed | Completed by | Time to complete | |
|---|---|---|---|
| _9/12_ | _Jared MacLemore_ | _2 hours_ | |

| Remarks: _Emphasis placed on completing any and all maintenance and equipment repairs during typical downtimes or before/after facility open hours to avoid interfering with client usage. A 2-hour completion time frame on this assignment was very acceptable and appreciated by staff and member clients._ |
|---|

**Figure 14.11**    Sample of a completed preventive maintenance order form.

## Key Terms

benchmarking

contract maintenance

needs assessment

preventive maintenance

preventive maintenance order (PMO)

purchase order system

strategic plan

# Understanding Legal and Insurance Issues

*John Wolohan*

## Learning Objectives

After studying this chapter, you will be able to

- identify the legal duty that health and fitness providers owe their clients,
- discuss the tort of negligence and its defenses,
- recognize potential danger areas in health and fitness clubs,
- explain the importance of contract law to health and fitness providers,
- understand the implications of employment law in managing employees, and
- discuss the importance of insurance to clubs.

The local health and fitness center operates a summer baseball camp. During the camp's lunch break one day, one of the participants, J.T., sustained a permanent eye injury when he was struck by a wood chip thrown by another student. The injury happened not on the baseball field but in one of the facility's courtyards. As a result of the injury, J.T.'s parents filed a claim of negligence against the center on behalf of their minor son.

In its legal defense, the center argued that the waiver contained in the camp's online enrollment form, which had been filled out and signed by J.T.'s mother, insulated it from liability. The form stated that the campers "agree to assume all liability with regard to the activities that make up the school."

Consider the following questions as though you were on the jury.

- Did the fitness center's negligence cause J.T.'s injury?
- Are there any defenses?
- Is the waiver valid?
- What impact, if any, does J.T.'s age have on the case?
- Does it matter that being hit by a wood chip is not a normal risk in baseball?

It is essential that health and fitness managers have at least a basic understanding of certain legal principles and how they relate to managing and operating a facility. After reading this chapter, managers should be able to identify and evaluate the risks involved in operating a health and fitness facility and determine when to obtain formal legal advice from competent counsel. In order to assist in identifying potential liability, a Legal Liability Checklist is included later in this chapter. Please note that the checklist is not intended to cover every legal area but to provide a framework for identifying major areas of risk.

Although the purpose of this chapter is to provide health and fitness managers with a basic understanding of the law, it is not meant to take the place of an attorney. Managers must seek competent legal counsel for periodic review of any documents or contracts used by the organization and for help with any legal questions that may arise.

# CIVIL VERSUS CRIMINAL LIABILITY

The difference between **civil liability** and **criminal liability** lies in the interests affected and in the remedy afforded (Keeton et al. 1984). In criminal law, a crime has been committed against society, and the state (as the protector of society) is responsible for bringing any criminal prosecution. The purpose of criminal law, therefore, is to protect society by punishing antisocial behavior. Civil cases, on the other hand, are filed by the injured party with the primary purpose of recovering money damages against the person who caused the harm. The purpose of civil cases, therefore, is to compensate the injured party by the payment of money. Even though the same action can give rise to both criminal and civil liabilities, a tort or civil wrong is legally not a crime.

For example, if during a basketball game, one of the players intentionally punched another player and caused physical injury, the injured party could file a civil lawsuit (tort of battery) to recover any damages, such as medical costs, pain and suffering, and lost wages. In addition, the state could also file a separate criminal complaint, resulting in jail or probation.

# TORT LAW

Generally, a **tort** is a private or civil wrong, other than a breach of contract, committed upon a person or property as the result of another person's conduct. The three main areas of tort law that health and fitness managers need to be aware of are negligence, intentional torts, and reckless misconduct.

## Negligence

The most common tort in the health and fitness industry is **negligence**. Negligence is an unintentional tort. Negligence cases are based on the legal theory that people are required to act in a way that avoids creating an unreasonable risk to others (Schubert, Smith, and Trentadue 1986). Therefore, any conduct or action that falls below a certain standard and creates an unreasonable risk is considered negligence.

In order to establish a claim of negligence, a person must establish all four of the following elements:

- Duty of care
- Breach of duty
- Causation
- Damages

**Duty of care** refers to the standard of care the law has established for the protection of others (Schubert, Smith, and Trentadue 1986). In determining whether one person owes another a duty of care, there needs to be a special relationship between the parties. Some examples of relationships in a health and fitness setting that create a legal duty of care include employer to employee; employee to guest or member; and instructor, coach, or trainer to student.

The law of negligence does not require that you ensure the safety of every person using the facility from every conceivable injury; it merely requires that you do not create an unreasonable risk and that you protect people from risks that are foreseeable. If the risk is not foreseeable, there is no liability. In determining whether someone breached his or her duty of care and created an unreasonable risk of injury, the courts use what is known as a *reasonable person test*. The reason-

## Legal Liability Checklist

☐ Do professional staff members have appropriate credentials?

☐ Are all staff CPR certified?

☐ Are adequate staff available in the exercise and activity areas?

☐ Do all new members go through a thorough orientation program?

☐ Is a standard health and fitness screening protocol used to check for certain medical conditions?

☐ Are safety notices clearly posted on or near all equipment?

☐ Are all public areas regularly inspected for unsafe conditions?

☐ Is all equipment inspected regularly?

☐ Is a standard procedure in place to respond to discovery of unsafe equipment or dangerous conditions?

☐ Are safety inspection records documented and kept current?

☐ Has the equipment layout been evaluated to determine safety concerns related to location and arrangement?

☐ Are internal and external lighting adequate to ensure safety?

☐ Does the facility have a written emergency plan available for review?

☐ Does the facility have adequate first aid supplies that are checked and refreshed regularly?

☐ Are all activity areas free from environmental hazards?

☐ Does the organization have written personnel policies that are available to all employees?

☐ Has the organization provided training for all staff in the areas of discrimination and harassment?

☐ Does management have clear procedures for responding to and documenting violations of personnel policy?

☐ Do all staff participate in safety training and review sessions for emergency procedures?

☐ Is a formal policy in place for making statements on behalf of the organization?

---

able person test examines whether a reasonable, prudent person in the same circumstances would have acted in the same manner. If someone fails to act in a way that a reasonable, prudent person would act in the same circumstances, that person is deemed to have breached the duty of care.

The standard of care is based on the qualifications or certification of a prudent professional in that industry, not on the individual's professional experience. Everyone, no matter how experienced or inexperienced, must meet the same standard of care. In determining the appropriate standard of care for the health and fitness industry, it is important to look at the guidelines developed and published by the AHA, ACSM, American Medical Association (AMA), and American Physical Therapy Association (APTA). Where appropriate, these standards should be incorporated into the written policies of the organization, including employee manuals, job descriptions, and training procedures.

Once injured parties are able to establish that the defendant breached his or her duty of care, they still must show that the conduct actually caused the injury. **Causation** is established when there is a causal connection between the negligent conduct and the injury.

The final element of any negligence claim is **damages**—the person must suffer some form of injury or harm for which he or she should be compensated. In awarding damages, the court will look at lost wages, pain and suffering, and medical expenses. In extreme cases, the court can also award punitive damages, which are designed to punish the party that caused the injury. If there is no injury or harm done, there is no liability.

## The Bottom Line

Negligence, the most common tort in the health and fitness industry, is based on the legal theory that people are required to avoid creating an unreasonable risk to others.

## Legal Status of Members and Nonmembers

To determine the duty of care that health and fitness facilities owe people using the facility, the courts examine the relationship between the user and the facility. These relationships can be divided into four groups: invitee, licensee, trespasser, and recreational user (Wolohan 2004).

**Invitees**    An **invitee** is any person whose presence produces a direct or indirect economic gain for the facility operator (Keeton et al. 1984). Members and guests of health and fitness facilities are generally classified as invitees. As a result, club operators have a legal duty or obligation to exercise reasonable care to keep members or guests safe, to protect them from unreasonable risk, and to avoid acts that can create risks. To meet the duty of care, the owner or occupier

- must warn of any known defects on the premises,
- is responsible for any unknown defects that could reasonably be discovered, and
- must make the premises safe and free from such defects or dangers.

The theory behind this rule is that the owner or occupier of the facility is in the best position to discover and control any risks or hazards. It is essential, therefore, that health and fitness man-

agers conduct frequent facility and equipment inspections.

**Licensee**    A licensee is any person who has the permission or consent of the operator to use the facility but provides no real or expected benefit to the facility owner. Unlike with an invitee, the facility owner has no duty or obligation to inspect the premises to discover dangers or to give any warnings of obvious dangers (Keeton et al. 1984).

**Trespasser**    A trespasser is any person who enters the facility without the permission of the operator. Generally, because no consent has been given to use the facility, the only obligation of the facility owner or operator is to refrain from any intentional conduct that would cause injury to the trespasser (Keeton et al. 1984).

**Recreational User**    A **recreational user** is any person who is on the premises specifically for recreational purposes. Generally, the owner's only obligation is to provide a warning of any known concealed danger that would not be apparent to the recreational user. The owner has no duty to warn of open and obvious hazards or of conditions that are unknown to the owner (Wolohan 2004). (For more information on recreational users, see the Immunity section later in this chapter.)

## The Bottom Line

The relationship between the user and the facility determines the duty of care that health and fitness facilities owe to people using the facility.

## Potential Danger Areas

Because providing a safe facility is the responsibility of the possessor or occupier of the property, health and fitness managers must take reasonable steps to protect members from any potential dangers. The following are just some of the potential danger areas.

### Floor Surfaces, Preparations, and Coverings

As stated, because members and guests using a club are invitees, health and fitness managers have an obligation to exercise reasonable care to

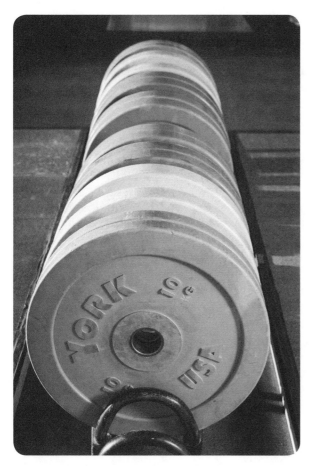

Returning weight plates to weight rack after use is one way to reduce physical hazards in health and fitness clubs.

keep them safe and to protect them from unreasonable risks. As a result of this duty, managers need to provide proper floor surfaces throughout the facility to avoid what are commonly called *slip-and-fall situations*. All slippery, oily, overwaxed, wet, dusty, or damaged floors must be cleaned or repaired to prevent serious falls, collisions, or other injuries.

Ignorance of the defect is not a defense, because facilities have a duty to inspect for dangerous conditions. It is essential that, upon discovering a dangerous situation, the club immediately either correct the condition or limit access to the location until the problem has been corrected.

**Equipment**  Health and fitness managers also have a legal duty to ensure that the equipment used in the facility is safe for its intended purpose. Therefore, it is critical that someone at the facility

visually inspect the equipment on a daily basis and replace or remove any equipment that is in disrepair or defective.

Besides inspecting the equipment, employees must teach members or anyone else using the equipment how to use it. This should be done as part of a new-member orientation, at the conclusion of which new members should sign an acknowledgment that they were provided proper instructions and warnings; the facility should also post the instructions. By posting instructions that are clear, concise, and easily understood in an area that is visible to all users, managers ensure consistent and accurate communication of not only the instructions but also adequate warnings of reasonably foreseeable and known risks.

**Equipment Design or Manufacturing Defects**
Because most, if not all, of the equipment used in a facility is not designed, manufactured, or built by program personnel, liability for injuries due to defective equipment will usually rest with the equipment manufacturers under the theory of product liability. However, even though product liability claims are usually against the manufacturers or sellers of the equipment, health and fitness organizations are not excused from inspecting the equipment, testing it for defects, and replacing any defective parts.

**Fitness Activities**  In addition to providing proper instructions on how to use equipment, facilities also have an obligation to provide adequate supervision during fitness activities and to warn people of any risks associated with an activity. In assessing the type of warnings necessary for a particular activity, managers must assess the nature of the activity and the skills and abilities needed to successfully and safely participate in the activity. For example, if the activity is difficult or potentially dangerous, direct supervision by experienced professionals is required. If, on the other hand, the activity is simple and safe, less direct supervision is required. It is the duty of the person supervising the activity to identify the inherent risks of the activity and warn the participant of these risks.

**Emergency Medical Care**  Another potential problem area is medical care. Generally, health and fitness clubs have a duty to provide timely and reasonable medical assistance. Additionally,

## CASE STUDY

Michael Smith was working out with a friend at the local fitness center. During their workout, the weight machine being used by his friend became jammed. As Michael tried to determine why the metal weight plates were jammed, the weights—approximately 140 pounds—suddenly dislodged and fell on his hand, which he had rested on the weight machine.

Consider the following questions as though you were on the jury.

- What other facts do you need to know to determine whether the fitness center is negligent?

- One of the key factors in the case is whether the fitness center had, or should have had, actual notice of the dangerous condition of the weight machine. How can you determine whether they had notice?

- If the fitness center custodian, who was responsible for cleaning and servicing the equipment, knew that the metal plates on the weight machine could easily become jammed if an accessory weight were improperly placed on the machine, does it matter if the fitness center's supervisor denies having knowledge of any problems with the weight machine prior to the accident?

- If the fitness center conducted regular risk management audits, would this problem have happened?

## CASE STUDY

After suffering an ankle injury, Jaime Gutierrez visited the local fitness facility to work out with an athletic trainer in order to improve his football skills. Kevin Jones, one of your certified athletic trainers, provided Gutierrez with an initial evaluation, which consisted of an interview, measurements, and some performance testing. Jones asked Gutierrez to estimate the maximum amount of weight he could lift while performing certain exercises, including bench press and squat lifts. Because they ran out of time, Jones never had Gutierrez do any squat lifts, even though this was part of a standard evaluation. Additionally, Jones did not ask Gutierrez when he had last exercised, which was important information to consider when designing a workout. He didn't realize, therefore, that Gutierrez had not done any lower-body workouts in the previous 12 weeks because of an ankle injury.

During one of his training sessions, Gutierrez felt a pop and a sharp pain in his lower back while doing a set of squat lifts. When immediately informed of the client's pain, Jones responded "no pain, no gain" and told Gutierrez to push through it. Gutierrez was able to finish the set, during which his pain increased significantly. Gutierrez eventually was diagnosed with a herniated disc in his back, which he had to have surgically repaired.

Consider the following questions as though you were on the jury.

- Is the fitness club negligent for failing to conduct a proper evaluation before designing a workout program for Gutierrez?

- Is the fitness club negligent for instructing Gutierrez to continue to work out after being advised of his back pain during the workout?

- Is the fitness club negligent for failing to discontinue the workout after being advised of Gutierrez's back pain?

they have a duty to refrain from taking any actions that could aggravate the injury. This means that the staff members have to be able to recognize when serious injury has occurred (Wong 2002).

As with supervision, the definition of reasonable medical care depends on the type of activity being performed. In addition, the duty to provide emergency care not only includes caring for injuries once they occur but also preparing for emergency care before the activity. For example, although a club does not need to have an ambulance in the parking lot, it does need to be able to contact one quickly in an emergency situation.

## Legal Documents

One of the best ways to protect your organization in the event of an injury is to keep detailed, written records on everything from facility and equipment repairs and maintenance to injury and treatment reports. In the case of a lawsuit, these records can be vital in demonstrating that the organization acted reasonably.

## Vicarious Liability

The owners and managers of health and fitness facilities need to be aware that under the theory

---

### CASE STUDY

While working out on a stair climber, one of Club XYZ's patrons, Judith Wolohan, suffered a heart attack. Hearing alarmed shouts from the other gym patrons, two employees ran to help Wolohan. One of the employees, who was certified in CPR, observed Wolohan lying on her back, bleeding from a cut on her head and shaking from small convulsions. When the employee knelt down beside her to assess her condition, he felt a faint pulse, which to him indicated a heartbeat. He also noted the red color of Wolohan's face and concluded that Wolohan had an oxygen supply. Based on these observations, he believed that Wolohan was having a seizure or stroke and therefore decided not to attempt CPR, which he believed might make matters worse. He testified that Wolohan had just begun to turn blue when the paramedics arrived.

Upon hearing the call for help, the other employee had instructed the receptionist at the front desk to call 911. It is estimated that it took the EMTs around 3 minutes after receiving the call to arrive, or a total of 4 to 6 minutes from the time the employees heard the cries for help. When the EMTs arrived, they found Wolohan lying on her back, not breathing and without a pulse. The EMTs quickly performed CPR and used a defibrillator to shock Wolohan's heart, but they were unable to reestablish a pulse, and Wolohan was pronounced dead at the hospital.

As a result of her death, Wolohan's estate has filed a wrongful death action against your club. In particular, Wolohan's estate alleges that the club breached its duty to render aid during a medical emergency because the employees failed to administer CPR, the club failed to have an AED on its premises, and the club failed to properly train its employees on how to handle medical emergencies.

Consider the following questions as though you were on the jury.

- Did the club have a legal duty to provide proper medical care to Wolohan?
- If so, why? If not, why not?
- If the club had a duty to render assistance, did it satisfy its duty by summoning professional medical assistance?
- Do clubs have a legal duty to have an AED on their premises?

of **vicarious liability**, they can be held accountable for the negligent actions of the people who work for them. There are three main exceptions to this rule.

- Employers are generally not liable for the negligence of independent contractors, unless they closely supervise the contractor's activities.
- Employers are generally not liable for intentional torts committed by employees.
- Employers are generally not liable for employee conduct that is outside the scope of employment.

## Defenses of Negligence

If someone is injured, a number of defenses are available to clubs. Following are five of the most common defenses:

- Assumption of risk
- Agreements to participate
- Waivers
- Immunity
- Contributory negligence

**Assumption of Risk**    Under the theory of **assumption of risk**, health and fitness managers are not liable for injuries resulting from risks that are inherent to the activity. In order for assumption of risk to apply, a person must voluntarily participate in an activity, knowing the inherent risks involved in an activity or event.

As a general rule, the assumption of risk defense does not apply to minors (children under the age of 18). Although there are limited exceptions to this rule, such as when a minor is highly experienced in the activity, managers should not depend on an assumption of risk defense when working with minors.

**Agreements to Participate**    One way to strengthen the assumption of risk defense is through the use of an agreement to participate. The **agreement to participate**, which is different from a waiver, is a document that helps managers inform participants of the nature of the activity, the risks involved in the activity, and the behaviors expected of the participant (Cotten and Cotten 2004).

**Waivers**    A **waiver** is a written contract between the facility or service provider and a club member or guest in which the person using the facility or services agrees to relinquish the right to pursue legal action in the event of an injury caused by the negligence of the provider.

Though waivers are not valid in Louisiana, and Virginia, in all other states a well-written, prop-

---

## CASE STUDY

During an adult soccer game, Sanjay Patel claimed that after he scored a goal, the goalkeeper from the opposing team charged him and tackled him by sliding into his leg. As a result of the sliding tackle, Patel suffered various injuries, including a broken right leg. Patel claimed that the opposing goalie could have avoided contact with his leg but that the goalie wanted to hit him. Two other people who saw the play, however, claimed that as Patel was striking the soccer ball, the goalie was falling down and sliding simultaneously while trying to grab the ball. As a result of his injuries, Patel sued the state soccer association and the local soccer complex for failing to properly train and properly supervise the officials that they provided to referee the game.

Consider the following questions as though you were on the jury.

- Is the referee negligent for not protecting Patel from injury?
- Does it matter whether Patel had previously complained about the goalie's play?
- What additional facts would be helpful in determining whether the referee was an independent contractor or an employee?
- If the referee is an employee, is the soccer complex liable for Patel's injury?
- If so, why? If not, why not?

erly administered waiver voluntarily signed by an adult is an effective tool in protecting health and fitness facilities and providers from liability for ordinary negligence (Cotton 2017).

The laws in each state are different; however, the following 12 guidelines should be used when developing a waiver (Cotten and Cotten 2004).

- The document should be titled properly: "Waiver" or "Waiver of Liability."
- The font size should be at least 10 point.
- The language should be clear and unambiguous.
- The waiver should be one page.
- The waiver should stand alone and not be part of another document.
- Because the waiver is designed to excuse negligence, the word *negligence* should be used in the document.
- The waiver should not contain any fraudulent statements.
- Because a waiver is a contract, it should state what the signer is receiving, such as "In consideration for waiving the right to sue for negligence, the signer is given the right to use the facility and equipment."
- The waiver should specify the parties covered under the waiver.
- The waiver should contain information covering the inherent risks of activity.
- The waiver should include a statement by which the signer confirms that he or she understands the risks and assumes responsibility for the risks.
- The waiver should include a statement indicating that the signer read the document.

Just as with assumption of risk, in most states, waivers are generally not enforceable with minors. However, because waivers show that the parties were aware of the risks associated with the activity, you should still require minors and their parents to sign waivers before participating in potentially dangerous activities. Likewise, even if you live in a state where waivers are unenforceable due to public policy or other reasons, it can still be useful to have an adult participant sign a waiver.

Just like paper waivers, online or electronic waivers provide health and fitness managers legal protection when a participant is injured due to the facility's negligence. When the sport or recreation provider's form asks participants to click on or check a box to accept the terms of the waiver, the participant has accepted the contract or waiver terms by clicking on the box, and he or she has entered into a legally binding agreement. If you plan to use online or electronic waivers, it is important that you always include a statement concerning which jurisdiction or state laws will apply in the case of a lawsuit. Otherwise, you could find your organization defending a lawsuit in an out-of-state court (Wolohan 2013).

**Immunity** Traditionally, there have been two types of immunity: sovereign immunity, which prevented an injured party from suing the government or its political subdivisions without consent, and charitable immunity, which prevented an injured party from suing charitable organizations. Due to the hardship the immunities caused to the injured people, most states have modified or abolished the two traditional immunities.

Although most states have modified or abolished the two traditional immunities, every state has created another immunity in an effort to make more land available for recreational use. The immunity, called a recreational user statute, is designed to encourage landowners to open their property to the public for recreational use by giving them immunity from liability if someone is injured while on the property for recreation.

Each state has its own variation of the recreational user statute, but most statutes have four common characteristics (Wolohan 2004):

- *Type of property.* Originally, immunity was designed to protect private landowners only. In some states, however, the owners of public lands (i.e., local, state, and federal government agencies) are also afforded immunity.
- *Free use of property.* Landowners cannot charge a fee for people to use the premises.
- *Condition of property.* The land must be unimproved or undeveloped rural land retained in its natural condition.
- *Obligations of the landowner.* The owner's only obligation is to provide a warning for any known concealed danger that would not be apparent to the recreational user.

In addition to recreational user statutes, most states have also enacted volunteer immunity statutes with the goal of protecting people who volunteer with not-for-profit organizations from liability for negligence.

**Contributory Negligence** Under contributory negligence, if the injured person's conduct contributed in any way to the injury, no matter how small, the person is barred from recovering any damages. Due to the injustices caused by the rule, most states have replaced it with comparative negligence. Under comparative negligence, damages are awarded according to the person's degree of negligence or fault. For example, if a person was 5% at fault in the injury, the courts will reduce the amount received in damages by 5%.

Only four states (Alabama, Maryland, North Carolina, and Virginia) and the District of Columbia still use contributory negligence as a valid defense. The rest of the states have adopted a form of comparative negligence either by statute or judicial decisions (Swisher 2011).

## Intentional Torts

**Intentional torts**, as the name implies, arise out of an intentional or willful action. For example, if a club member violently and intentionally strikes another member during an argument, the violent member has committed the intentional tort of battery. The legal remedy is to force the violent member to pay for any damage caused and possibly impose punitive damages to deter the activity from being repeated. Other intentional torts include assault (an apprehension of immediate harm), slander (false and defamatory verbal statements), libel (false and defamatory written statements), fraud (intentionally misleading someone for financial or material gain), false imprisonment (wrongful detention), trespass (unlawful use or injury of property), and conversion (unlawful taking and keeping of property).

## Reckless Misconduct

Although not as common as negligence or intentional torts, the tort of **reckless misconduct** can be important when someone is injured while participating in group activities. For example, if a softball player intentionally slides into another player in an attempt to break up the play, even though sliding is not permitted, that person is said to have acted with reckless disregard for the safety of the other person. The key to any reckless misconduct is that the intentional action must be done in a reckless, willful, or wanton manner, especially if it is in violation of an established and known safety rule. The conduct is not an intentional tort, however, because it is usually performed with no intent to harm or touch.

# CONTRACTS

Health and fitness managers use **contracts** on almost a daily basis. An exhaustive discussion of contract law is well beyond the scope of this brief chapter; this section simply outlines certain essential concepts of contract law.

## Contract Essentials

A contract is "a promise, or set of promises, for breach of which the law gives a remedy, or the performance of which the law in some way recognizes as a duty" (Restatement of Contracts 1979). However, not all promises are contracts, so it is important to understand how a promise is transformed into a legally binding contract. In order for a promise to become a valid contract, it must contain the following five elements:

- Offer
- Acceptance
- Consideration
- Intent
- Legality

An offer is a conditional promise made by one party, the offeror, to another party, the offeree, to do or refrain from doing something in the future (Calamari and Perillo 1998). To be valid, an offer usually must contain the parties involved, the subject matter, the time and place for performance, and the price or consideration to be paid.

In order for the offer to be binding, the offeree must accept the offer. *Acceptance* must be made in some positive form, whether in words or by conduct, and can only be made by the party to whom the offer was made. If an offer has been made and the offeree proposes to change one of the terms, such a counteroffer is considered a rejection of the original offer. In addition, an offer may no longer be accepted by the offeree in circumstances in which the offer has lapsed due to time or has been revoked by the offeror, or when either of the parties dies or loses mental capacity before acceptance (Calamari and Perillo 1998).

The next element of a valid contract is consideration. *Consideration* is the mutual exchange of value that induces a party to enter into a contract and may include money, services, goods, or any other thing of value. Therefore, although the parties may exchange promises, any agreement that does not contain a mutual exchange of value is void for lack of consideration. The final two elements require that all the parties have a genuine *intent* to create an enforceable contract and that the performance involved in the contract is for legal activity or does not violate public policy.

Although technically not a required element for a valid contract, the legal capacity of a person can also affect the enforceability of a contract. For example, the law seeks to protect people who lack the capacity to understand the essential terms of the contract by making such contracts, except for necessaries, voidable at the individual's option (but enforceable by the individual if he or she so chooses). The courts generally consider minors and other people with diminished mental capacity to lack the ability, competence, or capacity to enter into contracts. As a result, minors may often disregard their promises with impunity, as, for example, when a minor signs a waiver agreeing to relinquish the right to pursue legal action against a service provider. As discussed previously, in most circumstances, the waiver will be ineffective in shielding the provider from suit by the minor.

Finally, contracts in general do not need to be in writing to be legally enforceable, but the law does require that certain contracts must always be in writing. The three categories most relevant to health and fitness managers are

- contracts involving the sale, mortgage, or lease of an interest in land (e.g., facility lease agreements, land purchases);
- contracts that cannot be performed within 1 year from the date of their making (e.g., long-term vendor or employment contracts); and
- contracts for the sale of goods for $500 or more.

As a matter of good business practice, managers should put all contracts in writing in order to reduce future problems and misunderstandings over the actual terms of the contract.

## *The Bottom Line*

A contract is a promise that the law recognizes as a duty. However, not all promises are contracts, so it is important to understand what turns a promise into a legally binding contract.

# Types of Contracts

Some of the most common contracts found in the health and fitness industry are membership agreements, waivers and releases, independent contractor agreements, vendor contracts, and employment contracts.

## Membership Agreements

All relationships between a health and fitness organization and its members are based on contracts. This is true whether a written, signed agreement exists or members are merely paying a daily entry fee each time they visit the facility.

Because of the wide range of health and fitness settings, it is difficult to generalize about membership contract requirements. Some states have passed laws requiring fitness clubs to include certain terms related to duration of the contract, cancellation of the contract, refund of deposits, automatic billing of checking accounts and credit cards, and transferability of the contract. Because these laws are enacted at the state level, managers must obtain copies of their state's laws and regulations related to spas, fitness centers, and health clubs.

In general, it is to the mutual benefit of the health and fitness organization and the member to have a clearly worded, complete written agreement that identifies the obligations of the organization and of the member. Examples of issues that a membership contract should address include the following:

- Names and addresses of the parties
- Duration of the contract, with clearly stated starting and ending dates

- Signatures and dates
- Location of the facilities, facility access concerns such as time of day and days of the week, and facility use limitations (e.g., tennis only, cardiorespiratory areas only, classes only)
- Membership fees and terms of payment
- Rights, penalties, and fees associated with cancellation or transferability
- Renewal options
- Direct billing terms for checking accounts or credit cards

In addition, the agreement should contain the following obligations of members:

- Pay amounts due in a timely manner.
- Abide by all rules and regulations.
- Operate the equipment safely and cautiously.

- Notify the staff immediately about any observed unsafe condition, equipment, or practice.
- Notify the staff of any personal health or fitness conditions that affect the member's ability to participate in health or fitness activities, programs, or use of equipment.

The lifeblood of any health and fitness club is its members. However, very few relationships last forever. Therefore, it is not unusual for health and fitness clubs to include some type of termination or liquidated damages clause in their membership agreements. Although the goal of such clauses is to protect the club and to ensure a positive cash flow, health and fitness clubs need to be careful that these clauses are not unfairly punitive and therefore unenforceable.

In trying to determine whether the termination clause imposes an unenforceable penalty under

## CASE STUDY

On October 22, 2013, Nicole Wolf entered into a fitness services agreement with her local fitness club. The agreement entitled Wolf to four personal training sessions per month for a period of 12 months. In exchange for the promised services, Wolf made an initial payment of $170 and agreed to have 11 additional monthly payments of $120 each charged to her credit card. If at any time during the 12 months Wolf wanted to terminate the relationship, the agreement contained this termination clause:

Voluntary Termination: Client may voluntarily terminate this Agreement at any time by doing the following: (1) giving the club 30 days' written notice of cancellation, sent by registered mail, return receipt requested, and (2) paying a fee equal to 50% of the remaining balance as of the notice, in addition to any and all fees incurred, including, but not limited to, any late fees, return fees, collection fees, etc.

Wolf became dissatisfied with the personal training because the trainer did not adequately communicate to her how she should exercise and he missed scheduled personal training appointments. As a result, Wolf cancelled her membership based on what she viewed as poor performance by the club. Because of the club's termination clause, the club charged $660 to Wolf's credit card account. Upon receiving the charge, however, Wolf called to demand a full refund of the $660 fee. The club refused, and Wolf sued to recover her money.

Consider the following questions as though you were on the jury.

- Is the termination clause an unenforceable penalty?
- What impact should the club's own performance or, in this case, nonperformance have on the case?
- Does the termination clause have any relationship to the damages suffered by the club?
- If so, why? If not, why not, and what *would* be reasonable?

state law, one court held that a contract clause is an enforceable liquidated damages provision when (1) the actual damages from a breach are difficult to measure at the time the contract was made and (2) the specified amount of damages is reasonable in light of the anticipated or actual loss caused by the breach. A contract clause is unreasonable and is hence a penalty, the court held, when the amount required to be paid has no relationship to the injury suffered or the gravity of the breach. Put another way, a termination clause is a penalty clause if it specifies the same damages regardless of the severity of the breach or even who is at fault (Wolohan 2011).

## Waivers and Releases

As part of the membership contract—but on a separate, stand-alone form—health and fitness clubs should also require each member, or anyone just using the facility for the day, to sign a waiver. The purpose of the waiver is to expressly waive the member's right to sue the organization for any injury, damage, or loss suffered while on the premises as a result of negligence by the organization or its employees. (See the Defenses of Negligence section earlier in this chapter.)

## Independent Contractors

In order to keep costs low while at the same time providing a wide variety of services, it is essential to use the services of independent contractors. In addition to keeping employee costs down, using independent contractors can also cut down on liability. For example, as long as the organization uses reasonable care in selecting a qualified and competent independent contractor, the legal liability for any injuries that are caused by the independent contractor's ordinary negligence generally shifts from the organization to the independent contractor (Wolohan 2017).

In addition, in the United States the health and fitness organization is not required to pay FICA (Federal Insurance Contributions Act, or Social Security), FUTA (Federal Unemployment Tax Act), or state unemployment taxes on independent contractors. Also, employers do not provide independent contractors health care benefits, retirement benefits, vacation pay, sick-leave pay, or any other employee benefits.

To prevent organizations from classifying everyone as independent contractors and to ensure that employers are paying the appropriate unemployment and social security taxes, the IRS has developed guidelines to help identify who is an employee and who is an independent contractor. As a general rule, however, an individual is an independent contractor if the company for whom the work is being performed has the right to control or direct only the result of the work, and not what will be done or how it will be done. If an organization improperly designates an employee as an independent contractor, it is subject to back taxes, interests, and penalties. For more information go to the IRS website and search the term independent contractors.

## Vendor Contracts

In order to provide a wide range of services, health and fitness organizations are also required to enter into contracts for various services and products. To protect the organization, it is essential that these agreements be in writing. Although most of the agreements will be standard form contracts, managers should feel free to negotiate any of the terms found in the contract. Critical terms in vendor agreements include the rights to terminate the agreement without cause, return unused goods without charge, maintain a nonexclusive relationship that allows the organization to use other products or services, and be indemnified by the vendor for any loss or damage caused by the vendor's services or products.

In some cases, the organization may select a vendor to subcontract operation of one or more membership or operational services. Examples of operations frequently contracted out to vendors include pro shops, food and beverages, vending machines, specialty health services (e.g., massage therapy, health and beauty services, sports medicine services), facility maintenance (e.g., night janitorial services), and towel laundry service. Whenever subcontracting with a vendor, establish written contracts that outline the relationship of the parties.

## Employment Contracts

In most cases, the employer–employee relationship is based on contract law. Whenever one person agrees to work for another person or legal entity in exchange for wages and other benefits, an employment contract is in place. The rights and obligations of the employer and employee are governed by a combination of general contract law and state and federal regulations and statutes. In many states, unless a written employment contract is signed, employment is considered to be **employment at will**. Employment at will means that, absent a discriminatory motive, an employer may terminate an employee at will and without cause. Similarly, the employee is not required to give notice or reasons for quitting and may do so at any time without liability.

Because most employees in the health and fitness industry do not have employment contracts, employee manuals and handbooks take on the added importance of defining the employer–employee relationship. Many organizations require that all new employees sign a document stipulating that they have read or been provided with a copy of the employee handbook. Because of the importance of these issues in determining employer liability, the next section of this chapter reviews the subject matter that an employee handbook should include.

## EMPLOYMENT LAW

There are two distinct areas of employment law (van der Smissen 2004): employment process and workplace environment. Employment law deals with the rights, obligations, and responsibilities within the employer–employee relationship and encompasses issues of wages, workplace safety, discrimination, and wrongful termination.

### Employment Process

The employment process is concerned with fundamental concepts related to the recruitment, selection, and hiring process. Two of the most important items in the employment process are the employee handbook and the personnel policy manual.

**Employee handbooks** are addressed to employees and generally communicate in clear, direct terms the more important policies that govern employment, such as employment benefits, vacation, sick leave, holidays, and grievance and discipline procedures. In addition, hand-

books should also include guidelines defining inappropriate conduct that may result in disciplinary action and list the circumstances under which the company will consider an employee to have voluntarily terminated employment.

The main benefit of an employee handbook is that it informs employees what they may expect of their employer and what the organization expects of them. In the absence of written guidelines, an employer is more likely to encounter problems arising from ignorance of company policies and confusion about what is expected. An employee handbook can help avoid some of these problems.

**Personnel policy manuals** are addressed to managers and personnel professionals who must administer the employer's policies. The manuals not only describe the policies but also designate administration procedures. Personnel policy manuals, therefore, are more comprehensive. They address a larger number of policies, such as background and criminal checks for employees and volunteers, and address each in greater detail. Personnel policy manuals can be accessed by all employees, but they usually are not distributed to each employee.

Developing a personnel policy manual is a detailed and extensive process. Large organizations consider policy manuals necessary to maintain consistency and to ensure compliance. For all employers, personnel policy manuals are a two-edged sword. To the extent that the manual defines standards and procedures for discipline, performance evaluations, and payment of wages and to the extent that these policies and procedures are followed, it can help avoid legal problems. However, if the personnel policy manual is overly complex, not properly distributed, or not enforced, different legal issues and liabilities may arise.

See the Policies to Include in an Employee Handbook sidebar later in this chapter for a list of items that should be included in an employee handbook or personnel policy manual.

### Workplace Environment

In addition to making sure that the environment is safe for club members and guests, health and fitness managers also need to ensure that they do not violate any laws governing the workplace environment. Laws governing the workplace environment include those that deal with dis-

## Policies to Include in an Employee Handbook

- Introduction to the manual
- Equal employment opportunity
- Employment at will
- Orientation and probationary period
- Hours of work, overtime, and payday
- Vacation
- Holidays
- Sick leave
- Other leaves of absence, including disability and family and medical leave
- Internal complaint review procedure
- Termination, discipline, and rules of conduct
- Employee classifications
- Performance and pay review
- Personnel records
- Dress and grooming standards

- Smoking
- Recruitment and selection, employment of relatives, and rehires
- Safety program
- Security and confidential information
- Blood-borne and airborne pathogens in the workplace
- Employee benefits
- Nonfraternization
- Conflicts of interest
- Proof of right to work
- Medical examinations
- Inspections for prohibited materials or substances, including concealed weapons
- Drug-free workplace
- Harassment
- Employee assistance program

crimination, disabilities, sexual harassment, and workplace safety.

## Title VII of the Civil Rights Act of 1964

**Title VII of the Civil Rights Act of 1964,** which applies to organizations with 15 or more employees who are employed for at least 20 weeks a year, prohibits discrimination in employment by making it illegal for an employer "to fail to hire or to discharge an individual, or otherwise discriminate against any individual with respect to compensation, terms, conditions, or privileges of employment, because of such individual's race, color, religion, sex or national origin" (Title VII 2003).

Anyone who believes that he or she has been discriminated against under Title VII should file a claim with the EEOC. The EEOC will investigate all charges and attempt to resolve any disputes. If the discrimination continues and the organiza-

tion will not remedy it, the EEOC has the power to file suit in federal court (Masteralexis 2013).

## Americans with Disabilities Act of 1990

The **Americans with Disabilities Act of 1990 (ADA)** is divided into five sections covering the rights of people with disabilities in the areas of employment, public services, transportation, and telecommunications. Title I of the ADA, which covers employment, provides that "no covered entity shall discriminate against a qualified individual with a disability because of the disability of such individual in regard to job application procedures, the hiring, advancement, or discharge of employees, employee compensation, job training, and other terms, conditions, and privileges of employment" (Americans with Disabilities Act 2003).

Title I covers any organization with 15 or more employees who worked for 20 or more calendar weeks in the current or preceding calendar year.

If that criterion is met, the organization must make reasonable accommodations for any qualified person with a disability. (However, employers only need to do so if providing the reasonable accommodation does not result in undue hardship.) Examples of reasonable accommodation include the following (Hums 2013):

- Making existing facilities reasonably accessible to and usable by people with disabilities
- Job restructuring; part-time or modified work schedules; reassignment to a vacant position; acquisition or modification of equipment or devices; appropriate adjustment or modifications of examinations, training materials, or policies; the provision of qualified readers or interpreters; and other similar accommodations

When an employee's excessive absenteeism or tardiness is related to a disability, the organization may be required to make reasonable accommodations in the form of leave or a modified work schedule. Although *reasonable accommodation* is a term defined by courts, many courts have held that if regular attendance is an essential job component, an organization is not required to accommodate a disabled employee's high rate of unpredictable absences if it would result in an undue hardship. Organizations facing these issues should consult with legal counsel before disciplining a possibly disabled employee for absenteeism or tardiness.

## Age Discrimination in Employment Act of 1967

The **Age Discrimination in Employment Act of 1967 (ADEA)**, which was based on Title VII of the Civil Rights Act of 1964, makes it unlawful "to fail to hire or to discharge an individual, or otherwise discriminate against any individual with respect to compensation, terms, conditions, or privileges of employment, because of such individual's age" (Age Discrimination in Employment Act 2003).

As baby boomers age, ADEA, which covers all employees or potential employees over the age of 40 in the United States, has the potential to become extremely important to health and fitness professionals. However, like Title VII, ADEA applies only to those organizations with 20 or more employees who are employed for at least 20 weeks a year.

For more information on age harassment, see the EEOC website and search the term age harassment.

## Sexual Harassment

Title VII of the Civil Rights Act of 1964 prohibits sex discrimination and sexual harassment. **Sexual harassment** includes any unwelcome sexual advances, requests for sexual favors, or other verbal or physical conduct of a sexual nature imposed on the basis of sex.

There are two theories of sexual harassment: quid pro quo and hostile environment. **Quid pro quo sexual harassment** occurs when a manager grants or withholds employment opportunities or benefits as a result of another person's willingness or refusal to submit to the manager's sexual demands. Because the pressure may be either an explicit or implicit term or condition of the person's employment, the critical point is not whether the victim submits voluntarily but whether the conduct is unwanted.

**Hostile environment sexual harassment** exists when a manager or coworker's conduct

---

### Exceptions to the Law

People with disabilities have also used the ADA with varying degrees of success to force health and fitness facilities to accommodate their disabilities when providing recreational activities. As a general rule, if accommodating a person with a disability does not pose a direct threat to the safety of the other participants or require a fundamental modification of the activity, the organization must accommodate the individual.

For more information on the ADA, see the **U.S. Department of Justice** website at www.ada.gov.

has the purpose or effect of unreasonably interfering with an employee's work performance or when conduct creates an intimidating, hostile, or offensive work environment. Some examples of hostile environment sexual harassment are unwelcome verbal expressions of a sexual nature, including sexual comments about a person's body or dress; the use of sexually degrading language; and jokes, sexually suggestive objects, pictures, videotapes, audio recordings, or literature in the work area that embarrass or offend an individual (Wolohan 1995).

Sexual harassment does not necessarily involve people of different sexes. The U.S. Supreme Court has recognized that an individual of the same sex as the victim can be guilty of creating a hostile environment of sexual harassment, as long as the harassment is motivated by the victim's sex (Wolohan 1995).

To discourage such behavior and to protect the organization from costly lawsuits, all health and fitness organizations should proactively take the following steps:

1. Include a sexual harassment policy in all employee handbooks and make sure that the policy clearly communicates to employees that sexual harassment will not be tolerated and that no retaliation will be permitted against employees who file a complaint.

2. Provide all employees with sexual harassment training.

3. Establish an effective complaint or grievance process that encourages all employees to report any incident to an appropriate manager. To be safe, and to ensure that the person doing the harassing is not the person who receives the complaint, employees should be offered two different sources for reporting sexual harassment complaints.

4. Immediately review and investigate all complaints as thoroughly and confidentially as possible. If the facts are discovered to be true, the offending employee's relationship with the organization should be terminated.

For more information on sexual harassment, see the EEOC website and search the term sexual harassment.

## Employee Safety

The health and safety of all employees are regulated by OSHA. The areas affected by OSHA regulations include injury and illness records, employee safety posters, posting of signs, bloodborne pathogens, written plans and training, personal protective equipment, safety equipment, electrical safety, toilet facilities, regular inspections, housekeeping, safety conditions, emergency evacuations, machine guarding, hazard communication, and chemicals (van der Smissen 2004).

For more information on workplace safety, see the OSHA website and search the term health and safety regulations, www.osha.gov/pls/publications/publication.html.

## *The Bottom Line*

Health and fitness clubs must not only ensure a safe environment for club members and guests but also ensure that they do not violate any laws governing the workplace environment.

## INSURANCE CONSIDERATIONS

A health and fitness facility can present a number of potentially dangerous conditions for members, guests, and personnel. An environment with cardiorespiratory and weight training equipment, a locker room with showers, a sauna or steam room, and a pool all possess the potential for accidents and injuries. Combine these facilities with a clientele comprising men and women of every age range, fitness level, and health status, and the potential for injury seems almost endless.

The easiest way to protect yourself and your organization from the legal liability and financial loss associated with these risks is through insurance. Insurance allows the facility to trade the potentially devastating financial risk of a future loss for the cost certainty of a monthly or yearly payment (premium).

## Determining Insurance Needs

Because insurance is a vital part of any risk management plan, it is essential that the facility take the time to determine its specific insurance needs. The first step in determining insurance needs is identifying the potential risks within the facility. For example, if the facility has a pool, the potential risks include someone drowning or slipping and falling. Once the risks are identified, the next step involves analyzing the potential risks and weighing them against any potential financial loss. Using the pool example again, either type of incident could result in a lawsuit and potentially substantial financial losses, so it would be in the best interest of the club to obtain insurance, thereby transferring the risk of such losses to the insurance company.

In examining your insurance needs, it is important to not only identify potential problem areas in the facility but also evaluate all the programs, activities, and equipment used in the facility. Identifying and evaluating everything will ensure that proper coverage is given to the entire facility and help guard against possible gaps in the policy.

In addition, insurance policies should be tailored to the individual club, because every club is different. It is important to study each policy before signing it in order to determine the areas specifically covered by the policy and, more importantly, to identify areas not covered by the policy. Finally, after entering into an initial insurance contract or renewing a policy, it is necessary to take time during the year to evaluate the coverage and make changes or additions as needed.

## The Bottom Line

Insurance is the easiest way to protect a health and fitness center from legal liability and financial loss.

## Types of Insurance

Purchasing adequate and affordable insurance can be a frustrating task for health and fitness professionals. However, two types of insurance every facility should have are property insurance and general liability insurance. The following section examines some of the most common types of insurance in the health and fitness industry.

## Property Insurance

Property insurance is the primary means of protecting the facility from accidental losses resulting from damage or destruction. The two primary areas covered by property insurance are (1) the buildings and (2) business and equipment contents contained within the designated buildings.

There are three levels of property insurance: basic, extended coverage, and special form, sometimes referred to as *open perils* (Cotten 2013). The basic coverage protects against a limited number of hazards, such as fire, weather-related damage, and vandalism. Extended coverage not oly includes the same protections as the basic coverage but also covers additional hazards, such as ice, water, and smoke damage. Special form coverage is designed to protect against any losses except those specifically excluded (Cotten 2013).

Even with special form coverage, there will be some property risks that are not covered under the policy. If the facility believes that more coverage is needed, it can purchase additional endorsements. An example of one such endorsement is **business interruption**, or coverage for loss of earnings when disasters temporarily affect the daily operations of a facility. If a facility is damaged by a fire and cannot reopen for 12 days, for example, the cost of renovation is not the only financial loss; there is no revenue during this time to offset the expenses that are incurred even when the club is not operational (i.e., debt service, real estate taxes, insurance, the demand portion of utilities). In addition, in some situations, key employees will need to be retained during the reconstruction phase, and a temporary office and furniture may be required.

## General Liability Insurance

**General liability insurance** is designed to protect businesses from any financial losses due to the negligence of the owner and employees. General liability insurance is often referred to as *third-party insurance* because if a business is sued, the insurance company protects the owner against suit by a third party. A general liability insurance policy generally provides for investigating and negotiating private settlements. In addition, it covers the

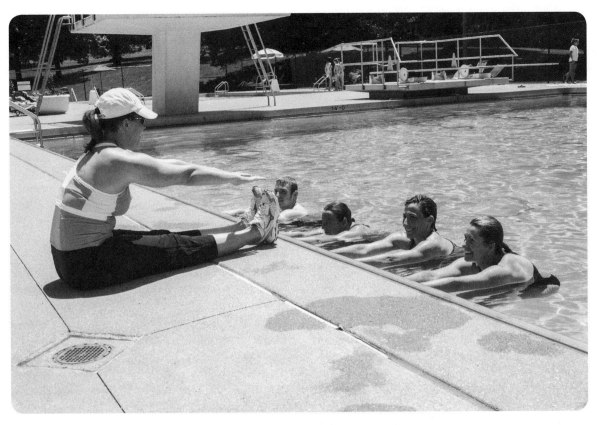

All wet areas pose potential risks to the health and safety of members and guests. Accidents could result in lawsuits and financial loss, and it's in the best interest of the club to obtain insurance.

defense of lawsuits brought against the owner and the payment of judgments up to the limit of the policy, usually $500,000 to $1 million.

## Umbrella Liability Insurance

Although general liability insurance covers most risks associated with running a health and fitness facility, the policies are subject to financial limits and ordinarily do not exceed $500,000 to $1 million in coverage. Therefore, in order to protect businesses from a catastrophic loss where liability may exceed the limits of the general liability insurance, the business must have an **umbrella liability** policy.

In addition to general liability coverage, an umbrella liability policy can allow a business to greatly increase its coverage in other key areas, such as auto liability, workers' compensation, and employer liability. Umbrella liability policies also usually provide broader coverage than most underlying policies, thus providing primary coverage for certain occurrences that would not be covered by an existing policy.

## Event Liability Coverage

When planning a special event or trip, it is essential that managers contact their insurance agents to determine whether the event is covered under the existing general liability policy. If not, the business should purchase additional event liability coverage. If a business offers off-site trips, it should ask the coordinating outside party to provide the necessary insurance. This applies to ski tour companies, white-water rafting companies, and even the charter bus company that transports members to an event. Generally, such companies do not have to pay anything extra to name the club on their insurance coverage for an outing or event. However, if the outside party chooses not to provide insurance coverage, it is the responsibility of the club to obtain an insurance rider on its liability policy to cover the event.

## Automobile Insurance

A significant liability exposure facing virtually all businesses comes from operating automobiles. In the United States, automobile accidents produce the greatest number of liability claims and account for most of the liability awards higher than $1 million. Even businesses that do not own a vehicle can be held liable for the operation of a vehicle by others. For example, an employee could take the day's cash deposit to the bank and have an accident on the way. If the employee is at fault, the business can be held responsible because the employee was acting on behalf of the business.

In addition to liability and physical damage coverage, several other endorsements can be added to a standard commercial auto policy, such as protecting employee-owned cars and rental vehicles while on company business. It is recommended that a club manager discuss all the vehicle-related situations that may exist in the operation of the club with the insurance agent to ensure that proper coverage is obtained at the best rate.

## Workers' Compensation

Most work-related accidents, diseases, and disabilities are subject to state **workers' compensation** statutes, which require employers to provide compensation for covered injuries without regard to fault. The scope of coverage varies in each state with respect to benefits payable in the case of early death, total disability, and partial disability due to specific injuries.

Every state has its own workers' compensation laws, but there are two requirements that injured employees must satisfy before they can recover workers' compensation benefits (Wolohan 2017):

- They must show that they were an employee of the organization.
- The injury must have occurred in the course of employment.

The benefits paid in a valid workers' compensation claim might include medical expenses, rehabilitation services to assist the employee in getting back to work, or disability income or death benefits to replace lost wages.

Although the U.S. government and all states have enacted workers' compensation laws, in Oklahoma and Texas workers' compensation is no longer mandatory. Instead, in these states, workers' compensation is elective and employers are able to opt-out of the state-run program. Even if an employer opts out of the state system, Oklahoma still requires employers to carry some form of insurance for their workers, as well as meet certain financial and other requirements established by the individual states. While Texas does not have the same protections for workers as Oklahoma, employees in Texas retain the right to sue their employers for negligence if they are injured on the job. However, this does not help the employee pay their bills while the case is being litigated. In addition, a number of employers in both Texas and Oklahoma have started to use arbitration clauses in their employee contracts, which keeps the employees out of court.

## Independent Contractor Liability

General liability insurance typically protects employers from liability due to the negligent acts of their employees, but such policies do not currently cover independent contractors working on the premises of a club. Consequently, club managers must require self-employed contractors to obtain their own insurance coverage.

Typically, the insurance agent requests copies of independent contractors' insurance certificates before underwriting the facility's liability insurance. Because the liability associated with being an independent contractor varies, insurance companies have established different policies for specific groups. For example, companies specializing in health and fitness insurance offer a separate personal trainer insurance policy.

## Key Terms

Age Discrimination in Employment Act of 1967 (ADEA)

agreement to participate

Americans with Disabilities Act of 1990 (ADA)

assumption of risk

business interruption

causation

civil liability

contracts

criminal liability

damages

duty of care

employee handbooks

employment at will

general liability insurance

hostile environment sexual harassment

intentional torts

invitee

negligence

personnel policy manuals

quid pro quo sexual harassment

reckless misconduct

recreational user

sexual harassment

Title VII of the Civil Rights Act of 1964

tort

umbrella liability

vicarious liability

waiver

workers' compensation

U.S. Department of Justice

# Strategic Planning and Evaluation

## Learning Objectives

After studying this chapter, you will be able to

- understand the purpose, structure, and benefits of a strategic plan;
- identify evaluation goals and processes to determine program efficiency;
- understand the importance of evaluation processes related to additional profit centers and how to implement them;
- acknowledge that what is measured is easier to manage; and
- determine the best evaluation method for a health and fitness facility and its programs.

As the owner of a moderate size multipurpose fitness club for 5 years, Shawna had experienced ups and downs, but the past 2 years had seen steady growth—up until the last 3 months. During this time, a new facility opened and began offering a number of programs not offered at Shawna's club, resulting in some members leaving for this competitor. Acknowledging that the new competitor's programs were one factor responsible for her club's falloff, she wanted to dig deeper to see whether there were other reasons members were leaving.

In order to better understand the club's decline, Shawna arranged some member focus groups and personally called some members who had left. The information gathered brought to light member issues that she was not aware of or hadn't realized were serious. Comments included the following:

- "The locker rooms have become dingy, worn, and drastically in need of upgrading."
- "My friends and I have been requesting new high-intensity training classes for the past 2 years; no one at your club seemed interested, but they are offered at the new club."
- "Personal training at the new club is fantastic, with helpful trainers and innovative training options."

The author acknowledges the significant contributions of Dave Hardy to this chapter.

Shawna was surprised by these comments; if she had known about these concerns, they could have been addressed. Perhaps the personal training at her club was too expensive or not beneficial, or maybe members had dissatisfactory experiences with her trainers. Shawna was not even aware that members were interested in high-intensity interval training, and she had thought members would prefer to see more treadmills and elliptical machines as opposed to upgraded locker rooms.

With this input from members, Shawna realized that she needed to spend more time paying attention to member preferences and needs. If she had been doing so, and addressing member concerns, the club would have been in a stronger position to compete against the new facility. A formal member feedback and evaluation program, along with informal member conversations on a regular basis, would have revealed that these issues.

This experience caused Shawna to wonder whether there were other issues at the club that needed similar attention. To find out, she decided to conduct a full evaluation of the entire operation, a time-consuming endeavor that she hoped would result in a more effective and efficient operation. Shawna first implemented both formal and informal evaluation methods that would take place throughout the year so that any substandard practices could be quickly addressed. The second phase would be to begin a comprehensive strategic planning process to set long-range direction for the club.

---

In the fitness industry, doing strategic planning to chart a course for a club or group of clubs has become a standard management practice. There is also an increased awareness of the need to develop meaningful operating standards and quality controls to evaluate and measure the extent to which a program or service has achieved its stated objectives. Because the industry has evolved significantly over the last 50 years, the planning and evaluation processes are important in setting business direction, priorities, and objectives as well as documenting the outcomes and processes involved in health and fitness services and successful club management.

## STRATEGIC PLANNING

It is difficult to grow any business and attain significant accomplishments without a plan. Defining a vision, goals, and objectives for your health club as part of a comprehensive management strategy is important to ensure its long-term growth and sustainability. This means analyzing the major initiatives that your company undertakes and putting them into reasonable and workable goals. The most common way to accomplish this is to develop a **strategic plan**, a document used to communicate an organization's vision and goals and the actions the organization will undertake over a defined period of time.

Strategic planning is the process of determining what an organization intends to look like in the future and the road it will take to get there. It is used to set priorities, assign resources, strengthen operations, confirm that the entire staff team is working toward common goals, and make sure everyone understands the projected outcomes and results. A good strategic plan will assess, adjust, and set an organization's direction in response to a changing environment. Having a strategic plan provides discipline to an organization as it makes fundamental decisions and actions that will shape and guide its future. Effective strategic planning will result in a clear vision for the organization and the action steps required to get there. Such planning will require an organization to determine or reaffirm some critical choices concerning where it is headed:

- The goals it intends to pursue
- The programs, services, or products it will offer to accomplish these goals
- The methods that will be used to attain, develop, and deploy the needed resources (e.g., people, skills, capacity, facilities, and funding)

When health clubs are interested in planning, there can be confusion about how to best go about the task as well as some skepticism about the value of planning. Strategic planning done poorly can be a waste of time and may do more harm than good. Planning can be problematic if the facility is using planning tools that don't fit the business, does not have the time to do a thorough job, or lacks the resources for doing it properly. However, with some common sense and basic tools, strategic planning does not have to be an overwhelming task and can prove to be a useful and pragmatic guide for organizational decision-making. One of the prerequisites for developing a strategic plan is commitment from the organization's leadership. If leadership commitment to the process is lacking, the process will be viewed as unimportant and ultimately be unproductive. Strategic planning can be transformative for an organization, but it has to be at the right time, with the right leadership, and the right process. The plan's timing and procedures should be adjusted to fit your organization's level of dedication to the process and its culture.

## Strategic and Operational Planning

A strategic plan looks out over an extended time horizon, typically 3 to 5 years, to develop a vision for the future of a business. Within every long-term strategic plan there are short-term operational or annual work plans. **Operational planning** is the common business activity of developing annual objectives, program plans, and budgets. The sum total of multiple years' operational plans should lead to the achievement of the strategic plan's goals. Operations management is responsible for achieving the objectives set forth in each annual plan, showing in specific terms what is intended for a given year. Annual plans set priorities for the day-to-day business operations, with short-term goals at 1 to 12 months that provide evidence of success in moving the organization closer to achieving the strategic plan vision. Although operational plans are for a 1-year period, a strategic plan takes a longer view. Strategic planning for more than 5 years is discouraged, however, because it is difficult to plan strategies, adapt to changing conditions, and predict outcomes beyond that time frame.

A distinction is sometimes made between long-range planning and strategic planning. Some say that long-range planning focuses on what an organization intends to look like at the end of a given time period and that strategic planning focuses on the action plan to get there. In practice, however, the two go hand in hand, because a good plan does both—it sets a vision as well as a roadmap to reach it. Operational plans then break down the longer-term strategic plan into annual actionable steps.

Sometimes companies are very good at designing a strategic plan but fail to execute a short-term operational plan. Likewise, having short-term plans without a long-term strategy results in a lack of direction or focus as to the vision of the company. By combining these two planning components, a company is able to set a general path based on company values, goals, and objectives while having the ability to adapt to changing environments annually.

Both long-term strategic and short-term operational planning are important to the future success of any organization. A strategic plan alone cannot account for the operational factors necessary in the short term to achieve the company's long-term objectives. Without a tactical short-term plan, operations management is unable to identify the milestones that are important to achieving the overall strategy set forth in the strategic plan. Therefore, it is necessary to coordinate operational short-term plans to ensure that they are effective in achieving the vision and goals of the company.

## Developing a Strategic Plan

The key to developing a successful strategic plan is to make sure that you create one that you will actually use—one that will become a roadmap for your organization's success. Strategic plans can be structured and organized in a number of different ways but most have the following critical elements:

1. Organization
   * Decide to develop a strategic plan
   * Obtain commitment from leaders and other stakeholders
   * Develop a planning outline that fits your organization
   * Form a planning team
2. Assessment
   * Describe organizational history and present situation
   * Identify opportunities and threats

- Identify strengths and weaknesses
- Develop an understanding of the current internal and external environments

3. Strategy formulation
   - Articulate critical issues
   - Identify alternatives
   - List goals
   - Develop strategy
   - Refine the plan
   - Adopt the plan
4. Strategy execution
   - Translate plan into operational plans and action steps
   - Implement plan
5. Evaluation
   - Monitor performance
   - Report results
   - Take corrective action
   - Update plan as required

Following is a list of tips to keep in mind during the process of developing a strategic plan:

1. Involve all the organization's key leaders in the planning process.
2. In meetings, establish ground rules and an environment where it is safe to speak freely and all ideas are considered.
3. Consider using an outside consultant as an unbiased facilitator to run the planning meetings.
4. Gather enough internal and external data on your club and the current operating environment to focus discussion and drive goal setting.
5. If part of a larger organization or company, consider how your club's goals and priorities align with the overall company strategy and vision.
6. Revisit your plan every year and adjust strategic priorities and goals as needed.

## Benefits of Strategic Planning

Although a health club may be able to grow or survive without strategic planning, most could benefit from a process that not only creates vision and goals but also builds constructive teams. Managers need to take time to plan to ensure they are acting responsibly for their organizations. Strategic planning can be a tool for changing a manager's mode of functioning from reactive to proactive. It stimulates creative thinking about the future. The plan can be an excellent public relations piece for potential investors or partners as well as a practical blueprint for growth. An important benefit of the process is team building that is nurtured by an inclusive process. By getting input from all segments of the organization, the planning process will do the following:

- Improve communication
- Increase everyone's commitment to the organization
- Align values and beliefs
- Solve organizational problems by looking at the whole
- Anticipate obstacles
- Develop a common vision
- Provide a framework for day-to-day decisions

## *The Bottom Line*

Setting a vision, goals, and objectives for a health club is important to ensure its long-term growth and sustainability. Strategic planning can help managers by providing an action plan to follow. Numerous planning and evaluation tools are available to provide short- and long-term direction and benchmark current performance to guide successful club management. Spending time doing strategic planning will help set business direction, priorities, and objectives as well as document the outcomes of a club's health and fitness services.

## EVALUATION

**Evaluation** is the process of determining the extent to which an organization has achieved its stated objectives. It measures the efficacy of programs and services as well as the overall performance of an organization based on performance goals and industry standards. If evaluation is performed honestly, it may yield negative rather than positive findings and may ultimately result in program modifications or elimination.

## Goals of Evaluation

Clearly defined goals and objectives are essential components of evaluation. You must measure each one to determine program effectiveness. Program participation rates, satisfaction, attrition, postprogram behavior changes (e.g., weight loss, fitness improvements, stress reduction), and staff satisfaction are examples of areas that must be measured to determine program success. Evaluation is part of the control function of club operations.

The overall goals of evaluation in the fitness industry are as follows:

- To determine how effective a program or service is in meeting predetermined goals and objectives
- To provide comprehensive information about the full range of program achievements as well as possible weaknesses
- To measure the quality of a program based on accepted standards and criteria
- To appraise the quality of organizational management, such as the performance of staff or the effectiveness of policies and procedures
- To provide feedback for improving programs and recommending a direction for future reference
- To provide information for internal and external marketing of program achievements

## Models of Evaluation

There are various evaluation methods that can be used in determining whether the goals and objectives of a fitness facility are being met.

### Summative and Formative Models

At one time, evaluation was primarily thought of as summative. **Summative evaluation** provides information on efficacy—that is, the ability of a program to do what it was designed to do. Summative evaluation is carried out at the end of a program to measure its success or failure and make recommendations for the future.

Now, however, there is a greater emphasis on an evaluation process that is formative, providing continual monitoring of a program while it is being planned and implemented. **Formative evaluation** is a method of judging the worth of a program while the program activities are forming or occurring. This type of evaluation establishes whether goals and objectives are being met, modifying them as necessary throughout the process.

In order to maintain a competitive edge, managers should routinely conduct evaluations on all aspects of the business and regularly adjust operations to fit the needs of the consumer.

### Process and Preordinate Models

**Process evaluation models** delineate a set of steps and procedures to use in conducting an evaluation without identifying the judgment criteria, whereas **preordinate evaluation models** provide a process and specify the criteria necessary in determining the worth of a program. Preordinate models begin with determining exactly how an evaluation should be carried out, the type of information that will be required, and the best way to gather it. Member participation, interest, feedback, and instructor evaluation are examples of preordinate evaluation.

No single approach is correct in all situations. A combination is often used in evaluating fitness facilities and the operations.

### *The Bottom Line*

Effective evaluation determines the extent to which a health club has achieved its goals and objectives and measures the effectiveness of programs and services, making it a valuable management tool. Various evaluation models exist and can be adapted for use in fitness facilities. Evaluation is a vital part of monitoring, controlling, and adjusting club operations.

## HEALTH AND FITNESS EVALUATION MODEL

Maintaining a competitive edge over other fitness facilities is a matter of survival. Whether a facility is small, medium, or large, striving to be the best should be the goal.

Elements of quality may be measured in various ways. Regardless of the measuring system used, the end result should be to identify those areas that meet or surpass acceptable industry standards and pinpoint areas that need further investigation and improvement. As an example, one of the most widely used systems for measuring quality in many businesses, including the fitness industry, is **total quality management (TQM)**. TQM involves observing and measuring everything occurring within an organization so you can identify weaknesses and improve operations. Operational procedures and policies must be reviewed and revised to examine how and by whom decisions are made and carried out within the organization. TQM may improve worker performance, productivity, customer service, and profitability.

The purpose of an evaluation model is to develop an awareness of the management policies and procedures used in various health and fitness settings, provide a means to measure the quality of those policies and procedures against proven methods, and point out the need to assess, improve, and change any areas deemed deficient. Evaluation is a vehicle for improvement and an indicator of where to concentrate efforts within the business.

Within most health and fitness settings, there are various levels of communication that are important to the success of the business. When conducting a facility evaluation, the groups involved in the evaluation process generally include management, an evaluation coordinator or consultant, an evaluation committee, and staff.

• *Management.* It is the responsibility of management to take the data obtained from the evaluation and use it to monitor established goals. Managers should look for areas considered deficient, establish a plan for improvement, implement the plan with the assistance of personnel, and regularly review the results. Having the support of management for short- and long-term planning is essential; consequently, there needs to be a strong line of communication between managers and other members of the evaluation group. You can obtain this interaction through regular presentations and reports that focus on

significant findings and recommendations for improvement.

• *Evaluation coordinator or consultant.* The role of the evaluation coordinator is to be the intermediary between management and staff. This task is often performed by an independent, impartial consultant who has no ties to the organization. If you use an in-house employee, we recommend that both management and staff approve the selection. The person chosen to manage this process will be responsible for analyzing data, reviewing results, comparing data with industry benchmarks, and determining pertinent conclusions.

• *Evaluation committee.* The evaluation committee usually consists of supervisors or personnel who have a vested interest in the evaluation process. They are responsible for developing and administering the evaluation, reviewing the results with the evaluation coordinator, and providing recommendations for improvement. The committee performs these tasks through regular meetings and brainstorming sessions for solving problems associated with the evaluation process. Committee members obtain input from other staff to incorporate their ideas and to make them feel a part of the operation.

• *Staff.* Staff members assist the evaluation committee in planning and conducting the evaluation. More importantly, though, they are responsible for administering the changes approved by management. Their involvement in the evaluation process is absolutely crucial. Providing a sense of ownership during the evaluation phase helps ensure that staff members implement planned program, facility, or operational changes in a positive manner. Staff members are also responsible for providing regular feedback on these changes so the organization can make refinements as needed.

Evaluation findings may be used as an external marketing tool. Promotional and advertising vehicles such as social media, websites, newsletters, and direct mailings may be used to communicate evaluation results to members. The fitness manager should know and fully understand how to measure the organization's marketing effectiveness. Here are some of the best ways to measure the effectiveness of marketing efforts using both quantitative and qualitative methods:

1. Marketing metrics
2. Marketing goals
3. Surveys
4. Social media analytics
5. Google analytics
6. Customer relationship management (CRM)

Review chapter 7 for a detailed description of the evaluation of a marketing plan. Some of the metrics and data analytics may require the services of a specialist to effectively analyze and draw conclusions based on the business intelligence information uncovered.

As shown in figure 16.1, an ongoing cycle for evaluation implementation will help define new goals and objectives, establish strategic planning, and follow up on plan implementation. This cycle allows for the continual evaluation of the business to ensure proper managerial techniques are incorporated.

## *The Bottom Line*

A health and fitness evaluation model can measure the quality and effectiveness of management policies and procedures and highlight areas to improve, further assess, and modify. Regular evaluation of services involving all levels of staff can help maintain a competitive edge over other facilities. Regardless of the measuring system used, the end result is to identify areas that meet or surpass acceptable industry standards and pinpoint areas needing further improvement. A popular system for measuring quality is TQM, which involves observing and measuring everything within an organization. Ongoing evaluation helps define new goals and objectives, establish strategic planning, and provide a check on plan implementation.

## LOCATION ANALYSIS

Many club operators believe a facility's financial future—one of losses or of profits—is determined the day the lease for the location is signed. As in most retail operations, the three most important

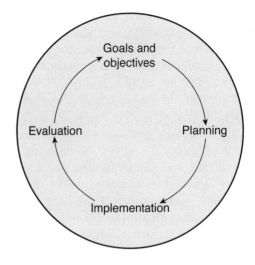

**Figure 16.1**  Implementation cycle of evaluation.

factors of success are location, location, location.

Four primary factors affect demand in the health and fitness industry:

- Population density
- Travel time to the health club
- Household income
- Educational attainment

In terms of population density, savvy club operators generally operate in markets where at least 50,000 people or more are within close proximity. Concerning travel time, the primary trading area should extend no more than 12 minutes from the point of departure. The **primary trading area** is the area closest to the club location and possesses the highest density of clientele. In suburban markets, in which the automobile is the primary means of commuting to a club, the primary trading area for clubs in competitive markets extends no further than a 12-minute drive from the club, which translates into a 5-mile radius around the club site (International Health, Racquet, and Sportsclub Association 2010).

Household income is a key determinant of member penetration rates and club pricing. There is a strong correlation between household income and club memberships. One out of six members of the general population is a health club member; however, member penetration rates among high-income segments are considerably higher. Individuals with annual household incomes exceeding $100,000 remain the largest member segment, accounting for 39% of the overall membership base (International Health, Racquet, and Sportsclub Association 2015). Educational attainment also dictates demand for memberships, because 52% of health and fitness facility members have earned a college degree or higher (International Health, Racquet, and Sportsclub Association 2015). In general, the higher the education attainment of the people in the primary trading area, the higher the membership penetration rates among that community.

The ultimate goal of location evaluation is to determine whether there is an available market to support the new facility and, for budgeting purposes, to estimate the number of monthly memberships the facility would likely sell. Both quantitative and qualitative approaches must be used in evaluating a location for a new fitness facility. **Quantitative research** refers to the collection of statistical data, whereas **qualitative research** refers to information based on opinions and values.

## Quantitative Methodology for Evaluating Locations

In evaluating a location, the following information should be researched:

- *Population density within the primary target trading area.* For example, if a facility is seeking to target 18 to 55 years old population density should be determined for everyone in this age range within the primary trading area. As mentioned, this is generally within a 12-minute travel time; however, it must be determined for the specific location.

- *Education attainment and average income.* This information helps determine whether the area will have a higher- or lower-than-average market penetration. Another influential factor is market positioning of the facility; for example, low-cost facilities would be more appealing to lower-income participants.

- *Traffic flow.* This should also be researched, because there is generally a positive correlation between traffic flow and the number of guests willing to drop in to the facility.

Once secondary data are collected, it is necessary to collect primary data on the existing market area in terms of over- or underfilled demand. **Secondary data** come from the collection, analysis, and interpretation of sources of primary data, whereas **primary data** are collected firsthand and include original materials, surveys, experiences, and so on.

To accomplish this, all potential competitors within the primary trading area should be plotted on a map. The following information should also be collected:

- A map of competitors' primary trading areas
- An estimate of competitors' current membership numbers
- The number of current competitor members who are within the proposed trading area of the new facility

Then, using the secondary demographic information of the population within the target market of the new facility, determine how many members would potentially purchase memberships at a fitness facility. A reasonable estimate should be made based on the available secondary data.

Finally, a calculation of the total potential market within the trading area less existing competition must be completed to determine whether the market has excess capacity for a new facility or whether excess supply already exists (see figure 16.2). A location analysis examines averages relevant to the primary trading area; most licensed real estate leasing agents are able to provide these averages based on a mapped primary trading area as laid out by the facility manager. Averages are dependent on the facility size, operating costs, and overall operating budget, and they determine whether the facility will be profitable as indicated by a mean average of attending members. This mean average does not take into account members who change facilities based on differences in services offered.

## Qualitative Methodology for Evaluating Locations

Real estate evaluation must also consider qualitative factors to determine the percentage of the market that the proposed facility will access. Some qualitative factors include the following:

|  | Target location | | Municipality averages | |
| --- | --- | --- | --- | --- |
| Total population | 114,080 | | 666,104 | |
| Under 20 years old | 44,532 | | 394,295 | |
| 20-34 years old | 25,443 | | 160,545 | |
| 35-54 years old | 39,003 | | 204,565 | |
| 55-59 years old | 5,102 | | 29,185 | |
| Completed university | 12.6% | | 19.2% | |
| Attending or attended university | 8.8% | | 8.0% | |
| Completed college | 15.8% | | 17.0% | |
| Attending or attended 2-year college | 7.5% | | 7.4% | |
| Trades certificate or diploma | 14.8% | 59.5% | 12.5% | 64.1% |
| Completed high school | 12.5% | | 10.8% | |
| Attending or attended high school | 24.5% | | 18.7% | |
| Completed less than grade 9 | 9.4% | | 6.5% | |
| Average household income | $52,816 | | $57,418 | |

**Target market penetration rates**

| | | | |
| --- | --- | --- | --- |
| Penetration rate, 20-34 years old | 20% | 5,089 | |
| Penetration rate, 35-54 years old | 15% | 5,850 | |
| Penetration rate, 55-59 years old | 10% | 510 | |
| Total potential members in market area | | 11,449 | |

**Total estimated members at competitors' locations**

| | |
| --- | --- |
| Competitor club A | 4,000 |
| Competitor club B | 3,500 |
| Competitor club C | 2,500 |
| Competitor club D | 500 |

**Percentage that infringe on market area of proposed facility**

| | |
| --- | --- |
| Competitor club A | 75% |
| Competitor club B | 85% |
| Competitor club C | 85% |
| Competitor club D | 25% |

**Number of members already serviced in market area**

| | |
| --- | --- |
| Competitor club A | 3,000 |
| Competitor club B | 2,975 |
| Competitor club C | 2,125 |
| Competitor club D | 125 |
| | 8,225 |
| Available market | 3,224 |

**Figure 16.2** Sample location analysis.

- *Brand awareness.* **Brand awareness** is a measure of how readily members of a target audience remember a product, service, company, or commercial brand and what the brand is about, as well as the consumer's level of trust in the brand.
- *Product offering.* This includes facility size, location, and amenities (e.g., types of equipment, pools, spas, courts for racket sports) as compared with competitors.

Qualitative factors will vary significantly by market area.

## The Bottom Line

Location analysis tools can be used to determine whether a market will support a new facility and to estimate the number of memberships the facility could expect to sell. The analysis should include the collection of statistical data as well as information based on opinions and values. A club's location is critical to its success. Factors that affect demand in health and fitness include population density, travel time to the club, household income, and educational attainment. Finally, a calculation of the total potential market can determine whether the market has excess capacity for a new facility or whether excess supply already exists.

## INDUSTRY EVOLUTION AND DIFFERENTIATION

The evolution of the fitness industry has been marked by increased sophistication in offerings and business practices. In the early days of the fitness industry, companies were typically focused on leasing space or providing equipment to members for an annual or monthly fee. The expansion of the fitness industry has been accompanied by significant increases in consumer expectations.

From a competitive perspective, the number of clubs has increased at a significant pace. Based on information from the International Health, Racquet, and Sportsclub Association (IHRSA), the number of adult commercial fitness clubs in the United States has increased significantly

since 2008, as shown in figure 16.3 (International Health, Racquet, and Sportsclub Association 2017). In addition, there has been a significant increase in not-for-profit and government facilities, including community centers, YMCAs, Jewish community centers, medical fitness facilities, and government-operated facilities.

The commercial fitness industry originated in the United States in the 1950s and 1960s, with the strongest growth happening in the last 30 years. There have been significant changes in the competitive landscape during this time. In previous years, competition was limited to other commercial entities, primarily traditional health clubs. Today, competition comes from a wide variety of sources, including boutique and specialty studios, warehouse gyms, home gyms, hospitals, hotels, community recreation centers, and not-for-profit organizations.

Increases in competition have forced businesses to focus on differentiation. Many clubs differentiate themselves by creating additional profit centers within their facilities (see chapter 11 for more details). These centers include the following:

- Food and beverage areas
- Group exercise
- Personal training
- Nutrition and weight loss
- Pro shops
- Fee-based group training in specialty areas such as Pilates
- Massage and other spa services
- Youth programming

Not all areas of differentiation are profit centers, but they are almost all cost centers, so they require an increased level of evaluation to ensure they are operating in the most efficient manner possible. Fitness facilities may have 5 to 10 cost or profit centers, each requiring a different level of expertise.

## Management of Multiple Profit Centers

The management of multiple profit centers within a fitness facility requires consistent terminology use and the identification of fixed and variable costs. Before evaluation can occur, subjective

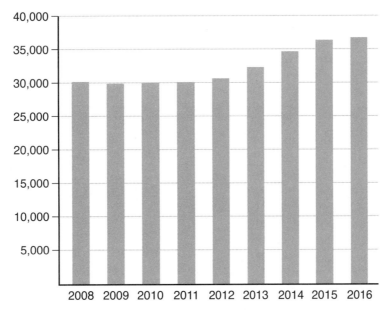

**Figure 16.3**    The number of operating fitness facilities in the United States has grown between 2008 and 2016.

Data from IHRSA, *Profiles of Success,* (Boston, MA: IHRSA, 2008-2016).

evaluations must be determined for the fixed and variable costs associated with that profit center. Management capital may be attributed to operating a profit center. This section will examine a few of the different types of profit centers, focusing on both possible financial returns and management costs.

## Food and Beverage Areas

Food service areas, such as juice bars, can be a point of differentiation and a selling feature used by fitness facilities to attract new members. The incorporation of a food and beverage area or juice bar into the operation of a fitness center followed a trend explosion in the 1980s that paralleled the growth of the fast-food industry across North America. Consumers would often request that fitness clubs provide beverages or other nutritional products, which eventually led to the evolution of the food service in health clubs. In addition to energy bars, snacks, bottled water, juice, sandwiches, and other such products, fitness clubs would also often provide nutritional or supplement products. This evolution continued as clubs looked for branded offerings, including franchises. These franchise offerings often resulted

in a significant increase in sales per square foot because of members' acceptance of the brand and interest in the products.

Many fitness operators complain that a food service operation is one of the most difficult to operate within a fitness facility. It is not uncommon for such operations to require hundreds of stock-keeping units (SKUs) for selling food and beverages. In addition to the large inventory that is required, staffing is also usually difficult to manage. Regulations for the operation of food services also place further restrictions on the operator of the fitness facility to ensure the proper and profitable operation of the profit center.

The primary evaluation reports used in profit and loss statements on a gross margin and net income basis, including a provision for rent, are as follows:

- Weekly or monthly food costs
- Weekly or monthly labor costs

One solution some health clubs are turning to is outsourcing the operation of food and beverage services to third-party operators. In many cases, the third-party operators are coordinated through franchise companies that are able to offer a branded product and, as a result of doing higher sales, are able to pay a higher rent to the club. Thus, many club managers are finding they are able to generate more income with fewer requirements for capital.

## Group Exercise

Group exercise is generally offered in fitness clubs as an included service. Some classes, however, are offered on a drop-in or fee-for-service basis.

When group exercise classes are included in the membership fee, the vast majority of facilities do not evaluate them based on performance or on return on investment. As a cost center, a free group exercise program may represent 5 to 10% of the overall operating costs of the facility. These costs should be controlled, and funds should be expended in such a way as to generate the highest return on investment for the operator. Although returns may not be quantified in terms of profit, the more people who take advantage of the service, the more likely those people are to maintain their membership and refer others, all of which will increase memberships and reduce attrition.

Since the early 2000s, there has been a movement to adopt branded and packaged group exercise programs by companies such as Zumba, Les Mills, YogaFit, and Beachbody. The classes are generally developed to appeal to a wider range of participants, thus increasing interest in the programs. These programs generally provide choreographed classes, including music, which allows clubs to outsource the development of programs. However, training instructors is often a challenge for fitness clubs because of labor shortages in these areas.

The primary selling feature of group exercise programs is the increased number of participants who attend group fitness classes, thus generating a greater return on investment. Evaluation techniques include the following reports:

- Cost per participant (This cost is calculated by dividing the cost of providing the class by the number of participants in each class. Managers should track the number of participants in each class and then use this information to track class trends in order to eliminate nonperforming classes and reward instructors who have high-performing classes.)

- Average number of participants per class
- Average number of participants per instructor

Both the second and third evaluation methods encourage the manager to focus on which classes are successful and which classes need to be revamped based on instructor or class. These results will be skewed based on time of day, club location, and so on; as such, they should not be the definitive method used to evaluate classes.

## Group Exercise Evaluation

The number and type of group exercise classes offered are determined based on the membership for the specific fitness facility. It is important to take into consideration the average age of the members for that specific location, patterns in traffic, and past participation rates.

In evaluating group exercise programs, it is essential to track the total number of classes taught per week, the total number of participants per club, and the percentage of participation based on class **capacity**. By tracking this information, the cost per participant can be determined. In tracking the average cost, you may determine the minimum cost per participant if and when the class is at 100% capacity. Capacity is based on room size and amount of equipment available. Figure 16.4 outlines three measurement devices used for evaluating the success of a group exercise program.

## Personal Training Evaluation

In many health clubs, personal training is a significant profit center operation, generating 8.4% of total revenue, the largest source of revenue after membership fees (International Health, Racquet, and Sportsclub Association 2017). In evaluating the effectiveness of a personal training program, it is necessary to compare the return on investment with the intrinsic value of the program. Fitness facilities sometimes offer personal training services on a break-even basis (or even with a negative return) simply because the intrinsic value of the program contributes to overall membership retention.

When evaluating the return on investment for a personal training program, the accrued gross margin should maintain at least a 30% contribu-

| | January | February | March |
|---|---|---|---|
| **1. How much does the class cost per person?** | | | |
| Total participants | 5,993 | 5,460 | 6,001 |
| Total program costs | $15,270.50 | $14,537.00 | $15,626.00 |
| Cost per participant | $2.55 | $2.66 | $2.60 |
| **2. How full is the class?** | | | |
| Maximum capacity | 30 | 30 | 30 |
| Average class attendance | 17.7 | 16.8 | 17.4 |
| Percentage of maximum class participation | 59% | 56% | 58% |
| **3. What is the participation?** | | | |
| Total number of visits that included participation in a group exercise class each month | 5,993 | 5,452 | 6,001 |
| Total club attendance (the total visits for each month) | 82,817 | 78,602 | 89,840 |
| Group exercise participation as a percentage of total attendance (participation divided by total attendance) | 7.2% | 6.9% | 6.6% |

**Figure 16.4**  Three ways to measure group exercise program success.

tion rate for the program to provide any return to the company. Depending on how the program is offered (for example, whether training sessions are offered on a pay-per-service delivery or pay-per-session basis), **bad debt**, or outstanding fees collected on a monthly or per session basis, must also be taken into account before calculating the gross margin contribution rate. See figure 16.5 for an example of the expense breakdown for personal training.

A personal training program must be evaluated by considering a number of **key performance indicators (KPIs)**. For instance, has the trainer maintained an average minimum number of hours of training per day? Has the trainer renewed a certain percentage of clients? Has the trainer recruited a certain number of new clients? Individual evaluation indicates consistency of service across the personal training program as a whole and ensures success of the program through maintenance of quality of service. See figure 16.6 for a sample form.

Personal training is one of the best ways to retain membership while providing clients with results-based training. A trainer's service allows for the success of members and is more likely to lengthen the life span of a membership. Having trainers on the facility floor also improves the overall optics of the facility—trainers are able to maintain the value of the overall facility by providing staff presence.

## The Impact of Technology

Advances in a wide range of technological tools have had a significant impact on the fitness industry in the past 10 years. Beyond computer systems, which are standard in clubs, available tools include smart fitness equipment, wearable technology devices, and software programs that allow tracking of member activity and services to provide managers with information to better engage and serve members, evaluate trends, and anticipate opportunities.

There are a number of fully integrated software programs and mobile tools that allow managers to track almost every area of their business. Many of these technology products include the following functions, the reports for which can be used in evaluation:

- Membership management and tracking
- Prospect management tracking and scheduling
- Sales-lead tracking and custom contracts
- Front-desk and facility access solutions

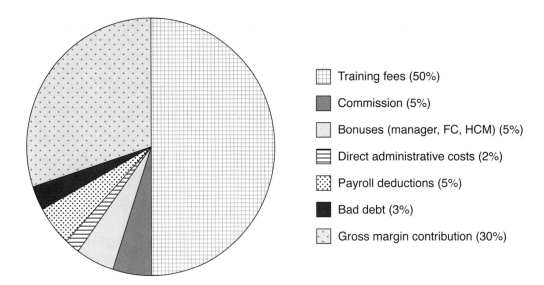

**Figure 16.5**   Sample business model for personal training.

- Website development tools
- Mobile app for members
- Member communications
- Tracking activity for those members eligible for insurance subsidies from health care companies
- Real-time feedback from equipment to improve service
- Workout administration for member fitness tracking
- Data entry for information management
- Performance reporting for club management
- Health club business modeling with artificial intelligence
- Billing and accounting system
- Cash or accrual financial reporting
- Payroll and commission modeling
- Collections solution for overdue payments

## *The Bottom Line*

As the health club industry has grown and evolved, operations have become more sophisticated to stay competitive and meet ever-increasing consumer expectations. Managers differentiate their business by creating multiple profit centers within facilities, such as food and beverage services, group exercise, and personal training. Advances in technological tools have had a significant impact on the industry; these tools include networked fitness equipment, wearable and mobile technology, and new member tracking software programs.

# KEY PERFORMANCE INDICATORS FOR PERSONAL TRAINERS

Personal trainer: _____

Month: _____

|  | Yes | No |
|---|---|---|
| 1. Trainer has performed 5 hours minimum (on average) of training per day. | ☐ | ☐ |
| 2. Trainer has attended and was on time for all appointments and staff meetings and the monthly review meeting. | ☐ | ☐ |
| 3. Trainer has thoroughly completed all paperwork and tracking forms this month and submitted them on time. | ☐ | ☐ |
| 4. For every day that the trainer hasn't had at least seven appointments, the trainer has done the required member assistance and passed the names of those members on to the club manager. | ☐ | ☐ |
| 5. Trainer has had 10% or fewer of their scheduled appointments not show up this month. If there were more no-shows than this, trainer has called the clients. | ☐ | ☐ |
| 6. Trainer renewed a minimum of 70% of clients who came up for renewal this month. If not, trainer placed follow-up calls with these clients to check progress, encourage renewals, and get referrals. | ☐ | ☐ |
| 7. Trainer has received and closed at least two referrals from existing clients. | ☐ | ☐ |
| 8. Trainer has worn the complete club uniform every day worked this month. | ☐ | ☐ |
| 9. If not completely booked up, trainer has sold packages to 20% of training demos. | ☐ | ☐ |
| 10. Trainer has recruited a minimum of two clients off the floor. | ☐ | ☐ |
| 11. Trainer has handed out client satisfaction surveys to at least 80% of active clients (and manager has received these from the clients). | ☐ | ☐ |
| 12. Trainer has worked a minimum of 40 hours per week (in appointments, doing member assistance, and doing follow-up calls—not working out). | ☐ | ☐ |
| 13. Manager has not received any complaints about the trainer from members. | ☐ | ☐ |

Trainer will receive 10 points for each indicator to which *yes* has been answered. Trainer is expected to receive a minimum score of 80% on the KPIs.

Personal trainer (signature): _____

Personal trainer coordinator (signature): _____

Date: _____

**Figure 16.6**  Sample form for key performance indicators for personal trainers

From M. Bates, M.J. Spezzano, and G. Danhoff, *Health Fitness Management*, 3rd ed. (Champaign, IL: Human Kinetics, 2020).

## Key Terms

bad debt

brand awareness

capacity

evaluation

formative evaluation

key performance indicator
(KPI)

operational planning

preordinate evaluation
models

primary data

primary trading area

process evaluation models

qualitative research

quantitative research

secondary data

strategic plan

summative evaluation

total quality management
(TQM)

# Appendix

## MEMBERSHIP AGREEMENT PART I

Membership number: _____

| | | | | |
|---|---|---|---|---|
| Name | Birth date | Marital status | Spouse's name | Birth date |
| Address | | Home phone | Teen 1 name | Birth date |
| City | State | Zip | Business phone | Teen 2 name | Birth date |

Occupation and employer                    Email

How did you hear about us?

Emergency contact                    Emergency phone number

## Buyer's Right to Cancel

If you wish to cancel your membership, you may cancel by delivering written notice in person or via certified mail, return receipt requested, to the Club. The notice must say that you do not wish to be bound by the Membership Agreement and must be delivered or mailed before midnight of the third business day after opening or if opened, by the third business day after you sign and receive a copy of the Agreement. The notice must be delivered or mailed to the Club. In some cases, as described in the Agreement, you may also cancel your membership if you sign the Agreement before the Club was completed, if the Club moves or goes out of business, if you become permanently disabled, or if you move from within a 30-mile radius. If you cancel, the Club may be entitled to retain a certain portion of the money you have paid. If the Club goes out of business or refuses to give you a refund, there may be a bond or letter of credit under which you are entitled to collect. For details, read the Agreement carefully. If you feel your rights have been violated, you may contact the Consumer Frauds and Protection Bureau of the state Attorney General's office.

## Notice

Any holder of this contract is subject to all claims and defenses which the debtor could assert against the seller of goods or services obtained pursuant hereto or with the proceeds hereof. Recovery hereunder by the debtor shall not exceed amounts paid by the debtor hereunder.

## Conditions

*Please see Membership Agreement Part II for all terms and conditions of this agreement.*

I have read and fully understand all the terms and conditions of this agreement.

Member's signature: _____ Date:_____

Club representative:_____ Date:_____

From M. Bates, M.J. Spezzano, and G. Danhoff, *Health Fitness Management*, 3rd ed. (Champaign, IL: Human Kinetics, 2020). Reprinted by permission from Island Health & Fitness (Ithaca, New York).

# MEMBERSHIP AGREEMENT PART II

1. *Terms.* The membership period is _____ months / month-to-month, beginning _____ _____. The Member may resign from the Club prior to the end of the Agreement if he or she meets any of the criteria outlined in the Buyer's Right to Cancel/Terminate section. The Member may resign from the Club after the initial _____-month term by providing a written notice to the Club. The Member's resignation becomes effective on the first day of the month following the expiration of the notice period. Notices must be received before the end of business hours on the 10th of the month in order to terminate the following month. If notice is received after the 10th of the month, termination will occur the 1st of the month after the following month. Prior to the effective date of termination, the Member shall be responsible for the payment of all fees, dues, and other charges due the Club.

2. Buyer's Right to Cancel/Terminate. The Member has the right to cancel this contract under certain circumstances:

   a. *Move.* The Member may cancel the contract if the Member provides written verification of having moved to a new permanent residence beyond a 30-mile radius from the Club, in which event the Club may make a prorated refund of prepaid dues if appropriate.

   b. *Disability or Death.* The Member may cancel if he or she becomes disabled, and the Member's estate may cancel in the event of the Member's death. The Club will make a prorated dues refund within 30 days of the written notice of this cancellation.

   c. *End of Term.* After the expiration of the initial _____ month term, the Member may terminate this agreement by written notice as indicated in Terms' section. Such notice must be delivered in person or by certified mail and will be effective on the first of the month as described above.

3. *Member Obligation.* Failure to use the facilities will not relieve the Member of the obligation to pay the monthly dues during the initial _____-month term or of monthly renewal term of the contract. If for any reason, the Member's bank or credit card does not honor any membership draft, the Member is responsible for said payment plus a penalty fee payable to the Club (currently $25.00). This will be in addition to any bank service charge fee(s).

My signature below indicates that I have read and fully understand the above (3) points relating to payment for membership.

## Enrollment Fee and Prorated Dues Payment

Primary member: _____

Associate member: _____

Teen member(s): _____

Fees paid by CHECK (or CASH)

Financial institution: _____

Check # _____

Payment amount $ _____

Enrollment fee $_____

Prorated dues $ _____

Total fees paid $_____

Fees paid by CREDIT CARD

Card type:   MC   VISA   AMEX   DISC

Credit card # _____

Credit card expiration date: _____

## Monthly Dues Draft Information

Bank debit     Credit card     Payroll deduction

Fees paid by BANK DEBIT

Check or savings acct. # _____

Financial institution: _____

Routing # _____

Fees paid by CREDIT CARD

Card type:   MC   VISA   AMEX   DISC

Credit card # _____

Credit card expiration date: _____

I have read and fully understand the contents of this document. I verify that the above financial information is accurate and understand that my monthly dues (and other fees as applicable) will be drafted each month following the terms and conditions of my membership agreement.

Member's signature: _____  Date: _____  Staff initials: _____

From M. Bates, M.J. Spezzano, and G. Danhoff, *Health Fitness Management*, 3rd ed. (Champaign, IL: Human Kinetics, 2020). Reprinted by permission from Island Health & Fitness (Ithaca, New York).

# TERMS AND CONDITIONS

1. The Club maintains a variety of services, including strength training, cardiovascular fitness, pools, and aerobic studios. From time to time mechanical problems, maintenance, or other issues may arise that cause these areas to be out of service. Should any of these major areas of the Club be unavailable to members for more than 90 consecutive days, an adjustment in monthly membership rates may be made.

2. The Club retains the right to suspend or cancel this membership and/or impose fines of $25.00 plus costs on any member for violation of the following rules:

   a. Theft, damage, or destruction of Club property or the property of other members

   b. Failure to pay dues or charges when due, or returned check or credit card payments

   c. Fighting with or harassing other members or guests

   d. Conduct of behavior found to be offensive or unacceptable

   e. Any other violation of the rules of conduct as described in the Membership Handbook and any subsequent policies that the Club issues

3. Members are responsible for the conduct, damages, and charges of their guests.

4. The Club reserves the right to amend its rules and regulations at any time. Changes will be posted on the Club bulletin board or communicated through other appropriate means.

5. The Member acknowledges and accepts the risk inherent in the use of Club services and facilities. By using the club, the Member hereby assumes the risk of injury, accident, death, disability, loss cost, or damage to his or her person or property that may arise from use of the Club's services or facilities. The Member, his or her heirs, executors, representatives, and assigns hereby release the Club from all claims or liabilities for personal injury or loss of or damage to property of any kind sustained by the Member while on the premises of the Club, except where this is the direct result of negligence or willful misconduct by the Club.

6. The Member certifies that he or she is in good physical health and is able to undertake and engage in the physical activities, exercise, or sports activities in which he or she has chosen to participate.

7. The Member shall dress in an appropriate manner while in all public areas.

8. By signing the Agreement, the Member agrees to adhere to and be bound by the Club's rules, to pay all fines levied for misconduct, and to forfeit membership without refund of dues or initiation/assessment fees if terminated by the Club for cause.

9. The Member agrees to pay, when due, all initiation/assessment fees, charges, and guest charges in accordance with this Agreement and in accordance with the rules and regulations of the Club. If the Member should fail to pay, when due, any amounts payable to the Club, then the unpaid balance will be assessed an interest charge at the rate of 1.50% per month until paid plus any penalty the Club imposes for nonpayment. Should collection efforts be required, the Member shall be fully responsible for payment of all costs of collection, including reasonable attorney fees.

10. *Membership Freeze.* Members may freeze their membership only for specific reasons and only by submitting their request in writing. For a Primary Member, freezes will only be allowed for medical reasons or temporary relocation in conjunction with their employment or vacation, more than 30 miles from their home. A doctor's letter or a letter from an employer is required to freeze a Primary Member. When a Primary Member freezes, all remaining family members are automatically frozen as well and are unable to use the Club. The exception is when Associate or Teen Members take over the responsibility of the Primary Member's dues. A minimum of one full calendar month notice is required to freeze a membership. The freeze shall be effective on the 1st of the month following the expiration of the previous calendar month. Associate and Teen Members may freeze their membership without providing a reason.

*(continued)*

## Terms and Conditions *(continued)*

The length of freeze for Primary Members may not exceed 5 months. A service charge of $25.00 for Primary and Associate, $10 for Associates or Teens, is required at the time of freeze. If the Primary and Associate Members freeze together, the charge is $25. Freezes by telephone or fax are not permitted. Any freeze must be in person or sent via certified mail, return receipt requested. The Club reserves the right to change this or any other policy at its discretion. For more information on this or any other Club policy, consult the Member Handbook. If you have signed for a 3-, 6-, or 12-month period, the frozen months are added at the end.

*Termination Policy.* Except for a doctor's official note contraindicating exercise, after you have completed your _____contract, a minimum of 20 days' notice (if received by the 10th of the month) is required to terminate a membership.

Initial and date

|  |  |
| --- | --- |
| Member | Member |

From M. Bates, M.J. Spezzano, and G. Danhoff, *Health Fitness Management*, 3rd ed. (Champaign, IL: Human Kinetics, 2020). Reprinted by permission from Island Health & Fitness (Ithaca, New York).

# References

## Chapter 1

Avolio, B.J., D.A. Waldman, and F.J. Yammarino. 1991. Leading in the 1990s: The four Is of transformational leadership. *Journal of European Industrial Training* 15:9-16.

Bass, B.M. 1985. *Leadership and performance beyond expectations.* New York: Free Press.

Bass, B.M., and B.J. Avolio. 1994. *Improving organizational effectiveness through transformational leadership.* Thousand Oaks, CA: Sage.

Buckingham, M. 2005. *The one thing you need to know.* New York: Free Press.

Buckingham, M., and C. Coffman. 1999. *First, break all the rules.* New York: Simon & Schuster.

Covey, S.R. 1989. *The seven habits of highly effective people.* New York: Simon & Schuster.

Covey, S.R. 2008. *The leader in me: How schools and parents around the world are inspiring greatness, one child at a time.* New York: Free Press.

Drucker, P. 1998. *On the profession of management.* Boston: Harvard Business School.

Evans, M.G. 1970. The effects of supervisory behavior on the path–goal relationship. *Organizational Behavior and Human Performance* 5:277-298.

Fiedler, F.E. 1967. *A theory of leadership effectiveness.* New York: McGraw-Hill.

Goleman, D. 1995. *Emotional intelligence: Why it can matter more than IQ.* New York: Bantam Books.

Gulick, L., and L. Urwick. 1937. *Papers on the science of administration.* New York: Institute of Public Administration.

Hersey, P., K.H. Blanchard, and D.E. Johnson. 2001. *Management of organizational behavior: Leading human resources.* 8th ed. Upper Saddle River, NJ: Prentice Hall.

Hersey, P., and P. Blanchard. 1969. The life cycle theory of leadership. *Training and Development Journal* 23(5): 26-34.

Herzberg, R. 1966. *Work and the nature of man.* Cleveland, OH: World.

House, R.J., and T.R. Mitchell. 1997. Path–goal theory of leadership. In *Leadership: Understanding the dynamics of power and influence in organizations,* ed. R.P. Vecchio, 259-273. Notre Dame, IN: University of Notre Dame Press.

Kirkpatrick, S.A., and E.A. Locke. 1991. Leadership: Do traits matter? *Academy of Management Executive* 5(2): 48-60.

Koontz, H., C. O'Donnell, and H. Weihrich. 1984. *Management.* 8th ed. New York: McGraw-Hill.

Likert, R. 1961. *New patterns of management.* New York: McGraw-Hill.

Lundin, S. 2000. *Fish: A remarkable way to boost morale and improve results.* New York: Hyperion.

Maslow, A.H. 1954. *Motivation and personality.* New York: Harper.

Mayo, E. 1933. *The human problems of an industrial civilization.* New York: Macmillan.

McGregor, D. 1960. *The human side of enterprise.* New York: McGraw-Hill.

Mintzberg, H. 1973. *The nature of managerial work.* New York: Harper and Row.

———. 1990. The manager's job: Folklore and fact. *Harvard Business Review* 68(2): 163-176.

Slater, R. 1999. *Jack Welch and the GE way.* New York: McGraw-Hill.

Taylor, F.W. 1911. *The principles of scientific management.* New York: Harper.

## Chapter 2

International Health, Racquet, and Sportsclub Association (IHRSA). 1998. *Why people quit.* Boston: IHRSA.

## Chapter 3

Boydell, J., Deutsch, B., and Remillard, B. 2006. *You're not the person I hired!: A CEO's survival guide to hiring top talent.* Bloomington, Indiana: Author House.

Andler, E.C. and Institute of Physics (Great Britain). 1998. The complete reference checking handbook: smart, fast, legal ways to check out job applicants. AMACOM, New York.

U.S. Small Business Administration. 2004. *Human resource management.* Washington, DC: Small Business Administration.

## Chapter 4

Avatech Solutions. 2007. Training return on investment: The real cost of not training. Retrieved April 19, 2007, from www.avat.com/training/trainingroi.asp.

Buckingham, M., and C. Coffman. 1999. *First, break all the rules.* New York: Simon & Schuster.

Carlaw, P., and V.K. Deming. 1998. *The big book of customer service training games.* New York: McGraw-Hill.

Carnegie, D. 1990. *How to win friends and influence people.* New York: Pocket.

Coelho, P. 1993. *The alchemist.* San Francisco: Harper.

Covey, S. 2004. *The seven habits of highly effective people.* New York: Simon and Schuster.

Cross, J., and T. O'Driscoll. 2005. New American workplace. *Training Magazine*, March.

eLogic Learning. 2017. 15 eLearning trends and statistics to know for 2017. Retrieved August 14, 2018, from https://elogiclearning.com/15-elearning-trends-and-statistics-to-know-for-2017.

Epstein, R., and J. Rogers. 2001. *The big book of motivation games.* New York: McGraw-Hill.

Gladwell, M. 2005. *Blink: The power of thinking without thinking.* New York: Little Brown.

Gallo, C. 2014. The Maya Angelou quote that will radically improve your business. Retrieved August 14, 2018, from www.forbes.com/sites/carminegallo/2014/05/31/the-maya-angelou-quote-that-will-radically-improve-your-business/#650c5c35118b

Hill, N. 1987. *Think and grow rich.* New York: Random House.

Jones, A. 2000. *Team-building activities for every group.* Richland, WA: Rec Room.

Murphy, J. 2001. *The power of your subconscious mind.* New York: Bantam.

Newstrom, J.W., and E.E. Scannell. 1997. *The big book of team building games: Trust-building activities, team spirit exercises, and other fun things to do.* New York: McGraw-Hill.

Scannell, E.E., and J.W. Newstrom. 1980. *Games trainers play.* New York: McGraw-Hill.

———. 1994. *The complete games trainers play.* New York: McGraw-Hill.

Sharma, R. 2004. *The monk who sold his Ferrari.* New York: Element.

Swanson, S. 2001. E-learning branches out. *InformationWeek*, 26 February.

Tamblyn, D., and S. Weiss. 2000. *The big book of humorous training games.* New York: McGraw-Hill.

Wetmore, D.E. 1999. Price of not training. Retrieved April 19, 2007, from www.balancetime.com.

Withrow, B. 2007. Corporate retreats: How to get the most out of them. Retrieved April 19, 2007, from www.facilitators.com/corporate_retreats.htm.

## Chapter 5

Collins, J.C., and J.I. Porras. 1994. *Built to last.* New York: HarperCollins.

Gostick, A., and C. Elton. 2001. *Managing with carrots.* Salt Lake City: O.C. Tanner.

## Chapter 6

IDEA Health and Fitness Association (IDEA). 2015. *2015 IDEA fitness industry compensation trends report.* San Diego: IDEA.

International Health, Racquet, and Sportsclub Association (IHRSA).

———. 2017. *Profiles of success.* Boston: IHRSA.

## Chapter 7

Ahmad, I. 2017. Internet users have average of 5 social media accounts. Retrieved August 5, 2018, from www.digitalinformationworld.com/2017/07/infographic-internet-users-average-social-media-accounts.html.

Bullas, J. 2017. 7 digital marketing trends that are transforming business. Retrieved August 5, 2018, from www.linkedin.com/pulse/7-digital-marketing-trends-transforming-business-jeff-bullas.

Davila, T., D. Oyon, P. Parmigiani, and M. Schnegg. 2015. Look outside your firm: A tool to sense what's coming. *IESE Insight* 25:58-65.

eMarketer. 2015. Social network ad spending to hit $23.68 billion worldwide in 2015. Retrieved June 30, 2017, from www.emarketer.com/article/social-network-ad-spending-hit-23680-billion-worldwide-2015/1012357#sthash.1BpDFob.dpuf.

Hiltbrand, T. 2015. Fire up your social media strategy with big data analytics. *Business Intelligence Journal* 20(3): 8-16.

Lake, A. 2011. Why Facebook fans are useless. iMedia Connection. Retried June 30, 2017, from www.imedia-connection.com/content/30235.asp.

Li, M., Pitts, B. G. and Quarterman, J. 2008. *Research methods in sport management.* Morgantown, WV: Fitness Information Technology.

Marketing Science Institute. 2013. MSI call for research proposals on social interactions and social media marketing. Retrieved August 5, from www.msi.org/uploads/files/2013-11-07_MSI_Social_Media_Competition.pdf.

McClue, T. 2013. Why infographics rule. *Forbes.* Retrieved August 5, 2018, from www.forbes.com/sites/tjmccue/2013/01/08/what-is-an-infographic-and-ways-to-make-it-go-viral/#250e52907272.

McKinsey and Company. 2014. McKinsey global survey results: The digital tipping point. Retrieved August 5, 2018, from www.mckinsey.com/insights/business_technology/the_digital_tipping_pointmckinsey_global_survey_results.

Mersey, R.D., E.C. Malthouse, and B.J. Calder. 2010. Engagement with online media. *Journal of Media Business Studies* 7(2): 39-56.

Morgan, B. 2015. Was Peter Drucker wrong? The modern purpose of a brand. Retrieved August 5, 2018, from www.forbes.com/sites/blakemorgan/2015/12/28/was-peter-drucker-wrong-the-modern-purpose-of-a-brand/#34ff81842349.

Powers, T., D. Advincula, M.S. Austin, S. Graiko, and J. Snyder. 2012. Digital and social media in the purchase decision process: A special report from the Advertising Research Foundation. *Journal of Advertising Research* 52(4): 479-489.

Rath, J. 2017. The 10 most powerful brands in the world. Retrieved August 5, 2018, from www.businessinsider.com/the-worlds-10-most-powerful-brands-2017-2.

Statista. 2018. U.S. fitness, health and gym clubs industry segmentation in 2016, by products/services. Retrieved August 5, 2018, from www.statista.com/statistics/242190/us-fitness-industry-revenue-by-sector.

Story, L. 2017. Anywhere the eye can see, it's likely to see an ad. Retrieved August 5, 2018, from www.nytimes.com/2007/01/15/business/media/15everywhere.html.

Syrdal, H. A., & Briggs, E. 2018. Engagement with social media content: A qualitative exploration. *Journal of Marketing Theory & Practice, 26*(1/2), 4-22. doi:10.1080/10696679.2017.1389243.

Whan Park, C., Eisingerich, A.B., & Pol, G. 2014. The power of a good logo. Retrieved August 5, 2018, from https://sloanreview.mit.edu/article/the-power-of-a-good-logo.

## Chapter 8

Centers for Disease Control and Prevention (CDC). 2015. Workplace health promotion. Retrieved June 25, 2018, from www.cdc.gov/workplacehealthpromotion.

International Health, Racquet, Sportsclub Association (IHRSA). 2018. *Health club consumer report.* Boston: IHRSA.

Mehrabian, A. 1972. *Non verbal Communication.* Chicago: Aldine-Atherton.

Peter Drucker Quotes. BrainyQuote.com, Xplore Inc, 2018. Retrieved July 25, 2018, from www.brainyquote.com/quotes/peter_drucker_142500.

## Chapter 9

Freeman, D. 2013. New customer-rage study out for holiday shopping season. Retrieved June 27, 2018, from https://asunow.asu.edu/content/new-customer-rage-study-out-holiday-shopping-season.

Gallo, Amy. 2014. *The value of keeping the right customers.* Boston: Harvard Business School Publishing.

Gautam, N. 2017. 50 Important Customer Experience (CX) Statistics You Need to Know. Retrieved June 27, 2018, from www.ameyo.com/blog/customer-experience-statistics.

Slowik, D. 2000. *Upset citizens and customers: How to deal with the angry, difficult, and demanding public.* Evergreen, CO: Evergreen Press.

## Chapter 10

International Health, Racquet, and Sportsclub Association (IHRSA). 2017a. 15 surprising facts about health club member retention. Retrieved August 20, 2018, from www.ihrsa.org/improve-your-club/15-surprising-facts-about-health-club-member-retention.

———. 2017b. *2017 profiles of success: The annual industry data survey of the health and fitness club industry.* Boston: IHRSA.

Reichheld, F., and W. E. Sasser Jr. Zero Defections: Quality Comes to Services. *Harvard Business Review* 68(5): 105–111.

## Chapter 11

American Council on Exercise. 2014. *American Council on Exercise Personal Trainer Manual.* 5th ed. American Council on Exercise. San Diego, CA: American Council on Exercise.

Centers for Disease Control and Prevention (CDC). 2015. Prevalence of childhood obesity among adults and youth: United States, 2011-2014. *NCHS Data Brief* 219.

ClubIntel. 2017. International fitness trend industry report: What's all the rage? Retrieved August 20, 2018, from www.club-intel.com/wp-content/uploads/2017-International-Fitness-Industry-Trend-Report-Whats-All-the-Rage.pdf.

IBISWorld. 2017. Personal trainers in the US: Market research report. Retrieved August 20, 2018, from www.ibisworld.com/industry/personal-trainers.html.

IDEA. 2015. *IDEA fitness programs and equipment survey.* San Diego: IDEA.

International Health, Racquet, Sportsclub Association (IHRSA). 2015. *Profiles of success.* Boston: IHRSA.

———. 2016a. *Health club consumer report.* Boston: IHRSA.

———. 2016b. *Profiles of success.* Boston: IHRSA.

———. 2017. *Health club consumer report.* Boston: IHRSA.

International Spa Association. 2017. *2017 ISPA industry study.* Lexington, KY: ISPA.

Landers, Linda. April 3, 2018. 4 Industries That Should Be Marketing to Baby Boomers. GirlPowerMarketing.com. Retrieved August 4, 2018, from https://girlpowermarketing.com/four-industries-that-should-market-to-baby-boomers.

Sports & Fitness Industry Association. 2016. *Pilates Training Participation 2016.* Silver Spring, MD.

Thompson, W.R. 2017. Worldwide survey of fitness trends for 2018: The CREP edition. *ACSM'S Health & Fitness Journal* 21(6): 10-19.

## Chapter 12

Caro, R. 1995. 35 cost-saving techniques to increase the club's bottom line. *Peak Performance,* August.

Fried, G. 2004. *Sport finance.* Champaign, IL: Human Kinetics.

Grantham, W., R.W. Patton, T.D. York, and M.L. Winickl. 1998. *Health fitness management.* Champaign, IL: Human Kinetics.

International Health, Racquet, and Sportsclub Association (IHRSA). 2006. *Profiles of success.* Boston: IHRSA.

International Health, Racquet, and Sportsclub Association (IHRSA). 2017. *Profiles of success.* Boston: IHRSA.

## Chapter 13

Abbott, A. 1989. Exercise science knowledge base of commercial fitness instructors in the State of Florida. Research study presented at the ACSM annual conference, 1990.

———. 2000. Are You Prepared? – Handling Emergency Situations. *Personal Fitness Professional Magazine*, November.

———. 2009. Fitness professionals: Certified, qualified and justified. *The Exercise Standards and Malpractice Reporter* 23(2): 17.

_____. 2015. A hot topic. *ACSM's Health & Fitness Journal.* 19(1): 35.

_____. 2017. Aquatic emergencies. *ACSM's Health & Fitness Journal.* 21(4): 35.

Alter, J. 1983. *Surviving exercise.* Boston: Houghton Mifflin.

American College of Sports Medicine (ACSM). 2012. *ACSM's health/fitness facility standards and guidelines.* 4th ed. Champaign, IL: Human Kinetics.

———. 2016. *ACSM's guidelines for exercise testing and prescription.* 10th ed. Philadelphia: Lippincott, Williams & Wilkins.

———. 2018. Legal structure and terminology. *Resources for the exercise physiologist.* 2nd ed. Philadelphia: Wolters Kluwer

American Heart Association. 1999. Recommendations for cardiovascular screening, staffing and emergency policies at health/fitness facilities. AHA/ACSM scientific statement. *Circulation* 97:2283-2293.

_____. 1999. *Basic life support for healthcare providers.* Dallas: AHA.

_____. 2001. *Basic life support for healthcare providers.* Dallas: AHA.

———. 2002. Automated external defibrillators in health/fitness facilities, AHA/ACSM scientific statement. *Circulation* 105:1147-1150.

_____. 2016. *Basic life support student manual.* Dallas: AHA

American Red Cross. 1993. *Oxygen administration.* St. Louis: Mosby Lifeline.

*Best's Review.* August 2002. *Need for Defibrillators Outweighs Potential Liability* 72.

Carnevale, A. P., N. Smith, and J. Strohl. 2011. Help wanted: Projections of jobs and education requirements through 2018. [Technical summary pdf file]. Georgetown University Center on Education and the Workforce. http://cew.georgetown.edu/JOBS2018.

Eickhoff-Shemek J., D.L. Herbert, and D.P. Connaughton. 2009. *Risk management for health/fitness professionals.* Philadelphia: Lippincott Williams & Wilkins.

Feigenbaum, M., and M. Pollock. 1999. Prescription of resistance training for health and disease. *ACSM's Medicine & Science in Sports & Exercise* 31(1): 38-45.

International Health, Racquet, and Sportsclub Association (IHRSA). 2005. *Guide to club membership conduct.* 3rd ed. Boston: IHRSA.

Malek, M., D.P. Nalbone, D.E. Berger, and W. Jared. 2002. Importance of health science education for personal fitness trainers. *NSCA Journal of Strength and Conditioning Research* 16(1): 19-24.

McInnis, K., W. Herbert, D. Herbert, J. Herbert, P. Ribisl, and B. Franklin. 2001. Low compliance with national standards for cardiovascular emergency preparedness at health clubs. *Chest* 120:283-288.

National Strength and Conditioning Association (NSCA). 2012. *Essentials of personal training.* 2nd ed. Champaign, IL: Human Kinetics.

_____. 2017. *Strength and conditioning professional standards and guidelines.* Colorado Springs, CO: NSCA.

U.S. Bureau of Labor Statistics. 2009. Fastest growing occupations. [Data file]. Retrieved August 20, 2018, from www.bls.gov/emp/ep_table_103.

## Chapter 14

*Cleaning and Maintenance Management.* 1995. 1995 in-house survey. 32(12): 2-8.

Feldman, E. 1991. *How to save time and money in facilities maintenance management.* Latham, NY: Cleaning Management Institute.

Fried, G. 2005. *Managing sport facilities.* Champaign, IL: Human Kinetics.

Grantham, W.C., R.W. Patton, T.D. York, and M. Winick. 1998. *Health fitness management.* 1st ed. Champaign, IL: Human Kinetics. Greenwood, M. 2000. Facility layout and scheduling. In *Essentials of strength training and conditioning,* eds. T.R. Baechle and R. Earle, 549-565. Champaign, IL: Human Kinetics.

———. 2004. Facility and equipment layout and maintenance. In *Essentials of personal training,* eds. T.R. Baechle and R. Earle, 587-601. Champaign, IL: Human Kinetics.

Greenwood, M., and L. Greenwood. 2000. Facility maintenance and risk management. In *Essentials of strength training and conditioning,* eds. T.R. Baechle and R. Earle, 587-601. Champaign, IL: Human Kinetics.

International Health, Racquet, and Sportsclub Association (IHRSA). 2006. *Global report: State of the health club industry.* Boston: IHRSA.

Patton, R.W., J.M. Corry, L.R. Gettman, and J.S. Graf. 1986. *Implementing health fitness programs.* Champaign, IL: Human Kinetics.

Patton, R.W., W.C. Grantham, R.F. Gerson, and L.R. Gettman. 1989. *Developing and managing health fitness facilities.* Champaign, IL: Human Kinetics.

Ray, R. 2000. *Management strategies in athletic training.* 2nd ed. Champaign, IL: Human Kinetics.

Rice, R. 1995. Housekeeping benchmarks. *Cleaning and Maintenance Management* 32(3): 62-65.

Tatum, R. 1995. How technology is reshaping facility management. *Building Operating Management* 42(1): 24-30.

Tharrett, A.J., and Peterson, J.A. 2012. *ACSM's health/fitness facility standards and guidelines.* 4th ed. Champaign, IL: Human Kinetics.

Williams, T. 1994. How top managers evaluate their facilities. *Cleaning Maintenance Management* 31(9): 40-42.

## Chapter 15

Age Discrimination in Employment Act, 42 U.S.C. §623 (4) (2003).

Americans with Disabilities Act, 42 U.S.C. § 12112 (2003).

Calamari, J., and J. Perillo. 1998. *The law of contracts.* 4th ed. St. Paul: West.

Cotten, D.J. 2013. Managing risk through insurance. In *Law for recreation and sport managers,* 6th ed., eds. D.J. Cotten and J.T. Wolohan. Dubuque, IA: Kendall/Hunt.

Cotten, D.J. 2017. Waivers and Releases. In *Law for recreation and sport managers,* 7th ed., eds. D.J. Cotten and J.T. Wolohan. Dubuque, IA: Kendall/Hunt

Cotten, D.J., and M.B. Cotten. 2004. *Waivers and releases of liability.* 4th ed. Statesboro, GA: Sport Risk Consulting.

Hums, M.A. 2013. Title I of the Americans with Disabilities Act. In *Law for recreation and sport managers,* 6th ed., eds. D.J. Cotten and J.T. Wolohan. Dubuque, IA: Kendall/Hunt.

Keeton, W., et al. 1984. *Prosser and Keeton on the law of torts.* 5th ed. St. Paul: West.

Masteralexis, L. 2013. Title VII of the Civil Rights Act of 1964. In *Law for recreation and sport managers,* 6th ed., eds. D.J. Cotten and J.T. Wolohan. Dubuque, IA: Kendall/Hunt.

Restatement (second) of Contracts §1 (1979).

Robertson, D., W. Powers, D. Anderson, and O. Wellborn. 2004. *Cases and materials on torts.* 3rd ed. St. Paul: West.

Schubert, G.W., R.K. Smith, and J.C. Trentadue. 1986. *Sports law.* St. Paul: West.

Swisher, P.N. 2011. Virginia Should Abolish the Archaic Tort Defense of Contributory Negligence and Adopt a Comparative Negligence Defense in Its Place. *University of Richmond Law Review* 46:359-371.

Title VII of the Civil Rights Act of 1964, 42 U.S.C. §§ 2000e *et seq.* (2003).

van der Smissen, B. 2004. Human resources law. In *Law for recreation and sport managers,* 3rd ed., eds. D.J. Cotten and J.T. Wolohan. Dubuque, IA: Kendall/Hunt.

Wolohan, J.T. 1995. Sexual harassment of student athletes and the law. *Seton Hall Journal of Sport Law* 5:339-357.

———. 2004. Land reform: Recreational-use statutes are expanding to include public fields, playgrounds and pools. *Athletic Business* 28:22-26.

———. 2005. Faulty waivers: A drowning death leaves all exculpatory agreements in state of Wisconsin under water. *Athletic Business* 29:20-26.

———. 2011. Wrongful termination: Court holds that a club that provided poor service is not entitled to a dissatisfied member's cancelation fees. *Athletic Business* 35:22-26.

———. 2013. Electronic waivers revisited. *Risk Management for Campus Recreation,* 8: 3- 6.

———. 2017. Workers' compensation. In *Law for recreation and sport managers,* 7th ed., eds. D.J. Cotten and J.T. Wolohan. Dubuque, IA: Kendall/Hunt.

Wong, G.M. 2002. *Essentials of sports law.* 3rd ed. Westport, CT: Praeger.

## Chapter 16

International Health, Racquet, Sportsclub Association (IHRSA). 2010. *IHRSA's guide to the health club industry for lenders & investors.* Boston: IHRSA.

———. 2016. *Profiles of success.* Boston: IHRSA.

———. 2017. *The 2017 IHRSA health club consumer report.* Boston: IHRSA.

# Index

*Note:* The italicized *f* and *t* following page numbers refer to figures and tables, respectively.

## A

acceptance stage of programming 187-188
accident reports 271, 272*f. See also* emergency management
accountability
  for customer service 171
  employee compensation and 105
  for member retention 185
accounting. *See* financial management
accounts receivable 234-236
accreditation organizations 203, 250-251
accrual accounting 224-225
ACE (American Council on Exercise) 204
ACE (alignment, capability, and engagement) model 16, 17*f*
achievement phase, of acceptance stage 188
ACSM (American College of Sports Medicine.) *See* American College of Sports Medicine (ACSM)
activation code, in emergency plan 270
active clients 201
ADA (Americans with Disabilities Act of 1990) 325-326
ADEA (Age Discrimination in Employment Act of 1967) 326
administrative (process) approach to management 4-5, 5*f*
administrative assistants 25-26. *See also* front-desk associates
advisory boards 177
AED (automated external defibrillator) 72, 274-275
aerobic capacity. *See* cardiorespiratory endurance
after-sales service and follow-up 159
Age Discrimination in Employment Act of 1967 (ADEA) 326
aged trial balance 235, 236*t*
agonal gasp 276
agreements to participate 318

AHA (American Heart Association) 249, 258, 275
alignment, capability, and engagement (ACE) model 16, 17*f*
amenities 289
American College of Sports Medicine (ACSM)
  accredited certification stance 203
  AED standards 274-275
  blood variable information 257
  certification quality 250
  fitness testing guidelines 260-261
  hazardous material advisory 248
  health history questionnaires 256
  risk classification guidelines 258
  screening recommendations 249
American Council on Exercise (ACE) 204
American Heart Association (AHA) 249, 258, 275
Americans with Disabilities Act of 1990 (ADA) 325-326
Ameyo statistics 165
analytics. *See* data analytics
appointment sheets 139
appraisals. *See* health risk appraisals
aquatic area risks and emergencies 268, 277-278
aromatherapy facial 210
aromatherapy massage 210
assets
  defined 225
  depreciation of 240-241
  employees and associates as 98, 102-104
associates. *See* employees and associates
assumption of risk 258, 318
attitude, in customer service 173
attrition. *See* membership attrition
automated external defibrillator (AED) 72, 274-275
automobile insurance 330

## B

babysitting services 217
background checks 58
bad debt 345
balance sheets 225-227, 226*f*
banks, as EFT providers 236
barrels (Pilates equipment) 208
*Basic Life Support Manual for Healthcare Providers* (AHA) 275
behavioral leadership theory 5
benchmarks, benchmarking
  club operations 233
  maintenance 306-307
  wage and salary 44-45
benefits, employee 100-102, 103*f*
BIA (bioelectrical impedance analysis) 261
bicycle ergometer tests 262
bioelectrical impedance analysis (BIA) 261
Blanchard, K.H. 4, 6
blood-borne pathogens standard 248
blood pooling 267
blood pressure 255, 256
blood profiles 257
body composition tests 261-262
body therapies 210
bomb threats 279
bonus plans
  approaches to 100
  incentive compensation plans 92-93
books, as training tools 73
boutique fitness studios 205
brainstorming, as training tool 70
brand awareness 342
branding, in marketing 125-126
brand mantra 127
break-even analysis 231
Buckingham, Marcus 7, 10
budgets and budgeting
  elements of 233-234
  guidelines for 230
  for incentive compensation 93
  in marketing plan 118
  preparation steps 231-233
  projecting profits and losses 232-233
  for repair work 287

budgets and budgeting *(continued)*
    sales forecasting 232, 232*f*
    types of budgets 230-231
*Built to Last* (Collins, Porras) 80
bundled class options 208
business entity, and tax liability 242
business identity 80-81
business interruption insurance 328
business plans, for profit centers 198

**C**
Cadillac (Pilates equipment) 208
calendars, for social medial marketing 130-131
capability, in ACE model 16
capacity, in group exercise evaluation 344
capital budgets 231
Cardiac Arrest Survival Act (2000) 274
cardiorespiratory endurance
    exercise program design 265
    fitness tests 262-263
cardiopulmonary resuscitation (CPR) 72, 276, 281
cardiovascular emergencies 273-276
career advancement, in job descriptions 47
career paths, of staff
    employee retention and 10
    training programs and 62
caretaking, vs. caring 12
Caro, Rick 233-234
case studies
    legal issue cases 316, 317, 318
    as training tool 70, 71
cash accounting 224
cash flows statement 227-229
causation, in negligence 313
certifications
    health and safety 281
    lacking or inadequate 249-250, 276
    of maintenance staff 299
    personal training and fitness 203-204
    Pilates instructors 209
    vs. qualifications 250
    third-party nationally accredited 28, 29, 203
    in training program 72-73
chairs, for Pilates 208
charitable immunity 319

checklists
    cleaning task assignments 292*f*
    health and safety 281-282, 283*f*
    programming development 193
chemical agent exposure 248
children
    childhood obesity 214-215
    child watch services 217
    emergencies involving 278
    youth programs 214-217
child watch services (babysitting) 217
cholesterol 256
civil liability 312
Civil Rights Act (1964) 48, 325
class capacity 344
*Cleaning and Maintenance Management* magazine 307
Cleaning Management Institute 307
cleanliness of facilities 168, 175, 289
clients. *See* members
clinical stress tests 257
closed-ended questions 52
closing the sale 158-160
club members. *See* differentiation
club operating benchmarks 233
club scorecard 79*f*
club tours
    closing the sale during 159-160
    creating desire during 151-153
    handling member concerns 156-157
    purpose of 151
    tour cards 140-141
    trial close questions during 153-156
Coffman, Curt 10
Collins, J.C. 80
colleges and universities, for recruitment 51
commercial organizations. *See* for-profit (commercial) organizations
commission-based pay 99, 139, 213
commitment stage of programming 188-190
communication
    of company goals 8
    in customer service 171-173
    in face-to-face sales 145-147
    with new members 182
    nonverbal 146, 172
    power talking (yes vs. no) 173
    in staff department partnerships 139

company names, and marketing 126-127
comparative negligence 320
compensation
    accountability to employees and 105
    average rates by position 109*t*
    compensation and benefits worksheet 103*f*
    employee benefits 100-102
    employee morale and 98
    fitness industry benchmarks 44-45
    forms of 98-100
    incentive programs 4, 92-94
    in job advertisements 50
    in job descriptions 46-47
    performance-based pay 110-113
    policy issues 104-105
compensation programs
    adaptive 105
    development process 107-110
    independent contractors in 105-107
    organizational structure and 105, 106
    review and revision of 109
    standards for development 108
    suggestions for 102-104
competition
    analysis of 121-122, 153, 154*f*-155*f*
    competitive strategy 80-81
    employee compensation and 102
    sustainable competitive advantage 7
competition analysis form 154*f*-155*f*
contests
    as employee incentive 94
    vs. focus groups 127
contingency model, Fiedler's 5-6
contract maintenance 298-300
contracts
    case study 322
    elements of 320-321
    employment 323-324
    independent contractor 323
    membership agreements 321-323, 349-352
    vendor 323
    waivers and releases 141, 259*f*, 318-319, 323
contributory negligence 320
conversion goals 199
Cooper 12-minute test 263

copyrighted material use 70
core values 14
corporate-based fitness organizations
    exercise physiologist 39-40
    general manager 37-39
    organizational chart 37f
    organizational design 36-37
corporate membership sales 160-161
corporate social responsibility (CSR) initiatives 125
corporation tax liabilities 242
cost centers 196
CPR (cardiopulmonary resuscitation) 72, 276, 281
crash bags 280
credit policies 235-236
criminal liability 312
CRM (customer relationship management) databases 119, 123, 133
cross-training 184
CSR (corporate social responsibility) initiatives 125
cultural heroes 8
culture, organizational 7-8
current assets 225
current liabilities 225
customer, defined 164
customer complaints 174
customer loyalty 164-165
customer relationship management (CRM) databases 119, 123, 133
customer satisfaction, defined 164
customer satisfaction surveys and inventories 177
customer service
    Ameyo statistics on 165
    best practices 174-176
    customer identification in 165-166
    customer survey cards 167f
    customer wants and needs in 166-168
    dealing with difficult customers 174
    exceptional, defined 164
    as fitness director responsibility 28
    importance of 164-165
    interview questions on 53
    monitoring effects of 176-178
    reasons for poor service 166
    staff pledge 170
    training staff for 66, 169-173

**D**
damages, in negligence 314
data analytics 118, 132, 133, 135
data-driven marketing 123-125
DEAC (Distance Education Accrediting Commission) 203, 250-251
deal breakers, in hiring process 52
decisional roles of managers 5
decision making, timely 14
defined behaviors 46
delegation 6, 16
demographics
    in health risk appraisals 255
    in location analysis 339-340
    of target markets 122, 125
demonstrations, as training tool 70
depreciation 240-241
DEXA (dual energy X-ray absorptiometry) 262
diagnosticians vs. suspecticians 255, 261
differentiation
    during club tours 152-153
    in competitive strategy 80-81
    industry evolution and 342
    in marketing 132
digital marketing 118. *See also* marketing and promotion
disaster plans 278
Distance Education Accrediting Commission (DEAC) 203, 250-251
diversified programming 184
documentation
    legal documents 317
    in risk management 271, 272f, 281-282
dual energy X-ray absorptiometry (DEXA) 262
duty of care 312-313

**E**
earnings before interest, depreciation, and amortization (EBITDA) 23
educational attainment, and market penetration 340
EEOC (Equal Employment Opportunity Commission) 48, 325, 327
efficiency, as customer need 168
EFT (electronic funds transfer) 236, 237
EI (emotional intelligence) 10
80:20 rule 15
e-learning 73

electronic funds transfer (EFT) 236, 237
electronic surveys 133-135
emergency management
    activation code 270
    aquatic emergencies 277-278
    bomb threats 279
    cardiovascular events 273-276
    child watch centers 278
    disaster plans 278
    documentation 281-282
    emergency drills 271-273
    emergency plan development 268-271
    employee training 280-281
    equipment and supplies for 277, 280
    fires 276-277
    incident and accident reports 271, 272f
    non-life-threatening incidents 279-280
    weather emergencies 279
emergency medical care 273-276, 315-316
emergency telephone numbers 270
emotional connections, in sales 147-148
emotional intelligence (EI) 10
employee benefits 100-102, 103f
employee handbooks 324, 325
employee recognition
    for customer service 171
    in performance management 91-92
employee safety 327
employees and associates
    accountability to 105
    as assets 98, 102-104
    benefits of new 45
    customer service best practices 175-176
    employee orientation 65
    empowerment of 16
    evaluation of 9, 86-87, 88f-90f
    expectations of 13-14, 81-82, 85
    feedback from 10, 12
    as friends 15
    health and safety role 248-251
    vs. independent contractors 106-107
    job satisfaction in 20
    membership attrition and 45
    motivation of 112-113
    operations evaluation role 338
    physical exercise in 64
    recruitment of 9-10, 202

employees and associates *(continued)*
  relationships with 10
  retention of 16-17, 20, 204-205
  termination of 94-96
  training. *See* training programs
  turnover costs and benefits 14, 16-17, 45
  use of club 149
employment at will 324
employment contracts 323-324
employment law 324-327
energy level, in face-to-face sales 145
engagement, in ACE model 16
Equal Employment Opportunity Act (1972) 48
Equal Employment Opportunity Commission (EEOC) 48, 325, 327
equipment
  customer service and 168, 175-176
  emergency 277, 280
  history cards 304, 305*f*
  monitoring via Internet 305
  for personal training 201
  Pilates 208
  pool 277
  potential dangers of 315
  preventive maintenance services 295-296
  repair and replacement of 287-288
  spa services 211
  warranty protection 295, 296
equity (net worth) 225-227
ergometer tests 262
evaluation committee 338
evaluation coordinator 338
evaluations
  customer service 176-178
  employee performance 9, 86-87, 88*f*-90*f*
  location analysis 339-342, 341*f*
  marketing and promotions 133-135, 338-339
  operations 337-339, 339*f*
  personal training 200, 344-345, 347*f*
  of profit centers 342-346, 345*f*
  of programming 191
Evans, M.G. 6
event liability insurance 329
exceptional customer service, defined 164
exclusive features of club 153

exercise contraindications 254
exercise physiologists 39-40
exercise prescription 264
exercise program design 264-266
exercise progression 265
expectations. *See* performance expectations
expenses
  expense management 237-241, 239*t*-240*t*
  on income statement 227
experiential questions 52
external customers 166
external equity 46

**F**
Facebook Insights 135
face-to-face selling process
  building trust and rapport 144-148, 147*t*
  closing the sale 158-160
  creating urgency 151-152
  differentiation in 152-153
  handling member concerns 156-157
  interview questions 148-151
  mental preparation for 149
  overview of steps in 144
  price presentation 157-158
  qualifying questions 150-151
  trial close questions 153-156
facial treatments 210
facilities. *See also* maintenance
  customer service and 168, 175-176
  health and safety in 247
  improvement projects 288, 293
  personal training location 199
  pro shops 218
  spa treatment rooms 211
  specialty group training location 207
  for youth activities 215
Fair Labor Standards Act 109
fango 210
federal taxes 242
feedback
  appropriate delivery of 12, 13
  on customer service 171
  from employees 10, 12
  employee termination and 95-96
  guidelines for 87-91
  in performance management 78-79, 86-87
  on training programs 71, 72*f*

Fiedler, F.E. 5-6
Fiedler's contingency model 5-6
fill-in-the-blank training exercise 70
financial management
  accounting systems 224-225
  accounts receivable 234-236
  budgeting 230-234
  expense management 237-241, 239*t*-240*t*
  financial statement analysis 229-230
  financial statements 225-230, 226*f*, 228*f*-229*f*
  income management 234
  questions to answer 224
  sales analysis 236-237, 238*t*
  tax considerations 241-243
financial pro forma 197-198
fires 276-277
first aid kits 280
*First Break All the Rules* (Buckingham and Coffman) 10
*Fish: A Remarkable Way to Boost Morale and Improve Results* (Lundin) 16
fitness assessments
  body composition 261-262
  cardiorespiratory endurance 262-263
  data evaluation 263
  flexibility 263
  informed consent for 260
  muscular strength and endurance 263
  preparation for 260
  purposes of 259
fitness director 28-29
fitness instructors
  certifications of 249-250
  incentives for 93-94
  job descriptions 35-36
  unqualified 249
fitness profiles 251, 260, 268
fitness specialists 54
fixed assets 225
flashlights, for emergencies 280
flexibility (range of motion)
  exercise program design 266
  fitness tests 263
floor supervision 267
floor surfaces, as potential danger 314-315
focus groups 127, 176-177
follow-up
  with new members 28, 159, 182
  in programming 192

food and beverage areas 343-344
formative evaluation 337
for-profit (commercial) organizations
    fitness director 28-29
    front-desk associates 25-26
    general manager 23-25
    membership consultants 27-28
    membership director 26-27
    organizational chart 24*f*
    organizational design 23
    personal trainers 29-30
Fried, G. 225, 231, 290
friendships, with employees 15
front-desk associates
    customer service best practices 174-175
    incentives for 94, 139
    as internal customers 166
    interview questions for 54
    job description 25-26
    membership staff and 138-141
    telephone skills 142-143
    tour card use 141
    training of 140
full range of leadership model 6
fun atmosphere, at work 15-16
fun phase, of commitment stage 189-190

**G**
general liability insurance 328-329
general maintenance 286-287, 293
general managers
    corporate-based fitness organizations 37-39
    for-profit organizations 23-25
Gerson, R.F. 290
Gettman, L.R. 290
glycolic peel facial 210
goals and goal setting
    communication of 8
    in compensation programs 107
    goal-setting worksheet 10, 11*f*
    for maintenance program 293-294
    in marketing plan 123-125
    of operations evaluations 337
    in performance management 85
    in profit center development 197
    for program development 190-191
    of programming 180, 184
    in sales preparation 149
    SMART goals 85, 123

GoodLife Fitness Clubs 8, 10
Good Samaritan law 274
Google Analytics 133, 135
Goslee, Georgia 253-254
graded exercise test (GXT) 263
Grantham, W.C. 290
Greely, Sean 3-4
Greenfield, Roz 61
Greenwood, L. 294
Greenwood, M. 294
group exercise
    as involvement programming 187
    as profit center 344, 345*f*
    specialty group training 205-209
group exercise supervisor 34-35
group fitness instructors 166
group membership sales 160-161
guest liability waiver form 259*f*
guest screening 258-259
*Guidelines for Exercise Testing and Prescription* (ACSM) 257, 258, 261
*Guide to Club Membership Conduct* (IHRSA) 277
Gulick, L. 4
GXT (graded exercise test) 263

**H**
hashtags, in social media marketing 130
hazardous materials 248
health and fitness evaluation model 337-338
health and safety. *See also* emergency management
    certifications 281
    employee training in 65
    fitness assessments 259-264
    guidelines for 247*f*
    as maintenance focus area 289
    manager's checklist 282, 283*f*
    member orientations 266-267
    member screening for 252-258
    personnel role in 248-251
    safe environments 246-248
    safe exercise programs 264-266
    supervision 267-268
    as workplace environment issue 327
health and wellness director 32-33
*Health/Fitness Facility Standards and Guidelines* (ACSM) 248, 256, 258

health risk appraisals 251, 254, 255-257. *See also* member screening
herbal wraps 210
Hersey, P. 4, 6
high blood pressure 255, 256
hiring process
    analyzing staffing needs 44-45
    applicant profiling 48
    background checks 58
    comparing applicants 58
    deal breakers in 52
    interviews 51-55, 56-57, 57*t*
    job application review 55-56
    job description use in 45-46
    job offers 58
    mistakes in 14
    new-hire packets 59
    in performance management 82-84
    recruitment vehicles 48-51, 49*t*, 51*t*
    reference checks 57-58
holiday pay 99, 100
Hootsuite 118-119, 129, 131
horizontal aspects of business 21
hospital-based fitness centers
    fitness instructors 35-36
    group exercise supervisor 34-35
    organizational chart 34*f*
    organizational design 33-34
hostile environment sexual harassment 326-327
hourly wages. *See* compensation
House, R.J. 6
housekeeping
    described 286
    infrequent 286-287
    interview questions for 54
    sample goal statement 293
    staff incentives 94
Houstonian Hotel, Club, and Spa 74-75
human relations management approach 4
hydrostatic weighing 262
hydrotherapy 210

**I**
icebreakers, as training tool 69
I-fees 27
IHRSA. *See* International Health, Racquet, and Sportsclub Association
immunity (negligence defense) 319-320

improvement phase, of commitment stage 188-190

improvement projects 288, 293

incentive compensation and rewards
 for customer service 171
 as element of budgeting 233-234
 management bonus plans 92-93
 in management theory 4
 for membership sales 139
 for nonsales staff 93-94, 199
 for sales staff 92

incident and accident reports 271, 272f

income, and market penetration 339-340

income management 234

income statements 227, 228f-229f

income taxes 242

increment-decrement budgeting 230

independent contractors
 advantages, disadvantages of 105-106
 contracts 323
 vs. employees 106-107
 food and beverage services 343-344
 liability insurance 330
 maintenance services 298-300

industry evolution and differentiation
 facility growth 342, 343f
 profit centers 342-345

industry metrics 201

industry-specific experts 72

informational roles of managers 5

informed consent 260

infrequent housekeeping 286-287

in-person interviews 56-57, 57t

instructional conferences 171

instruction phase, of integration stage 187

insurance considerations 327-330. See also employee benefits

integration stage of programming 186-187

intentional torts 320

interactive exercises 69-70

internal customers 165-166

International Health, Racquet, and Sportsclub Association (IHRSA)
 industry trend information 120
 *Profiles of Success* 29, 104, 196
 salary range information 44-45

interpersonal roles of managers 4-5

interruptions, managing 15

interview, of prospective members 148-151

interview process. See also hiring process
 in-person interviews 56-57, 57t
 job description use in 46
 job preview in 52
 lie detection in 53
 phone screening 56
 preparation for 51-52
 quality of answers in 54-55
 questions for specific positions 54
 questions to avoid 55
 question types and topics 52-53

introduction phase, of integration stage 186-187

inventory control 303-304

invitees (legal definition) 314

involvement phase, of acceptance stage 187-188

involvement programming 187

**J**

job advertisements 45-46, 49-51, 49t, 51t

job applications 55-56

job descriptions
 absence of 22
 developing 22
 exercise physiologist 39-40
 fitness director 28-29
 fitness instructor 35-36
 front-desk associate 25-26
 general manager 23-25, 37-39
 group exercise supervisor 34-35
 health and wellness director 32-33
 importance of 22, 40
 job expectations in 47, 81-82
 key elements of 46-48
 membership consultants 27-28
 membership director 26-27
 personal trainers 29-30
 positive profiling in 48
 reviewing and revising 27, 40
 use in hiring process 45-46, 48

job expectations. See performance expectations

job offer, in hiring process 58

job preview 52

job pricing 108-109

job satisfaction, in employees 20

Johnson, D.E. 4

Jurkiewicz, Dennis 295-296

**K**

key performance indicators (KPIs) 345, 347f

key performance numbers 79f

Kirkpatrick, S.A. 5

Koontz, H. 4

KPIs (key performance indicators) 345, 347f

**L**

laboratory tests 257

laissez-faire leadership 6

leaders
 characteristics of 7-9
 effective 6-7
 vs. managers 7

leadership skills training 65

leadership theory 5-6

leagues 187-188

legal issues
 avoiding litigation 251-252, 252f, 307
 case studies 316, 317, 318, 322
 civil vs. criminal liability 312
 contracts 320-324
 employment law 324-327
 health and safety 246
 intentional torts 320
 legal liability checklist 313
 negligence defenses 318-320
 negligence tort 312-318
 reckless misconduct 320
 in spa services 214

legal liability checklist 313

liabilities (financial) 225

liability insurance 328-329

liability waivers 141, 259f, 318-319, 323

licensee (legal definition) 314

licensure, of spa treatment providers 213-214

lie detection, in interviews 53

lifestyle questionnaires 256-257

liquidity, of assets 225

listening skills
 in customer service 172-173, 174
 in face-to-face sales 145-147

litigation. See legal issues

live video, in marketing 120, 129

location analysis 339-342, 341f

Locke, E.A. 5

locker-room amenities 289

locker room attendants 267-268, 297

logical progression of programming 184, 185-190, 186f

long-term liabilities 225

loofah scrub 210
Lundin, Stephen 16

**M**

magic circles (Pilates equipment) 208
maintenance
  activity categories 286-288
  cleaning task assignment checklist 292f
  contracting for services 298-300
  cost control 304
  defined 286
  as duty of care 314-315
  equipment and mechanical histories 304, 305f
  evaluating 304-307, 306f
  four-step management process 290, 290f
  goals and objectives for 293-294
  guidelines 300
  litigation risks and 307
  management focus areas 289
  needs assessment 290-293
  preventive 287, 293, 295-296, 307-310
  purchase order system for 303, 303f
  records and safety checklists 281-282
  scheduling 301, 302f
  of spa facilities 214
  staffing based on facility size 294-298, 297f, 298f, 299f
  strategic plan for 289-290
  work identification 300-301
  work-order request forms 301, 301f
  work tracking and monitoring 302
malpractice insurance 214
management plan, for profit centers 197
management support structure, in job descriptions 47
management theory 4-5
managers. *See also* performance management
  characteristics of 9-14
  health and safety role 248-249
  vs. leaders 7
  managing by wandering around 177
  networking opportunities 16
  in operations evaluation 338
  pitfalls to avoid 14-16
  of profit centers 198, 219-220

recruitment skills 9-10
  roles of 4-5
  talent management strategy 16-17
  training for 65
mantra, in branding 127
marketing and promotion
  best practices 131
  branding role in 125-126
  brand mantra 127
  company name and logo in 126-127
  data analytics in 118, 132
  differentiation in 132
  evaluation of 133-135, 338-339
  foundational questions 132
  goals and objectives for 123-125
  of profit centers 197, 198, 205, 209, 211-213
  program name and logo in 127
  of programs 184, 191
  shift to digital methods 118
  strategic plan development 118-119, 120
  target markets identification 122-123
  via social media 127-131
  why in 119-120, 125
  written plan guidelines 132-133
  written plan outline 134
marketing automation software 125
marketing communication 118
marketing metrics 133
marketing research
  competition analysis 121-122
  needs analysis 119-120
  trends analysis 120-121
massages 210
maternity leave, paid 100
mats, for Pilates 208
Mayo, E. 4
medical clearance 251, 252, 258
medical exams 257
Medical Fitness Association (MFA) 203
medical history questionnaires 254, 255-256
medical referrals 34
member recognition 188
member referral programs 27
members
  fitness assessments 259-264
  medical clearance 251, 252, 258
  orientations for 266-267
  as priority 15

risk classification 257-258
  screening of 252-258
  supervision of 267-268
member screening
  diagnosing vs. suspecting in 255, 261
  health appraisals 255-257
  medical exams and lab work 257
  preactivity screening 252-255
  risk classification 257-258
  use of screening data 257
membership agreements 321-323, 349-352
membership attrition
  employee attrition and 45
  profitability and 180
  rates of 197
  reducing 159, 180-181, 197
membership (sales) consultants
  interview questions for 54
  job description 27-28
  reception desk staff and 138-141
membership determinants 339-340
membership director 26-27
membership retention
  defined 181
  employee retention and 20
  incentive compensation and 93-94
  of new members 28, 159, 182
  program directors and 185, 192
  program implementation and 182
  programming best practices for 183
  programming by logical progression and 184, 185-190, 186f
  programming factors in 184-185
  as programming goal 180
  rate calculation 181
  tips for 181-182
membership sales. *See also* face-to-face selling process
  corporate and group sales 160-161
  front-desk staff role in 138-141
  sales skills and 138
  staff incentives 93, 139
  telephone skills 142-143
  tour cards for 140-141
  training in 65-66
mentors, of great leaders 9
MFA (Medical Fitness Association) 203

MI (myocardial infarction) 273-276, 280
micromanagement 15
Mintzberg, H. 4
Mitchell, T.R. 6
moisturizing facial 210
motivation
    of prospective members 148-150, 152
    in sales preparation 149
muscular strength and endurance
    exercise program design 265-266
    fitness tests 263
myocardial infarction (MI) 273-276, 280

**N**
National Athletic Trainers' Association (NATA) 250
National Commission for Certifying Agencies (NCCA) 203, 250-251
near-infrared interactance (NII) 261
needs analyses
    compensation needs 107
    maintenance 290-293
    in marketing research 119-120
    staffing needs 44-45
    training needs 62-63, 67f
negligence tort
    defenses 318-320
    documentation and 317
    elements of 312-314
    member, nonmember status and 314
    potential dangers 314-317
    vicarious liability 317-318
Net Profit Explosion (NPE) 3-4
networking events
    for managers 16
    as training tool 72
net worth (equity) 225-227
new-hire packets 59
NII (near-infrared interactance) 261
nondues revenue 23, 197-198, 234
nonexempt performance review 88f-90f
nonprescriptive emergency oxygen 273-274
nonverbal communication 146, 172
not-for-profit organizations
    fund-raising in 31
    health and wellness director 32-33

organizational chart 31f
organizational design 30-32
NPE (Net Profit Explosion) 3-4

**O**
obesity epidemic 214-215
Occupational Safety and Health Administration (OSHA) 327
O'Donnell, C. 4
off-site events 279
off-site training 64
Ojai Valley Racquet Club 101
1.5-mile test for time 263
1-repetition (1RM) maximum tests 263
online learning (e-learning) 73
online surveys 133-135
open book management 79, 79f
open-ended questions 52, 145
open perils 328
operating budgets 231
operating expenses 227
operational planning 335
operations evaluation 337-339, 339f
organizational charts
    business growth and 21-23, 21f
    corporate-based facility 37f
    for-profit organizations 24f
    hospital-based fitness center 34f
    maintenance staffing 297f, 298f, 299f
    not-for-profit community facility 31f
    redesign of 45
organizational culture 7-8
organizational design
    corporate-based fitness organizations 36-37, 37f
    for-profit organizations 23, 24f
    hospital-based fitness centers 33-34, 34f
    not-for-profit organizations 30-32
    reorganizing 45
    vertical, horizontal aspects of 20-21, 21f
orientation (integration stage) 186-187
orientation of members 266-267
OSHA (Occupational Safety and Health Administration) 327
outcome evaluation 306f
overtime pay 99
oxygen administration 273-274

**P**
PAD (public access defibrillation) program 274

paper screening, of job applicants 56
Pareto's Law 15
PAR-Q+ (Physical Activity Readiness Questionnaire) 258
participants. See members
participating (leader behavior) 6
partnerships
    business entity tax liabilities 242
    between staff departments 138-141
passion, in interview questions 53
Patchell-Evans, Dave 8
path-goal model 6
Patton, R.W. 290, 300, 306
payroll costs 99, 104
performance-based pay 110-113
performance evaluations
    expectations and 85
    formal process 86-87
    form for 86-87, 88f-90f
    ongoing feedback and 86, 87
    as talent assessment 9
    360-degree 87
performance expectations
    in job description 45-46, 47
    manager's role in 13-14, 81-82
    in measurement standards 85
performance management
    addressing problems 87
    clarifying job expectations 13-14, 81-82, 85
    defined 78
    employee recognition in 91-92
    employee termination 94-96
    giving feedback 78-79, 86-91
    goal of 81
    goal setting in 85
    hiring in 82-84
    incentive compensation plans in 93-94
    manager's role in 79-81
    training in 84-85
personal achievement, recognition for 188
personal appearance standards
    in job descriptions 47
    member perceptions and 145
    nonverbal communication and 172
personal days, paid 100
personality type, in interview questions 53
personal trainers
    certifications for 203-204, 249-250

incentive pay for 199
job description 29-30
key performance indicators for 347f
scope of practice 204
training for 66
personal training
defined 199
evaluation of 200, 344-345, 347f
increased demand for 198
marketing 205
policies and operations 201-202
pricing and profit margins 201
programs and packages 200-201
revenue from 198-199
sample business model 346f
selling 199-200
staffing 202-205
personal training revenue 202
personal training sales 202
personnel policy manuals 324
physical activity, vs. exercise 264
Physical Activity Readiness Questionnaire (PAR-Q+) 258
physical exams 257
physical fitness. See fitness assessments
physical inactivity, as risk factor 256
physical requirements, in job descriptions 47-48
Pilates 205-207, 209
plethysmography 262
PMO (preventive maintenance order) 308-309, 310f
points of difference (PODs) 121
points of parity (POPs) 121
population density, in location analysis 340
Porras, J.I. 80
positive profiling 48
power outages 279
power talking (yes vs. no) 173
preactivity screening 252-255
preordinate evaluation 337
pretour power questions 150-151
preventive maintenance
described 287
equipment service contracts 295-296
preventive maintenance order 308-309, 310f
program development 307-310
sample goal statement 293
sample schedule 309t
price presentation, in sales 157-158
primary data 340

primary target market 122
primary trading areas 339
priority of members 15
problem solving
in customer service 164-165, 168
interview questions on 53
process (administrative) approach to management 4-5, 5f
process evaluation 306f, 337
productivity and payroll costs 104
product offering 342
professional liability insurance 214
professional organizations 120, 214
professional speakers, as training tool 72
Profiles of Success (IHRSA) 29, 104, 196
profiling, of job applicants 48
profitability
attrition reduction and 180
of group training 201
of spa services 214
of specialty group training 207-208
profit and loss projections 232-233
profit and loss (income) statements 227
profit centers
benefits of 196
child watch facilities 217
defined 196
development of 197-198
food and beverage areas 343-344
group exercise programs 344, 345f
manager of 198
personal training 198-205, 344-345, 346f, 347f
pro shops 217-220
revenue contributions 197
spa services 209-214
specialty group training 205-209
youth programs 214-217
profit sharing 100, 101
program directors 185, 192
programming
development checklist 193
development of successful 190-192
evaluation of 191
factors in member retention 184-185
goals of 180, 184

implementation factors in retention 182
by logical progression 184, 185-190, 186f
member benefits 182-183
as member retention tool 183-184
promotion of 184, 191
safe exercise programs 264-266
program names, and marketing 127
program urgency 152
progression of exercise 265
progression of programming 184, 185-190, 186f
promotion. See marketing and promotion
property insurance 328
property taxes 242-243
pro shops 217-220
psychographics, of target markets 122
public access defibrillation (PAD) program 274
public seminars, as training tool 72
purchase order system 303, 303f

**Q**
qualifying (pretour) questions 150-151
qualitative research 340-342
quantitative research 340
quid pro quo sexual harassment 326

**R**
range of motion (ROM) tests 263
rapport building, in sales 144-148
rating of perceived exertion (RPE) 265
Ray, R. 290, 300
readiness level, of followers 6
reading aloud, as training tool 70
reasonable accommodation 326
reasonable person test 312-313
reception desk staff. See front-desk associates
reckless misconduct 320
recognition programs. See employee recognition; member recognition
Recommendations for Cardiovascular Screening, Staffing, and Emergency Policies (AHA) 258
recreational user (legal definition) 314
recreational user statutes 319

recruitment. *See also* hiring process
job advertisements 45-46, 49-51, 51*t*
job previews 52
as management skill 9-10
sources for 48, 49*t*
variables to consider 48-49
reference checks 57-58
referral programs 27
reflexology 210
Reformers 208
regional and local taxes 242-243
relationship building
with employees 10
in sales 144-148
reliability, of program schedules 184
repair work 287, 293
replacement, in maintenance 287-288
reporting structure 45
research, quantitative vs. qualitative 340
retention. *See* employee recognition; membership retention
retention-based incentives 93-94
revenue
income management 234
on income statements 227
nondues sources 23, 197-198, 234
from personal training 198-199
profit centers contribution 197
rewards. *See* employee recognition; incentive compensation and rewards; member recognition
risk assumption 258, 318
risk management. *See* emergency management; health and safety; insurance considerations
risk stratification 251
Rockport fitness walking test 263
role-play, as training tool 69-70, 71, 149, 169
ROM (range of motion) tests 263
RPE (rating of perceived exertion) 265

**S**
safety. *See* emergency management; health and safety
safety orientation 266-267
salaries 99. *See also* compensation
salary surveys 108
sales. *See* face-to-face selling process; membership sales

sales analysis 236-237, 238*t*
sales forecasting 232, 232*f*
sales meetings 149
sales representatives. *See* membership (sales)
salt glow 210
saunas 268, 307
SCA (sudden cardiac arrest) 273-276, 280
scientific management approach 4
scope of practice, for personal trainers 204
scoring, of job applicants 58
S corporation tax liabilities 242
screening. *See* guest screening; interview process; member screening
secondary data 340
secondary target market 122, 123
secret shoppers 143, 178
security, in child watch area 217
self-funding incentive programs 93
self-help books, as training tools 73
selfies, in social media marketing 129
self-talk, in sales preparation 149
selling (leader behavior) 6
selling styles 147-148
servant leadership model 80
service, defined 164
sexual harassment 326-327
sharps containers 280
shiatsu massage 210
sick leave, paid 100
signage
for health and safety 247-248, 268
out-of-order 287
situational analysis of marketplace 118
situational leadership model 6
situational leadership theory 5-6
situational questions 52
skin care therapies 210-211
skinfold testing 262
skits, as training tool 70
slip-and-fall situations 315
SMART goals 85, 123
SMM. *See* social media marketing
smoking, as risk factor 256
sociability
in fun phase 189-190
member retention and 182
social events 189-190
social media (data) analytics 118, 132, 133, 135

social media marketing (SMM)
best times to post 129
content for 128, 129
hashtags in 130
marketing calendar for 130-131
social media engagement in 127-128, 132
top mistakes in 129-130
software-supported EFT 236
sole proprietorship tax liabilities 242
sovereign immunity 319
spa services
facilities and equipment 211, 212, 214
industry trends 209-210
legal considerations 214
marketing 211-213
menu of services 210-211
profitability of 214
staffing 213
specialty group training 205-209
Sports and Fitness Ventures 61
sports massage 210
sprinkler system activation, accidental 279-280
stability chairs 208
staffing needs. *See also* employees and associates
analyzing 44-45
maintenance 294-298
personal training profit centers 202-205
spa facilities 213
staff meetings 68
staff pledge, for customer service 170
staff retreats 64-66
standard of care 252
statement of cash flows 227-229
steam rooms 268, 307
step tests 262-263
strategic planning
benefits of 336
maintenance plans 289-290
marketing plans 118-119
operational planning and 335
plan development 335-336
purposes of 334
StrengthsFinder profile 10
strength training. *See* muscular strength and endurance
subtenants 24
sudden cardiac arrest (SCA) 273-276, 280

suggestion boxes 177
summative evaluation 337
supervision, of members 267-268, 277, 315
surveys
    for customer service evaluation 177
    for marketing evaluation 133-135
    salary data 108
suspecticians vs. diagnosticians 255, 261
sustainable competitive advantage 7
Swedish massage 210
swimming pools 277
SWOTT analysis 120
systems, for great management 12-13

**T**
talent
    evaluating 9-10
    management strategy 16-17
    recruiting 9
target heart rate (THR) 265
target markets
    identification of 118, 122-123
    reaching with technology 125
tax considerations 241-243
Taylor, Frederick 4
team building 65
teamwork, in interview questions 53
technological tools 345-346
telephone screening, of job applicants 56
telephone skills 142-143, 175
telling (leader behavior) 6
termination clause, in member contracts 322-323
termination of employees 94-96
tertiary target market 122, 123
thalassotherapy 210
THR (target heart rate) 265
3D surface scans 262
360-degree evaluation 87
time management 14-15
Title VII, Civil Rights Act of 1964 48, 325
tort law. *See also* legal issues
    defined 312
    intentional torts 320
    negligence 312-318

negligence defenses 318-320
    reckless misconduct 320
total quality management (TQM) 338
tour cards 140-141
towers (Pilates equipment) 208
toxic material exposure 248
TQM (total quality management) 338
trade-outs 64
traditional marketing 118. *See also* marketing and promotion
traffic flow, in location analysis 340
training bundles 208
training programs
    cost assessment 73-75
    in customer service 168-173
    emergency training 280-281
    feedback on 71, 72$f$
    for front-desk staff 140
    Houstonian example 74-75
    information delivery 66-67, 69
    interactive exercises 69-70, 71
    keys to effective programs 67-68
    needs analysis 62-63, 67$f$
    outside resources for 72-73
    in performance management 84-85
    planning ideas 65-66
    provider of 64
    staff meetings and 68
    staff retreats 64-66
    testing effectiveness of 70-71
    topics for 63-64, 63$t$
    venue for 64
trait leadership theory 5
transactional leadership 6
transformational leadership 6
trapeze table 208
treadmill testing 262
trend-line budgeting 230
trends analysis, in marketing research 120-121
trespassers (legal definition) 314
trial close questions 153-156
trust
    as leader characteristic 8
    of prospective members 147-148, 147$t$
Twitter Analytics 135

**U**
umbrella liability insurance 329
undertraining 14

unique selling position 152
unique selling propositions 80
urgency, in sales 151-152
Urwick, L. 4
U.S. Department of Justice 326
utilities 288, 293

**V**
vacation pay 99, 100
Valsalva maneuver 267
vendor contracts 323
vertical aspects of business 20
vicarious liability 317-318
video, in marketing 120, 129
volunteer immunity 319-320

**W**
wage position 44
wages 99. *See also* compensation
waivers and releases 141, 259$f$, 318-319, 323
warranties 295, 296
weather emergencies 279
websites
    EEOC 327
    for industry trend information 120-121
    OSHA 327
    StrengthsFinder profile 10
    U.S. Department of Justice 326
Weihrich, H. 4
Welch, Jack 7, 9
welcoming atmosphere 168
wet area risks and emergencies 268, 277-278
wheel of logical progression
    acceptance stage 187-188
    commitment stage 188-190
    integration stage 186-187
    overview of 184, 185-186, 186$f$
whirlpools 268, 307
why, in marketing 119-120, 125
workers' compensation statutes 330
work-order request form 301, 301$f$
workplace environment 324-327
worst-case scenario budget 231
wunda chairs 208

**Y**
yes, vs. no 173
youth programs 214-217

**Z**
zero-based budgeting 231

# About the Authors

**Mike Bates** is the owner of Refine Fitness Studio, located in Windsor, Ontario. Bates has worked in a variety of positions in the fitness industry, including sales, front desk, personal training, and management. He was recognized as one of the top sales managers at GoodLife Fitness in Canada and achieved one of the club chain's highest retention levels. Bates is also a lecturer at the University of Windsor, teaching courses in sport management, human resource management, and strength and conditioning. He coordinates and teaches personal training and sports conditioning certification courses in Windsor and is a regular speaker at International Health, Racquet & Sportsclub Association (IHRSA), canfitpro, and Club Industry. He was the managing director of Human Kinetics Canada from 1999 to 2007. Bates holds BHK and MBA degrees from the University of Windsor.

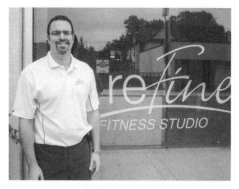

**Michael Spezzano** is a consultant in health, fitness, and healthy living program management and development, specializing in medical fitness programs and health care collaborations. Working with staff teams, he develops innovative and effective program solutions that respond to constituent needs and maintain organization health and vitality. Spezzano has extensive experience in developing and managing a broad range of adult and youth programming.

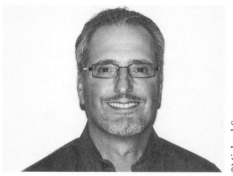

©Michael Spezzano

Prior to his consulting work, Spezzano had a 35-year career with the YMCA. As vice president of programs and membership at the YMCA of Greater New York, Spezzano managed delivery of health and fitness programs and membership services for the largest Y in the United States. He was responsible for $60 million in annual membership revenue and three annual marketing campaigns responsible for producing 20,000 new members a year. Prior to that, he was the national health and fitness director for the YMCA of the USA. In that position he provided national Y leadership in the field of health and fitness. His responsibilities included program design and development, certification training, resource development, and consultation to 2,600 YMCAs in the United States.

Spezzano has been featured in numerous national media outlets, including ABC TV online, *New York Times*, *USA Today*, Web MD, *Newsweek* online, Lifetime online, *Men's Health* magazine, *Weight Watchers* magazine, *Family Life* magazine, and *Wall Street Journal*.

**Guy Danhoff** has been teaching at Missouri Baptist University (MBU) in St. Louis, Missouri, since 2008. He currently serves as coordinator of the graduate fitness management program within the health and sport sciences division. Danhoff teaches courses in that division (fitness management, sport and social media, and sport marketing) as well as courses within the MBU School of Business (strategic management, entrepreneurial marketing, current issues in marketing, and introduction to marketing for health care systems). Danhoff completed all of his course work in 2018 and

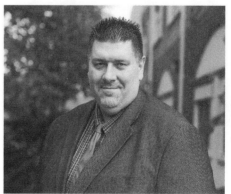

Courtesy of University Communications at Missouri Baptist University.

is slated to complete his business administration doctoral degree program at Walden University before 2020. His doctoral research capstone project is titled "Social Media Marketing Strategies to Increase Revenue in the Health and Fitness Industry." Danhoff also holds a master's degree in exercise science as well as a bachelor's degree in corporate fitness from Western Illinois University in Macomb, Illinois (magna cum laude).

Prior to teaching at in higher education, Danhoff spent 14 years in the fitness industry, with positions in sales, sales management, business development, and marketing. He was the director of fitness entertainment technology and operations for MYE Entertainment North America. He was recognized with the Top Producer of the Year award by multiple fitness equipment and fitness technology companies, including Fitness Warehouse, Tectrix, and Netpulse. He was later appointed by Precor to manage two national sales accounts: XSport Fitness and Power Wellness. Today, Danhoff consults with organizations—ranging from small businesses to large global brands—regarding their digital and social media marketing strategies and the use of data analytics to drive business intelligence and revenue generation. Since February 2018 Danhoff has served on the board of directors for the Missouri Association for Health, Physical Education, Recreation and Dance (MOAHPERD), overseeing the direction of the organization's digital marketing and communications.

# Contributors

*Anthony Abbott, EdD*
President, Fitness Institute International Inc.

*Mike Greenwood, PhD*
Professor, Texas A&M University

*John Wolohan, JD*
Professor, Syracuse University

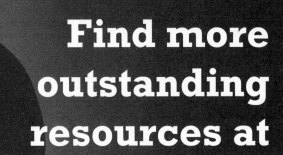

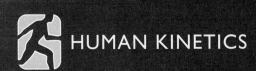